The Clinical Guide to Oncology Nutrition

Second Edition

Oncology Nutrition Dietetic Practice Group

Laura Elliott, MPH, RD, Laura L. Molseed, MS, RD,
and Paula Davis McCallum, MS, RD, Editors

With Barbara Grant, MS, RD, Technical Editor

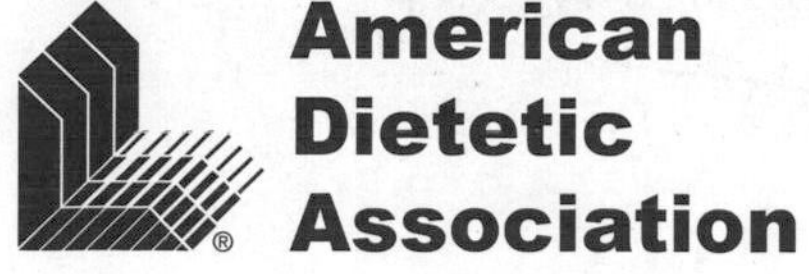

Diana Faulhaber, Publisher
Kristen Short, Development Manager
Elizabeth Nishiura, Production Manager

The views expressed in this publication are those of the authors and do not necessarily reflect policies and/or official positions of the American Dietetic Association. Mention of product names in this publication does not constitute endorsement by the authors or the American Dietetic Association. The American Dietetic Association disclaims responsibility for the application of the information contained herein.

10 9 8 7 6 5 4 3

Library of Congress Cataloging-in-Publication Data

The clinical guide to oncology nutrition / Oncology Nutrition Dietetic Practice Group; Laura Elliott, Laura L. Molseed, and Paula Davis McCallum, editors; with Barbara Grant, technical editor. — 2nd ed.
p. ; cm.
Includes bibliographical references and index.
ISBN-13: 978-0-88091-339-3
1. Cancer—Nutritional aspects. 2. Cancer—Diet therapy.
I. Elliott, Laura, 1955- . II. Molseed, Laura L. III. McCallum, Paula Davis. IV. American Dietetic Association. Oncology Nutrition Dietetic Practice Group.
[DNLM: 1. Neoplasms—diet therapy. QZ 266 C64147 2006]
RC271.D52C57 2006
616.99'40654—dc22

2006004165

Contents

Foreword

Maurice Shils, the father figure of the field of oncology nutrition, authored the foreword for the first edition of *The Clinical Guide to Oncology Nutrition,* and I am honored to follow in his footsteps. Since Shils's landmark 1979 article, "Principles of Nutritional Therapy," in the journal *Cancer* (1), the field of oncology nutrition and its leagues of health care professionals have observed many milestones. In the 1990s, for example, the interdisciplinary Society for Nutritional Oncology Adjuvant Therapy (NOAT) was founded; the scored Patient-Generated Subjective Global Assessment (PG-SGA) was developed and validated; and the Oncology Nutrition Dietetic Practice Group (ON DPG) of the American Dietetic Association (ADA) was established.

My relationship with the ON DPG is a very personal one. It was the joint alliance between NOAT and the ON DPG that advanced the awareness, acceptance, and use of the PG-SGA internationally. If it were not for two oncology dietitians in the Philadelphia area, Suzanne Kasenic and Susan DeBolt, who served as the co-investigators in the NOAT PG-SGA validation study, there never would have been a scored version of the form, a tool with which my name and work are often linked. I have had the honor of working with hundreds of registered dietitians, who daily improve the quality of care given to patients with cancer. I offer my sincere thanks to them, as well as to my RD colleagues and friends who served as chapter authors and editors for the second edition of this guide.

I congratulate the ON DPG on its accomplishments in this book. In this edition, the ON DPG provides readers with the most up-to-date review of the literature and evidence-based guidelines. Practical and easy to use, this text stands as a clinical guide that can be shared with all members of the interdisciplinary oncology team.

Faith D. Ottery, MD, PhD
Founding President, Society for Nutritional Oncology Adjuvant Therapy
(noatpres1@aol.com)
President, Ottery & Associates, Oncology Care Consultants
Senior Director, Medical Affairs, Savient Pharmaceuticals, Inc.

REFERENCE

1. Shils ME. Principles of nutritional therapy. *Cancer.* 1979;43:2093–2102.

Preface

Although the application of nutrition therapy in oncology care occurs in a variety of different settings, from small private practice offices and community hospitals to large academic institutions, what unites clinicians is the need for solid, up-to-date, scientifically based information. With the second edition of *The Clinical Guide to Oncology Nutrition,* dietetics and other health care professionals have a reliable resource for standards in oncology nutrition practice and professional performance.

A team of oncology nutrition experts collaborated on this revision, examining the most current nutrition research in oncology and the integral part that nutrition plays in cancer prevention, treatment, and recovery. This team has also expanded the scope of this guide, adding chapters on adult oncology, pediatric oncology, the Nutrition Care Process and medical nutrition therapy (MNT), reimbursement for MNT, and incorporating research into oncology practice.

As an essential resource, this text reflects the needs of clinicians at all levels of practice. For the basic-level practitioner, this text outlines the nutritional implications of cancer treatment and discusses specialty areas such as pediatric oncology and hematopoietic cell transplantation. For practitioners at all levels, this text examines enteral and parenteral nutrition support, pharmacological management of nutrition impact symptoms, and complementary and alternative medicine.

The Clinical Guide to Oncology Nutrition has been a critical tool in oncology nutrition practice for many years. It provides cutting-edge clinical information that practitioners need to deliver the best nutrition care to oncology patients throughout the continuum of their care. This revised edition takes this fine tradition one step further, offering even more information to develop and better define skills needed to improve the quality of nutrition care.

Together with the American Dietetic Association (ADA), the Oncology Nutrition Dietetic Practice Group (ON DPG) is working to create educational materials and educational opportunities to expand the knowledge base of the basic-level oncology nutrition dietitian, as well as the advanced-level practitioner. For the most comprehensive selection of material available from ON DPG, *The Clinical Guide to Oncology Nutri-*

tion, Second Edition, should be used in conjunction with *Management of Nutrition Impact Symptoms in Cancer and Educational Handouts,* which is also available through the ADA.

ON DPG has made a commitment to the continued education of dietetics professionals in oncology nutrition. We want to help demonstrate the need for trained dietitians in every health care setting where oncology patients are seen and treated. We are realistic, however, and understand that this need will not be recognized overnight. In the meantime, we will work to provide the best information on oncology nutrition for use by the existing practitioners in these settings.

Kathryn Hamilton, MA, RD
Chair, Oncology Nutrition Dietetic Practice Group
2005–2006

Contributors and Reviewers

CONTRIBUTORS

Christina K. Biesemeier, MS, RD, FADA
James Byron, RPh, BCOP
D'Nice Carden, MS, RN, CPNP, CPON
Carla Cartwright, RD, CNSD
Paula M. Charuhas, MS, RD, FADA, CNSD
Paula Davis McCallum, MS, RD
Robert S. DeChicco, MS, RD, CNSD
Laura Elliott, MPH, RD
Alice Fornari, EdD, RD, CDN
Carol Frankmann, MS, RD, CNSD
Dee Gabbard, RD
Anita L. Gallagher, MS, RD, CNSD
Barbara Grant, MS, RD
Sarah Harding Laidlaw, MS, MPA, RD
Jean D. Hurst, MS, RD, CNSD
Toni Isaacs, RD, CNSD
Sandra L. Luthringer, RD
Connie Mobley, PhD, RD
Laura L. Molseed, MS, RD
Terezie T. Mosby, MS, RD, IBCLC
Linda Nebeling, PhD, MPH, RD, FADA
Karen Ringwald-Smith, MS, RD
Kim Robien, PhD, RD, FADA, CNSD
Carrie A. Robinson, RD, CNSD
Ezra Steiger, MD, FACS, CNSP
Sheela Thomas, MS, RD, CNSD
Elaine Trujillo, MS, RD, CNSD
Jamie H. Von Roenn, MD

REVIEWERS

Abby Bloch, PhD, RD
Suzanne Dixon, MPH, MS, RD
Marianne Grandon, RD
Kathryn K. Hamilton, MA, RD
Dianne Kiyomoto, RD
Karen Kulakowski, MA, RD
Rhone Levin, MEd, RD
Karen Masino, MS, RN, RD, OCN, CNSD
Julie Meddles, RD
Jeannine Mills, MS, RD
Sharon Phillips, RD, CNSD

Section 1

Cancer Overview

Chapter 1

Adult Oncology

KIM ROBIEN, PHD, RD, FADA, CNSD

INTRODUCTION

The term *cancer* describes an assortment of neoplastic diseases that occur when abnormal cells exhibit uncontrollable growth, which can lead to devastating systemic and localized effects (1). This chapter reviews the incidence of cancer in the adult US population as well as cancer screening and classification methods. Because it is impossible to cover all that is currently known about cancer in adults, this chapter provides a general overview of adult oncology, focusing on the four most common cancer types and the appropriate risk factors, symptoms, screening, and treatment.

STATISTICS

The National Center for Health Statistics reports that cancer was the second leading cause of death in the United States in 2002 (2). Using data from the National Cancer Institute (NCI) Surveillance, Epidemiology and End Results (SEER) program, the American Cancer Society (ACS) estimated that 1.4 million new cases of cancer would be diagnosed in 2005 (3). Projected figures are published annually in the January issue of *CA: A Cancer Journal for Clinicians* (4), and are available as the *Cancer Facts and Figures* document on the ACS Web site (5).

Overall, men have a 1-in-2 lifetime risk of developing cancer, compared with women whose lifetime risk is a little more than 1 in 3 (5,6). Whites and African Americans have higher cancer incidence rates than other racial groups (3,7). Individuals from minority groups are more likely than whites to have their cancers diagnosed at an advanced stage (7). Overall, age-adjusted cancer incidence rates decreased by 4.8% per year from 1992 through 1995 and were essentially stable from 1995 to 2000 (8).

Overall, cancer death rates in the United States decreased beginning in 1994 and then stabilized from 1998 to 2000 (8). Specifically, cancer death rates for women stabilized, and cancer death rates for men continued to decline (8).

SCREENING

The most common cancer screening tests are based on physical examination or palpation, such as the breast or testicle self-exam, or examination of the skin to look for changes in pigmentation that may signal the development of skin cancer. However, when cancer is detected by these techniques, it is often fairly advanced. Early cancer detection refers to screening tests that can identify tumors before they become palpable. This is an active area of cancer research with the potential to significantly decrease cancer morbidity and mortality and health care costs (9).

Blood tests to determine levels of circulating tumor cell metabolites (biomarkers), such as prostate-specific antigen (PSA) testing, are being developed as early detection methods. Molecular techniques, such as genetics, gene expression assays, and proteomics, are also being explored for possible use in early cancer detection, as are many radiographic techniques. The ACS publishes yearly updates on cancer detection guidelines and reviews the current issues surrounding cancer screening and early detection (10). These guidelines are available on the ACS Web site (5).

STAGING

When a cancer is diagnosed, it must be staged to determine the most effective treatment plan and offer a prognosis. The TNM classification system (11,12), which stands for *T*umor, lymph *N*odes, and *M*etastasis, is the most common tumor staging tool, especially for solid tumors. Each tumor is assigned a *T* grade, which describes the size and location of the primary tumor; an *N* grade, which describes the degree of metastasis to regional lymph nodes; and an *M* grade, which describes the distant metastasis. In addition, a *G* grade describes the tumor's histopathology (see Table 1.1) (11,12). The SEER Registry uses a summary staging system to categorize cancers when collecting data for cancer statistics (see Table 1.2) (13).

Table 1.1 Summary of the TNM Classification System

Grade	*Definition*
Tumor*	
T0	No evidence of tumor
Tis	Carcinoma in situ or cancer that has not spread to the surrounding tissue
T1	Tumor not palpable or visible by imaging
T2	Tumor confined to the primary cancer site
T3	Tumor extending to the neighboring tissue
T4	Metastatic disease
Lymph Nodes	
N0	No involvement of the lymph nodes
N1	Metastasis to local lymph nodes
Metastasis*	
M0	No metastasis
M1	Distant metastasis
Histopathologic Grade	
G1	Well differentiated
G2	Moderately differentiated
G3	Poorly differentiated
G4	Undifferentiated

*Subcategories of the tumor and metastasis classification further define the stage of disease but are beyond the scope of this discussion.

Source: Data are from references 11 and 12.

COMMON ADULT CANCERS

The five most common cancer types for new cancer cases in US adults are prostate, lung, colorectal, bladder, and melanoma in men, and breast, lung, colorectal, uterine, and ovarian in women (3). Prostrate, breast, lung, and colorectal cancer are discussed here.

Prostate Cancer

The ACS estimated that 232,090 men would be diagnosed with prostate cancer in 2005 (3). The incidence of prostate cancer increased substantially in the late 1980s and early 1990s after the development of PSA testing. The incidence of prostate cancer has decreased somewhat since that time and is now relatively stable (5). Prostate cancer occurs primarily in men older than 50 years (14).

Risk Factors

Risk factors for prostate cancer include advanced age (older than 65 years), ethnicity, and family history of prostate cancer (5,14). Prostate cancer is more common in African American men than in white men, and it is less common in Asian and Native American men than in whites (14). Epidemiological studies have found that energy-dense diets and diets high in red meats and animal fat increase the risk of prostate cancer, whereas vegetable intake has been associated with a decreased risk of prostate cancer (15–17).

Table 1.2 SEER Registry Summary Staging System

Stage(s)	*Description*
0	In situ. Cancer that has not spread to surrounding tissues.
1	Localized. Cancer that is limited to the primary affected organ.
2–5	Regional. Cancer that affects the primary organ and its surrounding tissue but has not metastasized.
7	Distant. Cancer that has metastasized to other parts of the body.
9	Unknown if extension or metastasis. For cases in which there is insufficient information available to assign the cancer to another category.

Source: Data are from reference 13.

Symptoms and Screening

Symptoms of prostate cancer include difficulty starting or controlling urination, frequent need to urinate, pain or discomfort with urination, erectile dysfunction, pain on ejaculation, and the presence of blood in urine or semen.

The digital rectal exam (DRE), which feels for unusual lumps or other irregularities in the prostate, is commonly used to screen for prostate cancer. A blood test, the PSA, is also used to screen for prostate cancer. There is some controversy over the value of both these tests in screening men of average risk of prostate cancer (14,18). The tests are known to have high false-positive rates, and they may identify the presence of benign prostatic hypertrophy or infection of the prostate as well as prostate cancer (14). The ACS recommends that PSA and DRE testing be offered on an annual basis to all men 50 years and older who have a life expectancy of at least 10 years (10). Men of African descent and those with a family history of prostate cancer should begin annual DRE and PSA testing at age 45 (10).

Treatment

Treatment for prostate cancer depends on the stage of disease. It may include watchful waiting (for Stage 1, or for T1, N0, M0, or G1 disease), or surgery, radiation, or hormonal therapy to block the action of androgenic hormones (ie, androgen deprivation therapy) (6). For more information on radiation therapy and surgery, see Chapters 9 and 10. The NCI's Physician Data Query (PDQ) Cancer Information Summaries (19) offer the most current consensus statement on the treatment of prostate cancer.

Survival rates for prostate cancer vary, depending on the stage of disease at diagnosis. When the disease is contained to the prostate, the 5-year survival rate is 100% (6). Ten-year survival rates for all stages of the disease is 92%, and 15-year survival rates for all stages is 61% (5).

Breast Cancer

The ACS estimated that nearly 211,240 women and 1,690 men were diagnosed with invasive breast cancer in 2004 (3). In addition, an estimated 58,490 cases of in situ breast cancer would be diagnosed in 2005, most of which would be ductal carcinoma in situ (DCIS) (6). Overall, breast cancer incidence rates for women have been increasing since 1986 at a rate of less than 1% per year (8). This increase seems to be the result of better cancer screening and detection (20).

Risk Factors

Many factors have been evaluated for their influence on the risk of breast cancer in women. Women at increased risk of breast cancer include those with two or more relatives with breast or ovarian cancer, breast cancer occurring before age 50 in an affected relative, relatives with both breast and ovarian cancer, one or more relatives with two cancers (breast and ovarian cancer or two independent breast cancers), male relatives with breast cancer, or a family history of breast or ovarian cancer and Ashkenazi Jewish heritage (21). Women who carry BRCA1 or BRCA2 genetic mutations are also at increased breast cancer risk (22,23). Epidemiological studies have found that breast cancer risk increases as a woman ages (24). Women with dense breast tissue are at increased risk of breast cancer, as are women who have been diagnosed with atypical hyperplasia of the breast tissues or lobular carcinoma in situ (LCIS) (6).

Hormonal influences, especially those of estrogen, are thought to play a major role in the development of breast cancer. Women who begin menstruating at a young age or who go through menopause after age 55 have been found to have an increased risk, presumably because of prolonged exposure to estrogen (25). Similarly, women who have never had children and those who have children after age 35 are also considered to be at increased risk of developing the disease (5,24). Use of oral contraceptives or hormone replacement therapy (HRT) seems to modestly increase risk of breast cancer, although the risk seems to decrease as soon as oral contraceptives or HRT is stopped. At 5 or more years after discontinuation, the risk is the same as for women who never used contraceptives/HRT (24). Because the mesenchymal cells of adipose tissue produce estrogen (26), obesity is also thought to be a potential risk factor for the occurrence and recurrence of breast cancer in postmenopausal women (24,27). Epidemiological studies confirm that physical inactivity, weight gain, and obesity, especially after menopause, are associated with increased risk of breast cancer (28,29).

Studies investigating the links between diet and breast cancer risk have been inconclusive (24,30). Yet it seems prudent to suggest that the current general dietary guidelines (Chapter 4) to achieve and maintain a healthy weight; to limit alcohol intake; and to consume a plant-based, high-fiber diet may decrease the risk of breast cancer.

Symptoms and Screening

Symptoms of breast cancer may include changes in the size and shape of one or both breasts; nipple tenderness or discharge; one or more lumps in the breast; and scaly, red, or swollen skin of the breast or nipple (6). The current screening guidelines from the ACS call for clinical breast exams every 3 years for women in their 20s and 30s, and yearly for women 40 years and older (21). The guidelines call for yearly mammograms beginning at 40 years. Women at increased risk of breast cancer should discuss more frequent screening with their health care provider (21).

Breast self-exams (BSEs) are now considered optional for women at average risk for breast cancer. Several large studies have found that BSE does not result in decreased breast cancer mortality, but it increases the likelihood of the individual undergoing a breast biopsy for a benign lump (10,31).

Because breast tissue is comprised of a variety of different cell types, breast cancer is typically described by cellular classification: ductal, lobular, nipple, or undifferentiated. Staging for breast cancer follows the TNM classification system (see Table 1.1). Estrogen receptor status of the tumor, which assists clinicians in determining the most effective course of treatment, may also be determined (25).

Treatment

Treatment for breast cancer may include the use of chemopreventive agents (such as tamoxifen or raloxifene), chemotherapy, radiation, surgical resection, or a combination of therapies. For more information on chemotherapy, radiation therapy, and surgery, see Chapters 8 through 10. Refer to the PDQ Cancer Information Summaries (19) for the most current breast cancer treatment recommendations by stage of disease and survival rates associated with the various treatment options.

Current overall 5-year survival rates for breast cancer are estimated to be 97% for women whose cancer has not reached the lymph nodes, 79% for women with regional metastases, and 23% for women with distant metastases (6).

Lung Cancer

The ACS estimated that 172,570 Americans would be diagnosed with lung cancer in 2005 (3). Although cigarette use began to decline steadily after the release of the Surgeon General's report linking smoking and lung cancer in 1964 (32), lung cancer incidence and death rates did not begin to decline substantially for men until the early 1990s (6,33). Lung cancer incidence has continued to increase among women, although the rate at which new cases have been diagnosed has slowed since the late 1990s (6).

The median age range for individuals at diagnosis of lung cancer is 65 to 70 years (34). Symptoms usually appear late in the disease course; only 16% of lung cancers are diagnosed while the disease is still localized and easily resectable (6). Ninety percent of people diagnosed with lung cancer die of the disease rather than of other causes (33).

Risk Factors

The primary cause of lung cancer is exposure to tobacco smoke, whether from cigarettes, cigars, or pipes (32,34–36). Exposure to secondhand smoke is also known to be a significant risk factor for the development of lung cancer (37). Exposure to other environmental carcinogens, such as asbestos, radon, chromates, chloromethyl ethers, nickel, and polycyclic aromatic hydrocarbons, is also associated with increased risk of lung cancer (33).

Symptoms and Screening

Symptoms of lung cancer include coughing that fails to resolve or worsens, hemoptysis, shortness of breath, wheezing, hoarseness, repeated bouts of pneumonia or bronchitis, fatigue, and loss of appetite (6). Chest x-rays and sputum cytology have been used as lung cancer screening tests; however, several large prospective studies have failed to find that regular screening with these tests results in decreased mortality from lung cancer (38). The ACS does not currently recommend screening tests for lung cancer (10). The NCI-funded Prostate, Lung, Colorectal and Ovarian (PLCO) Cancer Screening Trial (39) and National Lung Screening Trial (NLST) studies (40) are in the process of evaluating the effectiveness of spiral CT screening in reducing lung cancer mortality.

Lung cancers are described by the type of lung tissue affected and are generally divided into two major histopathologic categories: non-small cell (75% to 90% of lung cancers) or small cell (20% to 25% of lung cancers) (6). Staging of lung cancer follows the TNM classification system (Table 1.1).

Treatment

Treatment for lung cancer may include surgery (if the tumor is localized), chemotherapy, radiation, photodynamic (laser) therapy, or a combination of these modalities (6). For more information on chemotherapy and radiation therapy, see Chapters 8 and 9. Refer to the PDQ Cancer Information Summaries (19) for the most current treatment recommendations by stage of disease. Improvements in surgical techniques for resection of lung cancers during the past 30 years have improved 1-year survival rates from 37% to 42%; however, the overall 5-year survival rate is only 15% (6).

Colorectal Cancer

The ACS estimated that, in 2005, more than 104,950 adults would be diagnosed with colon cancer and more than 40,340 would be diagnosed with rectal cancer (3). More than 90% of colorectal cancers are diagnosed in people older than 50 years (6).

Risk Factors

Risk factors for colorectal cancer include advanced age, family history of the disease, tobacco smoking, obesity, and physical inactivity (6). Dietary factors associated with increased risk of colorectal cancers include high intakes of dietary fat, well-cooked meats, and alcohol (16,41).

Symptoms and Screening

Symptoms of colorectal cancer typically do not occur until the later stages of the disease. They include rectal bleeding or blood in the stool, changes in normal bowel movement patterns, and crampy lower abdominal pain (6). Fecal occult blood testing (FOBT), flexible sigmoidoscopy, double contrast barium enema, and colonoscopy are the primary screening techniques for colorectal cancer. The ACS recommends annual testing with one or more of these techniques beginning at age 50 years (10).

The TNM classification system is currently the preferred method for staging colorectal cancer by most clinicians; however, some centers continue to use a modification of the Dukes classification system, which was first developed in the 1930s (42). The Dukes stages are A, limited to the colonic mucosa; B1, extending into, but not through, the muscularis propria; B2, extending through the entire wall, but no lymph node involvement; C1, limited to the colonic wall with lymph node involvement; C2, through all layers of the colonic wall, extending to the stromal surface with lymph node involvement; and D1, distant metastatic spread.

Treatment

Surgical resection of the affected segment of the colon or rectum is the primary treatment for colorectal cancer. However, chemotherapy or radiation may also be used (6). Chemotherapy, radiation therapy, and surgery are discussed in Chapters 8 through 10. Refer to the PDQ Cancer Information Summaries (19) for the most current treatment recommendations by stage of disease.

Overall 5-year survival rates of colorectal cancer are currently 62%. Individuals diagnosed in the earlier stages of disease, when the cancer is localized, have a 5-year survival rate of 90% (6).

REFERENCES

1. Shils ME. Nutrition needs of cancer patients. In: Bloch AS, ed. *Nutrition Management of the Cancer Patient.* Rockville, Md: Aspen Publishers, Inc.; 1990:3–10.
2. Kochanek KD, Smith BL. Deaths: preliminary data for 2002. *Natl Vital Stat Rep.* 2004;52:1–47.
3. Jemal A, Murray T, Ward E, Samuels A, Tiwari RC, Ghafoor A, Feuer EJ, Thun MJ. Cancer statistics, 2005. *CA Cancer J Clin.* 2005;55:10–30.
4. CA: A Cancer Journal for Clinicians. Web site. Available at: http://caonline.amcancersoc.org. Accessed April 11, 2005.
5. American Cancer Society Web site. Available at: http://www.cancer.org/docroot/home/index.asp. Accessed April 11, 2005.
6. American Cancer Society. *Cancer Facts and Figures 2004.* Atlanta, Ga: American Cancer Society, Inc.; 2004.
7. US Cancer Statistics Working Group. *United States Cancer Statistics: 2000 Incidence.* Atlanta, Ga: Department of Health and Human Services, Centers for Disease Control and Prevention and National Cancer Institute; 2003.
8. Weir HK, Thun MJ, Hankey BF, Ries LA, Howe HL, Wingo PA, Jemal A, Ward E, Anderson RN, Edwards BK. Annual report to the nation on the status of cancer, 1975–2000, featuring the uses of surveillance data for cancer prevention and control. *J Natl Cancer Inst.* 2003;95:1276–1299.
9. Etzioni R, Urban N, Ramsey S, McIntosh M, Schwartz S, Reid B, Radich J, Anderson G, Hartwell L. The case for early detection. *Nat Rev Cancer.* 2003;3:243–252.
10. Smith RA, Cokkinides V, Eyre HJ. American Cancer Society guidelines for the early detection of cancer, 2004. *CA Cancer J Clin.* 2004;54:41–52.
11. Sobin LH, Wittekind C, eds. *TNM Classification of Malignant Tumours.* 6th ed. New York, NY: Wiley-Liss; 2002.
12. Greene FL, Page DL, Fleming ID, Fritz A, Balch CM, Haller DG, Morrow M, eds. *AJCC Cancer Staging Manual.* 6th ed. New York, NY: Springer; 2002.
13. National Cancer Institute. SEER Summary Staging Manual—2000 Web site. Available at: http://seer.cancer.gov/tools/ssm/. Accessed April 11, 2005.
14. Crawford ED. Epidemiology of prostate cancer. *Urology.* 2003;62(6 Suppl 1):1–2.
15. Giovannucci E, Rimm EB, Colditz GA, Stampfer MJ, Ascherio A, Chute CC, Willett WC. A prospective study of dietary fat and risk of prostate cancer. *J Natl Cancer Inst.* 1993;85:1571–1579.
16. Glade MJ. Food, nutrition, and the prevention of cancer: a global perspective. American Institute for Cancer Research/World Cancer Research Fund, American Institute for Cancer Research, 1997. *Nutrition.* 1999;15:523–526.
17. Kristal AR, Cohen JH, Qu P, Stanford JL. Associations of energy, fat, calcium, and vitamin D with prostate cancer risk. *Cancer Epidemiol Biomarkers Prev.* 2002;11:719–725.
18. Caplan A, Kratz A. Prostate-specific antigen and the early diagnosis of prostate cancer. *Am J Clin Pathol.* 2002;117(suppl):S104-S108.
19. National Cancer Institute. PDQ®—NCI's Comprehensive Cancer Database. Available at: http://www.nci.nih.gov/cancerinfo/pdq/cancerdatabase. Accessed April 11, 2005.
20. Nasseri K. Secular trends in the incidence of female breast cancer in the United States, 1973–1998. *Breast J.* 2004;10:129–135.
21. Smith RA, Saslow D, Sawyer KA, Burke W, Costanza ME, Evans WP III, Foster RS Jr, Hendrick E, Eyre HJ, Sener S. American Cancer Society guidelines for breast cancer screening: update 2003. *CA Cancer J Clin.* 2003;53:141–169.
22. Miki Y, Swensen J, Shattuck-Eidens D, Futreal PA, Harshman K, Tavtigian S, Liu Q, Cochran C, Bennett LM, Ding W, Bell R, Rosenthal J, Hussey C, Tran T, McClure M, Frye C, Hattier T, Phelps R, Haugen-Strano A, Katcher H, Yakumo K, Gholami Z, Shaffer D, Stone S, Bayer S, Wray C, Bogden R, Dayananth P, Ward J, Tonin P, Narod S, Bristow PK, Norris FH, Helverig L, Morrison P, Rosteck P, Lai M, Barrett JC, Lewis C, Neuhausen S, Cannon-Albright L, Goldgar D, Wiseman R, Kamb A, Skolnick MH. A strong candidate for the breast and ovarian cancer susceptibility gene BRCA1. *Science.* 1994;266:66–71.
23. Wooster R, Neuhausen SL, Mangion J, Quirk Y, Ford D, Collins N, Nguyen K, Seal S, Tran T, Averill D, et al. Localization of a breast cancer susceptibility gene, BRCA2, to chromosome 13q12–13. *Science.* 1994; 265:2088–2090.
24. Key TJ, Verkasalo PK, Banks E. Epidemiology of breast cancer. *Lancet Oncol.* 2001;2:133–140.
25. Henderson BE, Pike MC, Bernstein L, Ross RK. Breast cancer. In: Schottenfeld D, Fraumeni JF Jr, eds. *Cancer Epidemiology and Prevention.* 2nd ed.

New York, NY: Oxford University Press; 1996: 1022–1039.

26. Simpson ER. Sources of estrogen and their importance. *J Steroid Biochem Mol Biol.* 2003;86:225–230.
27. Wasserman L, Flatt SW, Natarajan L, Laughlin G, Matusalem M, Faerber S, Rock CL, Barrett-Connor E, Pierce JP. Correlates of obesity in postmenopausal women with breast cancer: comparison of genetic, demographic, disease-related, life history and dietary factors. *Int J Obes Relat Metab Disord.* 2004;28: 49–56.
28. McTiernan A, Kooperberg C, White E, Wilcox S, Coates R, Adams-Campbell LL, Woods N, Ockene J. Recreational physical activity and the risk of breast cancer in postmenopausal women: the Women's Health Initiative Cohort Study. *JAMA.* 2003;290: 1331–1336.
29. Morimoto LM, White E, Chen Z, Chlebowski RT, Hays J, Kuller L, Lopez AM, Manson J, Margolis KL, Muti PC, Stefanick ML, McTiernan A. Obesity, body size, and risk of postmenopausal breast cancer: the Women's Health Initiative (United States). *Cancer Causes Control.* 2002;13:741–751.
30. Forman MR, Ballard-Barbash R, Kipnis V. Nutritional strategies for breast cancer prevention: what have we learned and where do we go from here? *Cancer.* 2003;98:1782–1785.
31. Thomas DB, Gao DL, Ray RM, Wang WW, Allison CJ, Chen FL, Porter P, Hu YW, Zhao GL, Pan LD, Li W, Wu C, Coriaty Z, Evans I, Lin MG, Stalsberg H, Self SG. Randomized trial of breast self-examination in Shanghai: final results. *J Natl Cancer Inst.* 2002;94: 1445–1457.
32. United States Public Health Service. *Smoking and Health: A Report of the Surgeon General.* Washington, DC: US Government Printing Office; 1964.
33. Alberg AJ, Samet JM. Epidemiology of lung cancer. *Chest.* 2003;123(suppl 1): S21-S49.
34. Bilello KS, Murin S, Matthay RA. Epidemiology, etiology, and prevention of lung cancer. *Clin Chest Med.* 2002;23:1–25.
35. Doll R, Hill AB. Smoking and carcinoma of the lung: preliminary report. *Br Med J.* 1950;2:739–748.
36. Wynder EL, Graham EA. Tobacco smoking as a possible etiological factor in bronchiogenic carcinoma. *JAMA.* 1950;143:329–336.
37. Hackshaw AK, Law MR, Wald NJ. The accumulated evidence on lung cancer and environmental tobacco smoke. *BMJ.* 1997;315:980–988.
38. Manser R, Irving L, Stone C, Byrnes G, Abramson M, Campbell D. Screening for lung cancer. *Curr Opin Pulm Med.* 2004;10:266–271.
39. Gohagan JK, Prorok PC, Hayes RB, Kramer BS. Prostate, Lung, Colorectal and Ovarian Cancer Screening Trial Project Team. The Prostate, Lung, Colorectal and Ovarian (PLCO) Cancer Screening Trial of the National Cancer Institute: history, organization, and status. *Control Clin Trials.* 2000;21(Suppl 6): S251-S272.
40. Recruitment begins for lung cancer screening trial. *J Natl Cancer Inst.* 2002;94:1603.
41. Sanjoaquin MA, Appleby PN, Thorogood M, Mann JI, Key TJ. Nutrition, lifestyle and colorectal cancer incidence: a prospective investigation of 10998 vegetarians and non-vegetarians in the United Kingdom. *Br J Cancer.* 2004;90:118–121.
42. Dukes CE. The classification of cancer in the rectum. *J Pathol Bacteriol.* 1932;35:323–332.

Chapter 2

Pediatric Oncology

D'NICE CARDEN, MS, RN, CPNP, CPON, AND TONI ISAACS, RD, CNSD

INTRODUCTION

This chapter reviews the incidence of cancer in the pediatric US population. It also examines common pediatric cancers and treatment considerations, including the importance of a multidisciplinary team and family-centered care.

STATISTICS

According to the National Cancer Institute (NCI) Surveillance, Epidemiology, and End Results (SEER) pediatric monograph, approximately 12,400 children younger than 20 years were diagnosed with cancer in 1998, and 2,500 children between the ages of 1 and 19 years died from cancer that same year (1). Cancer ranks fourth behind accidents, homicides, and suicides as a cause of death in children 1 to 19 years (2). A newborn male has a 1-in-300 chance of developing cancer by age 20; a newborn female has a 1-in-333 chance by age 20 (2). In children younger than 5 years and in those between the ages of 15 and 19, cancer occurs in 200 of every 1 million. In children between those two age ranges, the incidence rate is 110 to 120 of every 1 million (1).

SCREENING

There are no accepted screening guidelines for cancer in children. Screening for cancer in children is difficult because tumors originate from fetal-type cells, which occur deep within the child's body tissues and often become large and metastasize before they can be detected (3).

However, tumor markers, including tumor-specific antigens, catecholamines, and gene rearrangements, can be used for cancer diagnosis in children and to measure the efficacy of cancer treatment. Tumor markers also may be used to predict the likelihood of potential relapse and the need for more intensive therapy (4).

CANCERS FREQUENTLY DIAGNOSED IN CHILDREN

According to NCI, the three malignant cancers most frequently diagnosed in children between 1975 and 1995 were leukemia, tumors of the central nervous system (CNS), and lymphoma (1). These three cancer types are discussed in the sections that follow.

Leukemia

Leukemia is cancer of the bone marrow and blood and can be categorized as myeloid or lymphocytic. Both types can be further classified as acute or chronic. Between 1990 and 1995, leukemia accounted for nearly 25% of all cancers in children younger than 20 years (5). The most common cancer in children is acute lymphocytic leukemia (ALL) (5); it accounts for approximately 75% of all cases of leukemia (6). ALL occurs most frequently in children between the ages of 2 and 3 years, and white children are more likely to be diagnosed with ALL than other ethnic population groups (6–8). Children are four times more likely to develop ALL than acute myeloid leukemia (AML) (9). However, AML accounts for more than 30% of pediatric deaths from leukemia (9).

Chronic myeloid leukemia (CML) is very rare in children; it is a disease that almost exclusively affects the elderly. In CML, the bone marrow is affected slowly and by degrees. CML almost always evolves into an acute phase, which is similar to AML. At this time, prognosis for CML is poor for anyone diagnosed with the disease, even with aggressive treatment (10).

Risk Factors

ALL and AML occur more often in children with certain genetic conditions, such as Down syndrome, neurofibromatosis type 1, Bloom syndrome, ataxia telangiectasia, Fanconi's anemia, and Langerhans cell histiocytosis, than in other children (6,8). Some chemotherapeutic agents used to fight cancer during childhood and adolescence can be associated with the development of AML in adulthood (6).

Treatment

Current treatment strategies for acute leukemias are divided into two parts: induction therapy and postremission therapy (11). Induction therapy consists of dose-intensified combination chemotherapy. Postremission therapy can include bone marrow transplant with or without total body irradiation and additional high-dose chemotherapy.

The treatment course for ALL typically lasts 2.5 to 3 years (6–8). The survival rate for ALL is nearly 80% (6–8). Treatment for AML is aggressive and typically lasts 1 year (9). Most children with AML will have a bone marrow transplant if they have a sibling match for marrow or they will be given aggressive chemotherapy, which is associated with serious side effects and requires extended hospital stays. In children between the ages of 1 and 9, the rate of survival is 50% in AML compared with an 80% survival rate in ALL.

CML can be treated indefinitely with oral chemotherapeutic agents. However, the only cure is a bone marrow transplant, and the survival rate for children with CML who have a transplant is low (10).

Central Nervous System Tumors

CNS tumors are the second most common type of cancer in children (12,13). CNS tumors are classified as primary intracranial and spinal axis tumors. Examples of CNS tumors occurring in children include medulloblastoma, retinoblastoma, and meningioma.

Screening

No screening methods exist for CNS tumors. Symptoms of CNS tumors may include nausea and vomiting that occur upon arising; sudden changes in vision; evidence of interruption in cranial nerves; and changes in speech, memory, or balance (12).

Risk Factors

Certain rare syndromes, such as neurofibromatosis, Li-Fraumeni syndrome, tuberous sclerosis, Turcot's syndrome, and von Hippel-Lindau disease, place children at a markedly increased risk for developing brain tumors (13).

Treatment

Surgery is the primary treatment modality for brain tumors that are accessible and resectable (13). Radiation therapy is used as adjuvant therapy if the child is older than 3 years (13). Dietetics professionals should note that late effects of radiation therapy to the brain and spinal axis during childhood can cause neuroendocrine dysfunction, cataracts, dental problems, and diminished intellectual capacity, including mild to moderate learning problems, and attention-concentration changes (14). Chemotherapy is used for aggressive tumors when surgery is not possible because of the tumor location. It is also used when the child's age precludes radiation therapy, and it may be used to destroy malignant cells that were not removed in surgery, even when surgery is possible. At times, all three methods of treatment are used in conjunction with one another (11,12). Tumors of the CNS have the highest incidence of mortality of all cancers in children (11,12).

Lymphoma

Lymphoma is a disease of the lymphatic system that occurs in individuals of all ages. Because the lymphatic system stretches throughout the body, lymphoma-like leukemia is considered a systemic disease at onset (15,16). Lymphoma (including both Hodgkin's lymphoma and non-Hodgkin's lymphoma) is the third most common cancer in children; incidence in boys outnumbers girls 2 tol (16).

Non-Hodgkin's lymphoma accounts for approximately 7% of cancers in children younger than 20 years (17). There are approximately 800 new cases in US children each year (17). More than 70% of children and adolescents with non-Hodgkin's lymphoma survive at least 5 years with treatment. However, survival outcome is related to the extent of which the tumor has spread at diagnosis and whether or not the tumor is resectable (15,17).

Hodgkin's lymphoma in children resembles the disease in adults in terms of both biology and natural history. Hodgkin's lymphoma accounts for 6% of cancers in children. In preschool and school-age children, boys are more likely to have Hodgkin's lymphoma than girls. During adolescence, the incidence of occurrence equalizes (18,19).

Risk Factors

Although there are currently no proven risk factors for lymphoma, familial clustering is occasionally reported for Hodgkin's lymphoma when more than one family member develops the disease (19). Researchers are also investigating whether infection with Epstein Barr virus (EBV) is connected to the development of Hodgkin's lymphoma. However, the strongest evidence for such a link is seen in developing countries and is not a common finding in the cases diagnosed in the United States. Whereas EBV does not cause Hodgkin's lymphoma, patients in the United States who have had a documented case of mononucleosis will be four times more likely to have genetic material from the virus replicated within their cancer cells. Nonetheless, the association is, at best, correlational, and not causative (19).

Treatment

Treatment for non-Hodgkin's lymphoma generally includes combination chemotherapy, although treatment can vary. Treatment for non-Hodgkin's lymphoma is usually more aggressive, lasts longer, and requires more hospitalizations than treatment for Hodgkin's lymphoma (15–17).

Treatment for Hodgkin's lymphoma includes chemotherapy, which is primarily given in an outpatient setting, and usually lasts between 4 and 8 months (18,19). Radiation therapy may also be used but at a much lesser intensity than in adults, because of increased incidence of breast cancer among women who received radiation to their chest as a child or adolescent.

LESS COMMON CANCERS

Neuroblastoma, Wilms' tumor, and bone and soft-tissue sarcomas are considered "childhood" cancers, because of their all but exclusive occurrence in children or young adults. Although these malignant solid tumors are not seen as frequently as leukemia, brain tumors, or lymphoma, they are important in a discussion of pediatric oncology and are outlined in the following sections.

Neuroblastoma

Neuroblastoma is a disease of early childhood. Two-thirds of the cases are diagnosed in children younger than 5 years (20), with the overall incidence rate of 9.5 per million children. Among children younger than 15 years with cancer, 7.8% have neuroblastoma (1). Neuroblastoma is connected to the sympathetic nervous system and frequently originates in the adrenal medulla or along the spinal cord (21,22). In rare cases, a prenatal ultrasound may show neuroblastoma. In those cases, chemotherapy may be initiated immediately after birth if the infant is in distress related to the tumor (20).

Screening

When a diagnosis of neuroblastoma is suspected, 10 mL of urine are tested for specific catecholamines. However, this is not a practical screening tool because the disease is rare and the test is expensive and may have false-positive results (21,22).

Risk Factors

There are no known risk factors for neuroblastoma at this time.

Treatment

Children younger than 1 year have a very favorable prognosis regardless of the amount of tumor present and may require no treatment whatsoever other than frequent evaluations from a pediatric oncologist. Remarkably, in children younger than 1 year, neuroblastoma tumor cells seem to experience spontaneous regression, maturing from malignant to normal cells within less than 1 year. These children may not require any treatment if the size of the tumor does not cause distress. If the tumor size does interfere with normal organ function, such as an abdominal tumor pressing against the diaphragm and restricting lung expansion, chemotherapy can be used to shrink the tumor. However, in older children, the situation changes drastically. Children older than 1 year who have advanced disease at diagnosis have a poor prognosis and require extensive, aggressive treatment, including surgery, radiation, chemotherapy, as well as autologous stem cell transplant. It is estimated that only 20% of children older than 1 year with advanced neuroblastoma will survive disease free for 2 years (21,22).

Wilms' Tumor

Like neuroblastoma, Wilms' tumor (nephrobastoma) is highly specific to children. It is a cancer of the kidney and is considered highly treatable, with more than 90% of children surviving 4 years after diagnosis (22). Approximately 500 cases are diagnosed annually in the United States (22). Wilms' tumor occurs most frequently in younger children, with the incidence of occurrence being greatest—18 per million—in children younger than 5 years. The incidence drops sharply as age increases, with only 1 per million by age 20. At this age, kidney cancers are more likely to be the same as those found in older adults (1).

Screening

No specific screening tools exist for Wilms' tumor. However, symptoms such as hematuria should be investigated. The most obvious evidence of Wilms' tumor is a particularly prominent abdomen, which can be screened by visual observation, assessment, and investigation (23).

Treatment

Treatment for Wilms' tumor consists of chemotherapy before and after surgery to remove the diseased kidney. Radiation therapy may also be used. If there are tumors in both kidneys, more aggressive chemotherapy will be used to shrink the tumors as much as possible before surgery. This approach saves as much kidney function as possible. Overall, survival rates for Wilms' tumor are greater than 90% (23,24).

Bone and Soft-Tissue Tumors

Bone tumors, such as osteogenic sarcoma and Ewing's sarcoma, are seen in adolescents more than in any other age group. Less often, they are found in preadolescents; rarely are these diagnoses seen in persons older than 25 years (25). Osteogenic sarcoma accounts for 5% of tumors in children; Ewing's sarcoma, which can occur in the bone and soft tissues, accounts for 4%. With both types of tumors, individuals with localized disease and completely resectable tumors have the greatest chance of a good outcome (25). Individuals with metastatic disease at diagnosis have a 20% to 30% chance of survival. For both diseases, as many as 20% of patients will have metastases evident at time of diagnosis (25).

Rhabdomyosarcoma (RMS) is a soft-tissue tumor that originates in the skeletal muscle. It accounts for less than 4% of all cancer in children younger than 14 years and only 2% in those between 15 and 19 years. The survival rate depends on how far the disease has spread at time of diagnosis, with a 70% cure rate seen in children with localized disease. For children with metastatic disease at diagnosis, there is a 30% chance of survival (26).

Screening

Because these tumors may originate from so many different areas, a thorough radiographic examination, including ultrasound, conventional scanning (eg, computed tomography and plain films), and radionuclide bone scanning, is usually required. Diagnosis may also include bone marrow aspiration and biopsy (27).

Treatment

Treatment for bone tumors and soft-tissue tumors requires a combination of chemotherapy drugs given in recurring cycles. Treatments last for 1 year, with most of the therapy given in the hospital because of the complexity of treatment and the high incidence of nausea, vomiting, and possible dehydration. Surgery is also an important component, but it may not be utilized until after chemotherapy has been initiated and several treatments have been undertaken to shrink the size of the tumor, because complete resection of the tumor is extremely important in the overall outcome.

Radiation may also be used with soft-tissue tumors but is not effective in osteogenic sarcoma (25).

CONSIDERATIONS IN TREATING CHILDHOOD CANCER

The Multidisciplinary Team

A multidisciplinary team of cancer specialists, including oncologists, surgeons, pathologists, radiologists, nurses, child-life specialists, dietetics professionals, social workers, religious/spiritual advisers, and physical, speech, and occupational therapists, is recommended for the treatment of children with cancer. This approach is currently a requirement for institutional membership to the Children's Oncology Group (COG), an international cooperative group of centers that provide access to clinical trials for children with cancer (28).

Family-Centered Care

In family-centered care, the interdisciplinary team includes the family in planning and in providing patient care and respects the family's care decisions (29,30). Family-centered care is emphasized in the treatment of cancer in children, especially in palliative care settings. For more information on the principles and application of family-centered care, see the Institute for Family-Centered Care Web site (31).

Developmental Stages

Medical practitioners working with children should familiarize themselves with the stages in child development to understand how cancer treatment can affect a child's development. The physical stressors of cancer and its therapy may affect development. Extended hospitalizations, the treatment itself, or complications of treatment may also delay achievement of developmental milestones or cause a child to regress to an earlier developmental stage (32). There may be little that can be done to alter the course of treatment, but staff interactions with the child can affect his or her development.

Medication Dosages

Chemotherapy and radiation therapy dosages need to be carefully monitored in children to suit their body surface area (33–36). Depending on the age of the child patient, kidney and liver function may be immature and therefore metabolism and excretion of powerful chemotherapeutic agents may be very different from those of adult patients. When administering medication to a child, the margin of error for the dosage is narrow. A small mistake can result in a devastating outcome (33,34).

Internal Devices

Internal devices, such as a subcutaneously implanted vascular access device or a tunneled external multilumen intravenous catheter, are commonly used in the treatment of childhood cancer. Use of a permanent venous access system is the standard for children in the United States (37). Use of the central access devices, rather than peripherally inserted, temporary, intravenous catheters, results in fewer painful needle sticks, less trauma with treatment, and decreased risk for chemotherapeutic agents to leak into surrounding tissue (33). The most common complication of central access devices is infection (37).

Nutrition Impact Symptoms

Children and preadolescents typically do not experience as much nausea and vomiting as older individuals in undergoing chemotherapy (35). It is unknown whether children experience fewer nutrition impact symptoms because they receive smaller doses of chemotherapy or because children do not have preconceived expectations about the effects of treatment.

Adolescents frequently experience anticipatory nausea and vomiting before chemotherapy. They may become ill when they are en route to the treatment center, think about going for treatment, or have any type of sensory reminder of treatment—such as a smell, sound, or sight (35). Refer to Appendix A for suggestions for managing treatment-related side effects.

Children who experience severe nausea and vomiting after chemotherapy can become rapidly dehydrated (35). Younger children seldom have sufficient adipose reserves to withstand long bouts of loss of appetite, changes in taste, refusal to eat, or mucosal ulcers (35). If children need nasogastric or intravenous nutrition support, they may require hospitalization or complicated home health care (35).

The intensity of certain types of cancer treatment can result in protein-energy malnutrition (38). However, not all treatment regimens cause protein-energy malnutrition; approximately 50% of survivors of acute lymphoblastic leukemia become obese young adults (39).

Disease states that are managed with intense regimens, such as aggressive combination chemotherapies, radiation, and surgery, include the following (38):

- Advanced diseases during initial intense treatment
- Wilms' tumor stages III and IV
- Neuroblastoma stages III and IV
- Pelvic rhabdomyosarcoma
- Ewing's sarcoma
- Non-Hodgkin's lymphoma
- Acute myeloid leukemia
- Relapse acute lymphocytic leukemia
- Medulloblastoma

For a discussion of nutrition therapy recommendations in pediatric oncology, see Chapter 11.

REFERENCES

1. Ries LAG, Smith MA, Gurney JG, Linet M, Tamra T, Young JL, Bunin GR. *Cancer Incidence and Survival Among Children and Adolescents: United States SEER Program 1975–1995*. Bethesda, Md: National Cancer Institute; 1999.
2. Thiele CJ, Kastan MB. Biology of childhood cancer. In: Pizzo PA, Poplak DG, eds. *Principles and Practice of Pediatric Oncology.* 4th ed. Philadelphia, Pa: Lippincott Williams & Wilkins; 2002:45–88.
3. Ruccione K. Biologic basis of cancer in children and adolescents. In: Baggot CR, Kelly KR, Fochtman D, Foley GV, eds. *Nursing Care of Children and Adolescents With Cancer.* 3rd ed. Philadelphia, Pa: WB Saunders; 2002:24–65.
4. Sondel PM, Mackall CL. Tumor immunology and pediatric cancer. In: Pizzo PA, Poplak DG, eds. *Principles and Practice of Pediatric Oncology.* 4th ed. Philadelphia, Pa: Lippincott Williams & Wilkins; 2002:121–148.
5. Jemal A, Murray T, Samuels A, Ghafoor A, Ward E, Thun MJ. Cancer statistics, 2003. *CA Cancer J Clin.* 2003;53:5–26.
6. Margolin JF, Steuber CP, Poplack DG. Acute lymphoblastic leukemia. In: Pizzo PA, Poplak DG, eds. *Principles and Practice of Pediatric Oncology.* 4th ed. Philadelphia, Pa: Lippincott Williams & Wilkins; 2002:489–544.
7. National Cancer Institute. Childhood Acute Lymphoblastic Leukemia (PDQ®): Treatment. Childhood Acute Lymphoblastic Leukemia. Available at: http://www.nci.nih.gov/cancerinfo/pdq/treatment/childALL/healthprofessional. Accessed May 9, 2005.
8. Westlake SK, Bertolone KL. Acute lymphoblastic leukemia. In: Baggot CR, Kelly KR, Fochtman D, Foley GV, eds. *Nursing Care of Children and Adolescents With Cancer.* 3rd ed. Philadelphia, Pa: WB Saunders; 2002:466–490.
9. Golub TR, Arcessi RJ. Acute myelogenous leukemia In: Pizzo PA, Poplak DG, eds. *Principles and Practice of Pediatric Oncology.* 4th ed. Philadelphia, Pa: Lippincott Williams & Wilkins; 2002:545–590.
10. Altman AJ. Chronic leukemias of childhood. In: Pizzo PA, Poplak DG, eds. *Principles and Practice of Pediatric Oncology.* 4th ed. Philadelphia, Pa: Lippincott Williams & Wilkins; 2002:591–614.
11. Scheinberg DA, Maslak P, Weiss M. Acute leukemias. In: DeVita VT, Hellman S, Rosenberg SA, eds. *Cancer: Principles and Practice of Oncology.* 6th ed. Philadelphia: Pa: Lippincott Williams & Wilkins; 2001:2404–2433.
12. Ryan-Murray J, Petriccione MM. Central nervous system tumors. In: Baggot CR, Kelly KR, Fochtman D, Foley GV, eds. *Nursing Care of Children and Adolescents With Cancer.* 3rd ed. Philadelphia, Pa: WB Saunders; 2002:503–523.
13. Strother DR, Pollack IF, Fisher PG, Hunter JV, Woo SY, Pomeroy SL, Rorke LB. Tumors of the central nervous system. In: Pizzo PA, Poplak DG, eds. *Principles and Practice of Pediatric Oncology.* 4th ed. Philadelphia, Pa: Lippincott Williams & Wilkins; 2002:751–824.
14. Offinger KC, Hudson MM. Long term complications following childhood and adolescent cancer: foundations for providing risk-based health care for survivors. *CA: Cancer J Clin.* 2004:54:208–236.
15. Hussong MR. Non-hodgkin's lymphoma. In: Baggot CR, Kelly KR, Fochtman D, Foley GV, eds. *Nursing Care of Children and Adolescents With Cancer.* 3rd ed. Philadelphia, Pa: WB Saunders; 2002:536–544.
16. Magrath IT. Malignant non-hodgkin's lymphomas in children. In: Pizzo PA, Poplak DG, eds. *Principles and Practice of Pediatric Oncology.* 4th ed. Philadelphia, Pa: Lippincott Williams& Wilkins; 2002:661–705.
17. National Cancer Institute. Childhood Non-Hodgkin's Lymphoma (PDQ): Treatment. Available at: http://www.nci.nih.gov/cancerinfo/pdq/treatment/child-non-hodgkins/healthprofesssional. Accessed May 9, 2005.
18. Liebhauser P. Hodgkin's disease. In: Baggot CR, Kelly

KR, Fochtman D, Foley GV, eds. *Nursing Care of Children and Adolescents With Cancer.* 3rd ed. Philadelphia, Pa: WB Saunders; 2002:24–63.

19. Hudson MM, Donaldson SS. Hodgkin's disease. In: Pizzo PA, Poplak DG, eds. *Principles and Practice of Pediatric Oncology.* 4th ed. Philadelphia, Pa: Lippincott Williams & Wilkins; 2002:637–660.
20. National Cancer Institute. Neuroblastoma (PDQ): Treatment. Available at:http://www.nci.nih.gov/cancerinfo/pdq/treatment/neuroblastoma/healthprofessional. Accessed May 9, 2005.
21. Brodeur GM, Maris JM. Neuroblastoma. In: Pizzo PA, Poplak DG, eds. *Principles and Practice of Pediatric Oncology.* 4th ed. Philadelphia, Pa: Lippincott Williams & Wilkins; 2002:895–938.
22. Dadd G. Neuroblastoma. In: Baggot CR, Kelly KR, Fochtman D, Foley GV, eds. *Nursing Care of Children and Adolescents With Cancer.* 3rd ed. Philadelphia, Pa: WB Saunders; 2002:545–567.
23. Drigan R, Androkites AL. Wilms' tumor. In: Baggot CR, Kelly KR, Fochtman D, Foley GV, eds. *Nursing Care of Children and Adolescents With Cancer.* 3rd ed. Philadelphia, Pa: WB Saunders; 2002:568–574.
24. Grundy PE, Green DM, Coppes MJ, Breslow NE, Ritchey ML, Perlman EJ, Macklis RM. Renal tumors. In: Pizzo PA, Poplak DG, eds. *Principles and Practice of Pediatric Oncology.* 4th ed. Philadelphia, Pa: Lippincott Williams & Wilkins; 2002:1–12.
25. Betcher DL, Simon PJ, McHard KM. Bone tumors. In: Baggot CR, Kelly KR, Fochtman D, Foley GV, eds. *Nursing Care of Children and Adolescents With Cancer.* 3rd ed. Philadelphia, Pa: WB Saunders; 2002: 575–588.
26. National Cancer Institute. Childhood Rhabdomyosarcoma (PDQ): Treatment. Childhood Rhabdomyosarcoma. Available at: http://www.nci.nih.gov/cancerinfo/pdq/treatment/childrhabdomyosarcoma/healthprofessional/. Accessed May 9, 2005.
27. Ebb DH, Green DM, Shamberger RC, Tarbell NJ, Offinger KC, Hudson MM. Solid tumors of childhood. In: DeVita VT, Hellman S, Rosenberg SA, eds. *Cancer: Principles and Practice of Oncology,* 6th ed. Philadelphia: Pa: Lippincott Williams & Wilkins; 2001:2169–2214.
28. Baggot CR, Kelly KP. Interdisciplinary collaboration. In: Baggot CR, Kelly KR, Fochtman D, Foley GV, eds. *Nursing Care of Children and Adolescents With Cancer.* 3rd ed. Philadelphia, Pa: WB Saunders; 2002: 626–639.
29. Holm KE, Patterson JM, Gurney JM. Parental involvement and family-centered care in the diagnostic and treatment phases of childhood cancer: results from a qualitative study. *J Ped Onc Nurs.* 2003;20:301–313.
30. Walker CL, Wells LM, Heiney SP, Hymovich DP. Family-centered psychosocial care. In: Baggot CR, Kelly KR, Fochtman D, Foley GV, eds. *Nursing Care of Children and Adolescents With Cancer.* 3rd ed. Philadelphia, Pa: WB Saunders; 2002:365–390.
31. Institute for Family-Centered Care Web site. Available at: http://www.familycenteredcare.org/about-us-frame.html. Accessed May 9, 2005.
32. Algren C. Effect of hospitalization on the child and family. In: Hockenberry MJ, Wilson D, Winelstein ML, eds. *Wong's Essentials of Pediatrics.* 7th ed. St. Louis, Mo: Mosby; 2005:673–786.
33. Ettinger AG, Bond DM, Sievers TD. Chemotherapy. In: Baggot CR, Kelly KR, Fochtman D, Foley GV, eds. *Nursing Care of Children and Adolescents With Cancer.* 3rd ed. Philadelphia, Pa: WB Saunders; 2002: 133–176.
34. Balis FM, Holcenberg JS, Blaney SM. General principles of chemotherapy. In: Pizzo PA, Poplak DG, eds. *Principles and Practice of Pediatric Oncology.* 4th ed. Philadelphia, Pa: Lippincott Williams & Wilkins; 2002:237–308.
35. Panzarella C, Baggot CR, Comeau M, Duncan JM, Groben V, Woods D, Stewart JL. Management of disease and treatment-related complications. In: Baggot CR, Kelly KR, Fochtman D, Foley GV, eds. *Nursing Care of Children and Adolescents With Cancer.* 3rd ed. Philadelphia, Pa: WB Saunders; 2002:279–318.
36. Tarbell NJ, Kooy HM. General principles of radiation oncology. In: Pizzo PA, Poplak DG, eds. *Principles and Practice of Pediatric Oncology.* 4th ed. Philadelphia, Pa: Lippincott Williams & Wilkins; 2002:369–380.
37. Wallace JW. Central venous access. In: Kline N, ed. *Essentials of Pediatric Oncology Nursing: A Core Curriculum.* 2nd ed. Glenview, Ill: Association of Pediatric Oncology Nursing; 2004.
38. Rickard K, Grosfeld J, Coates T, Weetman R, Baehner R. Advances in nutrition care of children with neoplastic diseases: a review of treatment, research, and application. *J Am Diet Assoc.* 1986;86:1666–1676.
39. Didcock D. High incidence of obesity in young adults after treatment of acute lymphoblastic leukemia in childhood. *J Pediatr.* 1995;127:63–67.

Chapter 3

Changes in Carbohydrate, Lipid, and Protein Metabolism in Cancer

ELAINE TRUJILLO, MS, RD, CNSD, AND LINDA NEBELING, PHD, MPH, RD, FADA

INTRODUCTION

The presence of malignant cancer cells and the mediators that are triggered in the presence of cancer may result in a number of metabolic changes. This chapter examines the effects of malignant tumor growth on carbohydrate, lipid, and protein metabolism. Cancer-related cachexia and the effects that cytokines and mediators have on wasting associated with cancer-related cachexia are also discussed. Because there is variation among types of cancer, not every metabolic alteration described will apply in all cases.

CANCER AND METABOLIC RESPONSE

The presence of cancer can affect a patient's biochemical and metabolic functions. Malignant tumors can result in changes in energy expenditure and basal metabolism (1). Malignant tumors also can alter enzyme activity and the immune system (1). The results are changes in carbohydrate, lipid, and protein metabolism that can contribute to fluid imbalance, acid-base imbalance, and changes in the concentration of electrolytes, vitamins, and/or minerals (see Table 3.1) (2,3). These metabolic abnormalities can impair nutritional status and contribute to cancer-related cachexia by depleting fat, protein, water, and mineral stores (4). Figure 3.1 (5) identifies the mediators that are responsible for the cascade of metabolic disturbances associated with cancer-related cachexia.

CANCER-RELATED CACHEXIA

Derived from Greek words meaning "bad condition," cachexia is a clinical syndrome that occurs in many disease states. It is characterized by weight loss, muscle wasting, anorexia, asthenia, depression, and chronic nausea (6). Cancer-related cachexia occurs in approximately two-thirds of patients with malignant disease (7). Regardless of the level of energy and nutrient intake, cancer-related cachexia can occur in individuals with tumors less than 0.01% of total body weight (8).

Cancer-related cachexia is inversely correlated with length of survival and implies a poor prognosis (7). Causes of cancer-related cachexia include the following (9):

- Pain
- Depression
- Anxiety
- Hypogeusia
- Hyposmia
- Taste and food aversions
- Chronic nausea and vomiting
- Gastrointestinal dysfunction
- Metabolic shifts
- Iatrogenic causes (ie, chemotherapy and radiotherapy)

Although anorexia and decreased food intake occur in cancer-related cachexia, they are not the only factors contributing to the cachectic state. Even with an adequate nutrient intake through the use of nutri-

Table 3.1 Metabolic Changes in Cancer

Macronutrient	*Metabolic Changes*
Carbohydrate	• Increased gluconeogenesis from amino acids and lactate • Increased glucose synthesis • Decreased glucose tolerance and turnover • Insulin resistance
Lipids	• Increased lipolysis • Decreased lipogenesis • Decreased lipoprotein lipase activity • Elevated triglycerides • Decreased high-density lipoproteins • Increased venous glycerol • Decreased glycerol clearance from plasma
Protein	• Increased muscle catabolism • Increased whole-body protein turnover • Increased liver and tumor protein synthesis • Decreased muscle protein synthesis

Source: Data are from references 2 and 3.

tion support and pharmacological agents, individuals with cancer may be unable to restore lean body mass (10). The degree of malnutrition in individuals with cancer-related cachexia is not explained by their level of energy intake. In the malnourished individual with cancer, loss of muscle and adipose tissue occurs before a decline in food intake (8).

Metabolic Effects of Cancer-Related Cachexia vs Starvation

The normal physiological conservation mechanisms seen during periods of acute starvation do not occur in the presence of a malignant tumor. Starvation is characterized by loss of body fat and preservation of muscle mass. In contrast, cancer-related cachexia is characterized by the equal loss of fat and muscle, a loss of adipose tissue, and increased energy expenditure (10). During the first 12 to 24 hours of a starvation state that is not cancer-related, glucose is mobilized by hepatic glycogen stores (11). Thereafter, glucose production is increased in the liver, and to a lesser extent in the kidney, by gluconeogenesis (11). The process of gluconeogenesis, which utilizes amino acids derived from catabolism of muscle, is wasteful because large amounts of proteins must be broken down. Thus, in

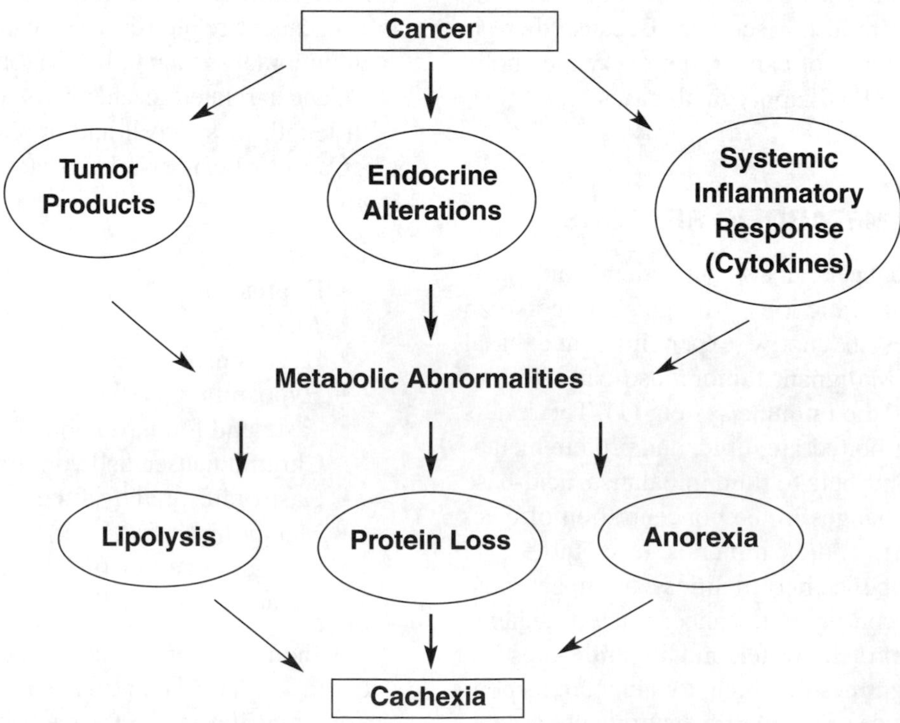

Figure 3.1. Factors contributing to cancer-related cachexia. Reprinted with permission from Argiles JM, Busquets S, Lopez-Soriano FJ. Cytokines in the pathogenesis of cancer cachexia. *Curr Opin Clin Nutr Metab Care.* 2003;6:401–406.

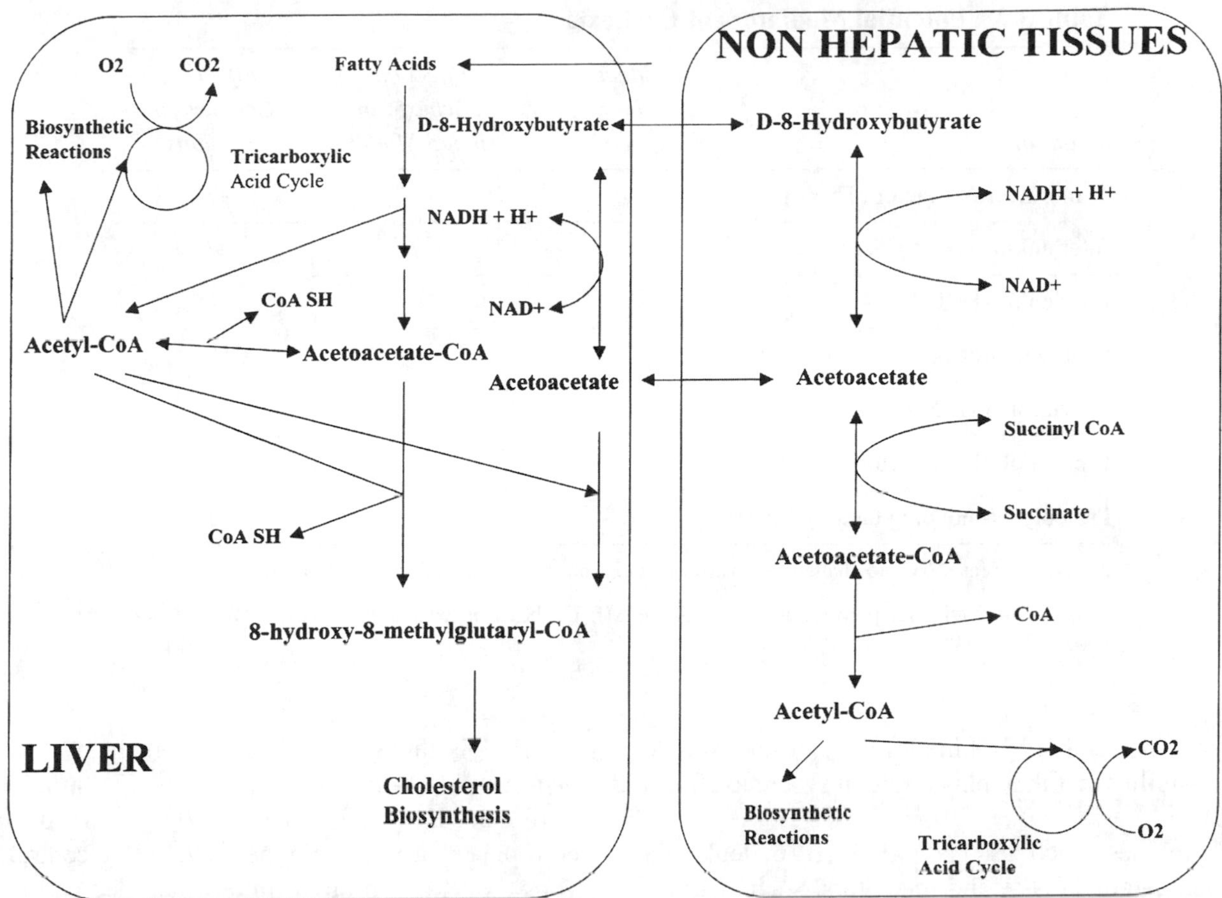

Figure 3.2. Metabolic pathways of synthesis of the ketone bodies (D-B hydroxybutyrate and acetoacetate) in the liver and their utilization in the brain and muscle (non-hepatic tissues). Ketones are transported from the liver to non-hepatic tissues via the circulation system. COA = coenzyme A; NAD+ = nicotinamide anenine dinucleotide; NADH = the reduced form for NAD+.

long-term starvation, gluconeogenesis is replaced by the use of fat as a fuel.

Free fatty acids are converted into ketone bodies (β-hydroxybutyrate and acetoacetate), which are used for energy by the peripheral tissues and the brain (Figure 3.2) (8,12). Acting as a glucose substitute, ketone bodies signal the body to inhibit glucose utilization and induce protein and adipose tissue conservation mechanisms (2). The rates of gluconeogenesis and protein breakdown from muscle mass decline along with insulin levels (2). Ketone bodies serve as an important alternative energy source during periods of starvation.

Effect of Cytokines and Other Potential Mediators on Cachexia

Cytokines are soluble glycoproteins and low-molecular weight peptides. They mediate interactions between cells and regulate cell and tissue functions (3). Cytokines contribute to the growth and spread of cancers by causing normal cells to produce additional cytokines that continue the malignant process (3,13). Cytokines and other mediators play a major role in the biological responses that lead to the wasting associated with cancer-related cachexia (see Table 3.2) (10). In cancer-related cachexia, cytokines affect gastric motility and emptying by altering the signals that regulate satiety (14).

Increased levels of cytokines, such as interleukin-1 (IL-1), interleukin-6 (IL-6), tumor necrosis factor (TNF)-α or -β, fibroblast growth factors, transforming growth factors, and granulocyte colony stimulating factor, have been found in blood, ascites, pleural effusions, and urine of individuals with cancer (3). No single cytokine has been shown to be present in all individuals with cancer (3). However, the absence of

Table 3.2 Potential Mediators of Cachexia

Mediator	*Effect on Appetite*	*Effect on Cachexia in Animal Models*	*Effect on Cachexia in Humans*
Tumor necrosis factor (TNF)-α	↓	+	+/–
Interleukin-6 (IL-6)	↓	+	+/–
Interleukin-1 (IL-1)	?	+	–
Ciliary neurotrophic factor (CNTF)	↓	+	?
Interferon-γ (IFN-γ)	↓	+	–
Lipid-mobilizing factor (LMF)	NC	+	+
Proteolysis-inducing factor (PIF)	NC	+	+

Key: ↓, decrease; NC, no change; +, positive association; –, no association; ?, not known.

Source: Adapted with permission from Tisdale MJ. Cachexia in cancer patients. *Nat Rev Cancer.* 2002;2:862–871.

clinically detectable cytokine levels does not exclude the possibility that they play a role in systemic effects (3,15).

Cytokines, such as TNF, IL-1, IL-6, leukemia inhibitor factor, IFN-γ, and mediators, such as lipid-mobilizing factor, proteolysis-inducing factor, neuropeptides, leptin, and uncoupling proteins (UCP), are the focus of many research studies. These studies are examined in the sections that follow.

Tumor Necrosis Factor and Interleukin-1

The initial studies of the role of cytokines in cancer-related cachexia in mice focused on TNF because mice with tumors producing TNF developed cachexia and because it was found that weight loss could be reversed with TNF-neutralizing antibodies (3,16). Tumor-bearing mice with paraneoplastic syndromes of hypercalcemia, leukocytosis, and cachexia who were injected with polyclonal neutralizing antibodies against TNF had a rapid and reproducible decrease in blood calcium and white cell count and an increase in body weight. In addition, the plasma TNF levels increased by almost fourfold in the tumor-bearing mice with the paraneoplastic syndromes compared to control tumor-bearing mice who did not have the paraneoplastic syndromes and mice without tumors. The results suggest that TNF was responsible for the hypercalcemia and cachexia found in the tumor-bearing mice with paraneoplastic syndromes (16).

IL-1 is thought to initiate anorexia by blocking neuropeptide Y-induced feeding (14,17). In addition, TNF and IL-1 may increase the levels of corticotropin-releasing hormone (5,7,14), a central nervous system neurotransmitter that decreases food intake (14). TNF also suppresses lipoprotein lipase activity in adipocytes (18).

Interleukin-6, Leukemia Inhibitor Factor, and Interferon-γ

There is evidence that IL-6 and leukemia inhibitor factor are produced by some cancers and may cause cachexia (3,18,19). In studies with tumor-bearing mice, ciliary neurotrophic factor, which is in the same cytokine family as IL-6 and leukemia inhibitor factor, induced cachexia and acute-phase proteins (14,18,20).

Interferon-γ (IFN-γ) also may be related to cancer-related cachexia. In tumor-bearing mice, the provision of monoclonal antibodies against IFN-γ reversed the wasting syndrome, which supports the evidence that endogenous production of IFN-γ causes metabolic changes that occur in cancer-related cachexia (14,21).

Lipid-Mobilizing Factor and Proteolysis-Inducing Factor

Animal studies show that lipid-mobilizing factor and proteolysis-inducing factor may contribute to cancer-related cachexia. In studies on mice, lipid-mobilizing factor was associated with cachexia-inducing tumors, and administration of lipid-mobilizing factor caused catabolism of skeletal muscle and loss of adipose tissue (3,15,22,23). In studies of individuals with cancer, the presence of lipid-mobilizing factor, which induces lipolysis, in urine was correlated with weight loss (15,24).

Proteolysis-inducing factor does not affect appetite, but it is associated with cachexia. This is because proteolysis-inducing factor is directed by tumor cells to induce protein breakdown in skeletal muscle and to decrease protein synthesis (10,25,26). Proteolysis-inducing factor may also be involved in cancer-related cachexia, by increasing cytokines and acute-phase proteins (10,27,28).

Neuropeptides, Leptin, and Uncoupling Proteins

Two types of neuropeptides, orexigenic (feeding-stimulatory) neuropeptides and anorexigenic neuropeptides, regulate energy expenditure by activating thermogenesis in brown adipose tissue and possibly in other sites, such as white adipose tissue and muscle (29). Orexigenic neuropeptides decrease sympathetic nervous activity, whereas anorexigenic neuropeptides increase sympathetic nervous activity (27). Neuropeptide-Y is thought to restore normal energy balance and body fat stores under conditions of energy deficit, the signals of which are falling leptin and/or insulin levels (29). Other feeding-stimulatory neuropeptides that may be interconnected with neuropeptide-Y include galanin, opioid peptides, melanin-concentrating hormone, orexin, and Agouti-related peptide, although it is not yet known whether these peptides are involved in cancer-related cachexia.

Leptin is a hormone that acts to control food intake and energy expenditure within the hypothalamus (30). A decreased food intake would normally suppress leptin levels and result in a compensatory mechanism of increased feeding. However, animal studies demonstrate that TNF, IL-1, and leukemia inhibitor factor increase leptin levels despite decreased food intake, thereby blocking the normal feeding compensatory mechanism and contributing to anorexia (29,31–33). These cytokines also have been shown to cause anorexia even in the absence of leptin, and failure to see elevated leptin levels was reported in tumor-bearing rats and in humans with cancer-related cachexia (34–36). On the other hand, very low levels of leptin were associated with high levels of inflammatory cytokines in individuals with advanced stage cancer (37). Although studies have explored the relationship between leptin and anorexia and weight loss, further research is needed to understand the relationship between cytokines, leptin, and cancer-related cachexia (29).

Studies show that the UCP 1 and the more recently identified UCP 2 and UCP 3 may play a role in the initiation of energy expenditure regulation (29,38,39). UCP 1, 2, and 3 are thought to be involved in the control of energy metabolism through the generation of heat instead of adenosine triphosphate (ATP) (10). UCP 1 is expressed only in brown adipose tissue; UCP 2 is widely distributed and expressed in most tissues; and UCP 3 is expressed in brown adipose tissue and skeletal muscle (10). The increased thermogenesis in brown adipose tissue can increase total energy expenditure and contribute to tissue wasting in cachexia. However, there is little brown adipose tissue in adult humans. UCP 3 in skeletal muscle may be of substantial importance in energy expenditure, and changes in UCP expression may be induced by tumor products or by cytokines (10). In one study, the injection of TNF-α in rats increased UCP 2 and UCP 3 levels in skeletal muscle (40). In another study, the administration of lipid-mobilizing factor in mice increased UCP 1, UCP 2, and UCP 3 in brown adipose tissue, and increased UCP 2 in skeletal muscle and liver (41).

CANCER-RELATED CACHEXIA CHANGES IN ENERGY EXPENDITURE

The presence of tumor may alter the individual's ability and desire to eat, and the adverse effects of traditional treatment modalities can act to further impair nutritional status. Glucose intolerance, impaired insulin sensitivity, muscle and fat wasting, and poor energy intake due to anorexia exacerbate changes in energy metabolism in people with cancer-related cachexia (42).

A substantial increase in the rate of glucose turnover, combined with increased energy demand by the tumor, may contribute to the increased energy expenditure and depletion of body fat stores that are observed in some individuals with cancer (42). Gluconeogenesis from lactate uses six ATP molecules for every lactate-glucose cycle and is very energy inefficient for the host. This futile cycle may add to an increase in energy expenditure (43).

The type of tumor seems to be correlated with the level of energy expenditure in individuals with cancer.

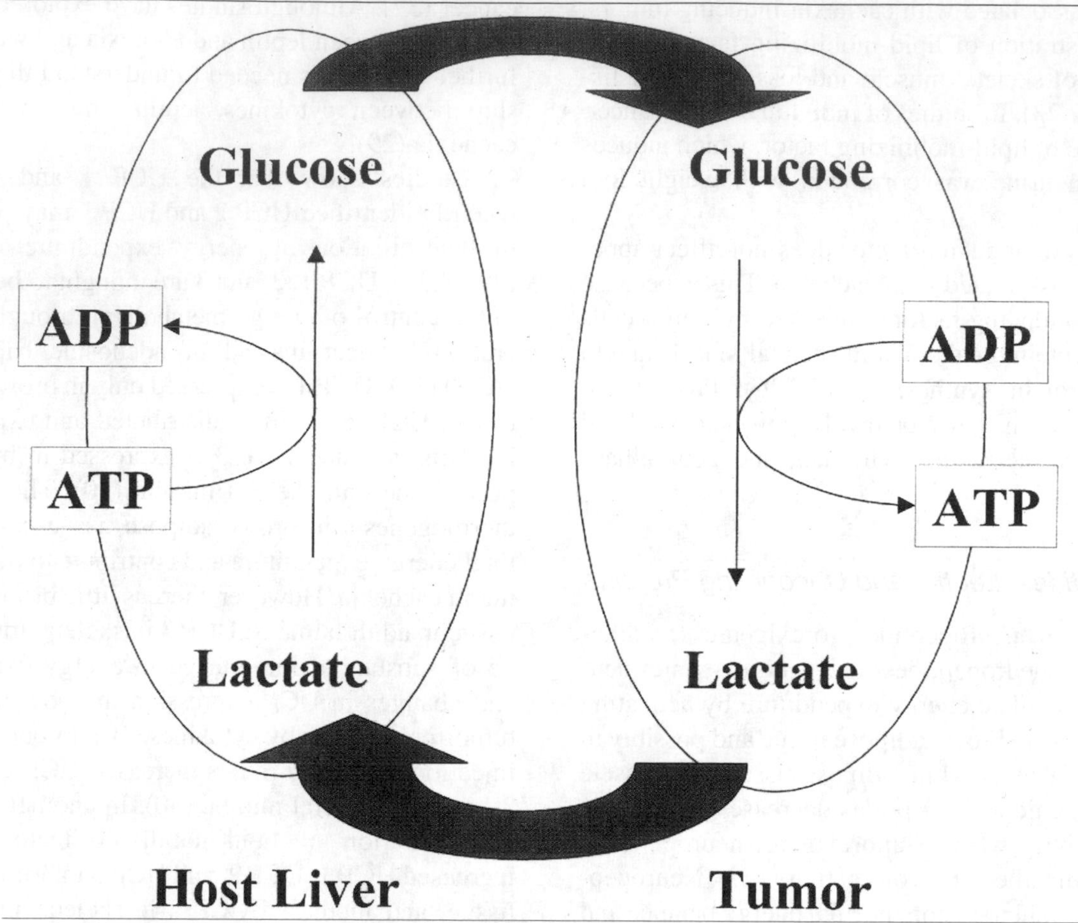

Figure 3.3. Cori-type cycling of glucose and lactate between the tumor and the host.

Resting energy expenditure (REE) is elevated in people with pancreatic or lung cancer and unchanged in people with gastric or colorectal cancer (10,44). In a study of almost 300 subjects with various types of cancer, about one-half had increased REEs. Importantly, this increase was not associated with a different dietary intake compared with normometabolic subjects. There was no up-regulation of dietary intake in response to elevated energy expenditure in the subjects with cancer (45).

In animals with cancer, the pattern of energy expenditure changes with time. An initial hypermetabolic phase is followed by a brief transition through a period of relatively normal energy expenditure. Finally, there is a preterminal hypometabolic phase (18,46). It is not known whether humans follow a similar pattern over time, because such longitudinal studies in humans have not been done. Energy expenditure in people with cancer does vary from person to person, from 60% to more than 150% of predicted normal expenditure (18).

CHANGE IN CARBOHYDRATE METABOLISM

Abnormal Elevations in Cori Cycle Activity

A well-nourished healthy adult in the basal or resting state will use 140 g (560 kcal) of glucose per day, 75 g (375 kcal) of protein per day, and 130 g (1,170 kcal) of fat per day (47). In the resting state, approximately 20 g of lactate are formed daily in adults. This lactate is normally resynthesized back to glucose (47). This cyclic metabolic pathway, referred to as the Cori cycle, converts glucose to lactic acid by glycolysis and then reconverts it to glucose in the liver (see Figure 3.3) (47).

Abnormal elevations in Cori cycle activity have been noted in malnourished people with cancer, and this increased activity accounts for energy losses ≤ 300 kcal/day (10,48). Glucose is the main energy source for tumors, and the demand for glucose by the tumor can increase glucose production by the liver. Thus, some individuals with cancer have increased Cori cycle activity and increased glucose production that is caused by the body's inability to effectively oxidize glucose (48).

Increased Glycolysis and Lactate Production

The increased lactate level and plasma lactate production rate in people with cancer is due to (*a*) increased glycolysis and lactate release by the tumor tissue, and (*b*) increased lactate release by skeletal muscle tissue (43). When glucose is used in high concentrations by the tumor and host, this stimulates the release of large amounts of lactate (43). Amino acids, primarily alanine and glutamine, which are released from skeletal muscle, are the precursors for glucose synthesis (7).

Increased Gluconeogenesis

Increased gluconeogenesis is critical in maintaining glucose homeostasis in people with cancer. Gluconeogenesis uses amino acids and glycerol, which are derived from muscle and fat breakdown (8). Individuals with cancer-related cachexia have reduced plasma levels of alanine, glycine, and glutamine (49), which may be related to an increase in their utilization by the liver for glucose production (49).

Increased Insulin Sensitivity

Glucose intolerance in people with cancer was reported as early as 1919 (50). Individuals with cancer often have increased glucose intolerance and insulin resistance with an increase in hepatic glucose production (42). Insulin resistance, which may be influenced by the counterregulatory hormones, glucocorticoids, or glucagon, causes a reduction of glucose utilization by the skeletal muscle (7).

The cause of insulin resistance in people with cancer is not known. Insulin resistance is not related to nutritional status in people with cancer. The amount of glucose metabolized is not related to the tumor site or stage (51). Insulin resistance seems to be caused, at least in part, by the tumor itself or by the tumor-influenced host, and the acute-phase response seems to enhance insulin resistance in individuals with cancer (51).

CHANGES IN LIPID METABOLISM

Individuals with cancer-related cachexia often lose a dramatic amount of adipose tissue. This loss may be related more to the increase in lipolysis than to the decrease in lipogenesis (Table 3.1). The adipose tissue loss may be caused by the higher turnover of glycerol and free fatty acids, and the increased mobilization of free fatty acids is often evident before weight loss is observed (10,52). The decrease in lipoprotein lipase activity and lipogenesis are thought to be due to cytokines, in particular TNF, IL-1, and IFN-γ (7,53). The lipid profile of individuals with cancer is characterized by decreased high-density lipoprotein cholesterol, decreased LDL cholesterol, and relatively high serum triglycerides (54). The hypertriglyceridemia is a consequence of the decreased lipoprotein lipase activity, which causes a decrease in the plasma clearance of both endogenous and exogenous triglycerides (7). Cytokines such as TNF, IL-1, IL-6, and IFN-α may influence liver lipogenesis and cause hypertriglyceridemia (7).

Lipid-mobilizing factor may induce lipolysis by stimulating an elevation of cyclic adenosine monophosphate production (44). Lipid-mobilizing factor has been found in the serum of individuals with cancer-related cachexia, but it is not found in the serum of healthy subjects, even under conditions of starvation. Interestingly, studies have found that circulating concentrations of lipid-mobilizing factor were proportional to the degree of weight loss (8,44,55).

CHANGES IN PROTEIN METABOLISM

Muscle wasting is caused by increased protein breakdown and, to a lesser extent, by decreased protein synthesis (8). Other protein alterations associated with cancer include nitrogen depletion and abnormal plasma amino acid levels in the host (Table 3.1). In cancer, there is a shift from normal muscle protein and other tissue protein synthesis to increased hepatic protein synthesis, which is reprioritized with an increased production of acute-phase proteins (18,25,56).

Negative nitrogen balance may be present in individuals with cancer, because of the increased turnover of whole-body protein and amino acid (25,57). Studies on protein metabolism in subjects with cancer demonstrated that muscle tissue degradation is elevated in the entire body and that this response is similar to other conditions, such as infection and injury (58).

TNF seems to mediate many of the changes in nitrogen metabolism associated with cancer-related cachexia. Studies of cancer in animals found an increased release of protein from skeletal muscle, which enhances muscle protein breakdown and activates the ATP ubiquitin-dependent pathway—one of the main pathways responsible for protein catabolism in skeletal muscle (7,59,60). Proteolysis-inducing factor is also linked to the ubiquitin-dependent pathway in humans (10,43).

NUTRITIONAL IMPLICATIONS

Effects of Metabolic Changes on Individuals With Cancer

A malignant tumor may alter body composition by initiating a sequence of events that leads to altered carbohydrate, lipid, and protein metabolism. This alteration in metabolism increases the likelihood that body stores will be depleted. The presence of tumors increases the rate of anaerobic glycolysis and increases the consumption rates of glucose or gluconeogenic precursors during phases of active growth (8). These changes in glucose and lactate metabolism may encourage tumor growth. Insulin resistance, glucose intolerance, and increased gluconeogenesis may help to maintain the glucose levels even when there is increased demand by the body and the tumor and a concomitant decrease in food intake (43,51).

Dietary Modulation and Tumor Growth Stimulation

Dietary modulation may be beneficial for individuals with cancer. However, the dietary manipulation can stimulate tumor growth (61). Studies continue to identify effective ways to supply adequate nutrition to the body without stimulating tumor growth (62,63). Data suggest that dietary modulations may be used to improve nutritional status and to prevent cachexia (63–65); however, further research is needed to confirm this. In some instances, tumor growth can be used to the individual's advantage, because the stimulation of the cells' proliferative phase may make certain chemotherapeutic agents work more effectively. The biochemical relationships between tumor-host interactions must be understood if nutrition intervention is to offer therapeutic benefits.

The following is a summary of findings on cancer and diet manipulation:

- Arginine supplementation may stimulate the immune system, enhance wound healing, improve recovery time from trauma, and inhibit tumor growth rates (58,64).
- Using ketone supplementation as the primary energy source may lower body urinary nitrogen levels and conserve protein (63).
- The provision of adequate energy in a form that cannot be utilized by the tumor may inhibit tumor growth by decreasing catabolism of body stores (63,66,67). Many tumors specifically metabolize glucose; therefore, the administration of a concentrated lipid source, such as MCT oil, may reduce the glucose substrate available to the tumor (68).
- In animal studies, polyunsaturated fatty acids promote cell growth both by stimulating cell proliferation and by inhibiting cell death or apoptosis (8).
- In animals, fish oil reduces tumor growth rate and decreases body weight loss (69). In mice, body weight loss and tumor growth rate were inhibited when fish oil replaced some carbohydrate and total energy, whereas nitrogen intake was not changed. These results did not occur with the use of gamma-linolenic acid (69).
- Interestingly, in a small pilot trial of 20 human subjects with pancreatic cancer, the addition of an oral diet enriched with eicosopentanoic acid reversed cachexia and increased body weight at 3 and 7 weeks (65). However, these results could not be replicated in a follow-up study of 200 subjects with pancreatic cancer, possibly because several subjects in the control group were taking eicosopentanoic acid (70).

The muscle wasting that occurs in cancer-related cachexia decreases whole-body nitrogen and increases total tumor nitrogen (71). Therefore, protein catabolism may favor tumor growth by providing the necessary nitrogen for tumor proliferation, and specific amino acids may be required for the growth of certain neoplasms (8). Glutamine is known to be an essential nutrient for tumor cells, and physiological concentrations of glutamine are required for optimal growth of malignant cells in culture. The altered protein metabolism may be affected by the glutamine requirements of the tumor, which may favor tumor growth and decrease protein synthesis (8). However, experimental models demonstrated that glutamine supplementation improved the effectiveness of methotrexate while reducing its toxicity (72,73). This phenomenon may be due to glutamine increasing the number of tumor cells in the S-phase, a cell-cycle phase during which tumor cells are particularly susceptible to chemotherapy (73,74).

REFERENCES

1. Knox LS, Crosby LO, Feurer ID, Buzby GP, Miller CL, Mullen JL. Energy expenditure in malnourished cancer patients. *Ann Surg.* 1983;197:152–162.
2. VanItallie T, Nufert T. Ketones: metabolism's ugly duckling. *Nutr Rev.* 2003;61:327–341.
3. Dunlop RJ, Campbell CW. Cytokines and advanced cancer. *J Pain Symptom Manage.* 2000;20:214–232.
4. Bloch A. Cancer. In: Matarese L, Gottschlich M, eds. *Contemporary Nutrition Support Practice.* 1st ed. Philadelphia, Pa: WB Saunders; 1998:475–495.
5. Argiles JM, Busquets S, Lopez-Soriano FJ. Cytokines in the pathogenesis of cancer cachexia. *Curr Opin Clin Nutr Metab Care.* 2003;6:401–406.
6. Bruera E, Sweeney C. Cachexia and asthenia in cancer patients. *Lancet Oncol.* 2000;1:138–147.
7. Argiles JM, Lopez-Soriano FJ. New mediators in cancer cachexia. *Nestle Nutr Workshop Ser Clin Perform Programme.* 2000;4:147–162.
8. Cravo ML, Gloria LM, Claro I. Metabolic responses to tumour disease and progression: tumour-host interaction. *Clin Nutr.* 2000;19:459–465.
9. Plata-Salaman C. Anorexia during acute and chronic disease. *Nutrition.* 1996;12:69–78.
10. Tisdale MJ. Cachexia in cancer patients. *Nat Rev Cancer.* 2002;2:862–871.
11. Corssmit EPM, Romijn JA, Sauerwein HP. Regulation of glucose production with special attention to nonclassical regulatory mechanisms: a review. *Metabolism.* 2001;50:742–755.
12. Berger M, Chiolero R. Trauma and burns. In: Rombeau J, Rolandelli R, eds. *Clinical Nutrition Parenteral Nutrition.* 3rd ed. Philadelphia, Pa: WB Saunders; 2001:304–334.
13. Negus R, Balkwill F. Cytokines in tumour growth, migration and metastasis. *World J Urol.* 1996;14: 157–165.
14. Argiles JM, Moore-Carrasco R, Busquets S, Lopez-Soriano FJ. Catabolic mediators as targets for cancer cachexia. *Drug Discov Today.* 2003;8:838–844.
15. Todorov P, Cariuk P, McDevitt T, Coles B, Fearon K, Tisdale M. Characterization of a cancer cachectic factor. *Nature.* 1996;379:739–742.
16. Yoneda T, Alsina M, Chavez J, Bonewals L, Nishimura R, Mundy G. Evidence that tumor necrosis factor plays a pathogenetic role in the paraneoplastic syndrome of cachexia, hypercalcaemia, and leucocytosis in a human tumor in nude mice. *J Clin Invest.* 1991;87:977–985.
17. Plata-Salaman C. Central nervous system mechanisms contributing to the cachexia-anorexia syndrome. *Nutrition.* 2000;16:1009–1012.
18. Barber MD, Ross JA, Fearon KC. Cancer cachexia. *Surg Oncol.* 1999;8:133–141.
19. Yasumoto K, Mukaida N, Harada A, Kuno K, Akiyama M, Nakashima E, Fujioka N, Mai M, Kasahara T, Fujimoto-Ouchi K. Molecular analysis of the cytokine network involved in cachexia in colon 26 adenocarcinoma-bearing mice. *Cancer Res.* 1995;55: 921–927.
20. Wang M, Forsberg N. Effects of ciliary neurotrophic factor (CNTF) on protein turnover in cultured muscle cells. *Cytokine.* 2000;12:41–48.
21. Matthys P, Heremans H, Opdenakker G, Billiau A. Anti-interferon-gamma antibody treatment, growth of Lewis ling tumours in mice and tumour-associated cachexia. *Eur J Cancer.* 1991;27:182–187.
22. Khan S, Tisdale M. Catabolism of adipose tissue by a tumour-produced lipid-mobilising factor. *Int J Cancer.* 1999;80:444–447.
23. McDevitt T, Todorov P, Beck S, Khan S, Tisdale M. Purification and characterization of a lipid-mobilizing factor associated with cachexia-inducing tumors in mice and humans. *Cancer Res.* 1995;55:1458–1463.
24. Islam-Ali B, Khan S, Price SA, Tisdale MJ. Modulation of adipocyte G-protein expression in cancer cachexia by a lipid-mobilizing factor (LMF). *Br J Cancer.* 2001;85:758–763.
25. Strasser F, Bruera ED. Update on anorexia and cachexia. *Hematol Oncol Clin North Am.* 2002;16: 589–617.
26. Ripamonti C, Twycross R, Baines M, Bozzetti F, Capri S, De Conno F, Gemlo B, Hunt TM, Krebs HB, Mercadante S, Schaerer R, Wilkinson P. Clinical-practice recommendations for the management of bowel obstruction in patients with end-stage cancer. *Support Care Cancer.* 2001;9:223–233.

27. Lorite MJ, Smith HJ, Arnold JA, Morris A, Thompson MG, Tisdale MJ. Activation of ATP-ubiquitin-dependent proteolysis in skeletal muscle in vivo and murine myoblasts in vitro by a proteolysis-inducing factor (PIF). *Br J Cancer.* 2001;85:297–302.
28. Watchorn TM, Waddell I, Dowidar N, Ross JA. Proteolysis-inducing factor regulates hepatic gene expression via the transcription factors NF-(kappa)B and STAT3. *Faseb J.* 2001;15:562–564.
29. Inui A. Cancer anorexia-cachexia syndrome: are neuropeptides the key? *Cancer Res.* 1999;59:4493–4501.
30. Mantovani G, Maccio A, Massa E, Madeddu C. Managing cancer-related anorexia/cachexia. *Drugs.* 2001; 61:499–514.
31. Sarraf P, Frederich RC, Turner EM, Ma G, Jaskowiak NT, Rivet DJ III, Flier JS, Lowell BB, Fraker DL, Alexander HR. Multiple cytokines and acute inflammation raise mouse leptin levels: potential role in inflammatory anorexia. *J Exp Med.* 1997;185: 171–175.
32. Grunfeld C, Zhao C, Fuller J, Pollack A, Moser A, Friedman J, Feingold KR. Endotoxin and cytokines induce expression of leptin, the ob gene product, in hamsters. *J Clin Invest.* 1996;97:2152–2157.
33. Finck BN, Kelley KW, Dantzer R, Johnson RW. In vivo and in vitro evidence for the involvement of tumor necrosis factor-alpha in the induction of leptin by lipopolysaccharide. *Endocrinology.* 1998;139: 2278–2283.
34. Chance WT, Sheriff S, Moore J, Peng F, Balasubramaniam A. Reciprocal changes in hypothalamic receptor binding and circulating leptin in anorectic tumor-bearing rats. *Brain Res.* 1998;803:27–33.
35. Jensen PB, Blume N, Mikkelsen JD, Larsen PJ, Jensen HI, Holst JJ, Madsen OD. Transplantable rat glucagonomas cause acute onset of severe anorexia and adipsia despite highly elevated NPY mRNA levels in the hypothalamic arcuate nucleus. *J Clin Invest.* 1998;101:503–510.
36. Wallace AM, Sattar N, McMillan DC. Effect of weight loss and the inflammatory response on leptin concentrations in gastrointestinal cancer patients. *Clin Cancer Res.* 1998;4:2977–2979.
37. Mantovani G, Maccio A, Mura L, Massa E, Mudu MC, Mulas C, Lusso MR, Madeddu C, Dessi A. Serum levels of leptin and proinflammatory cytokines in patients with advanced-stage cancer at different sites. *J Mol Med.* 2000;78:554–561.
38. Fleury C, Neverova M, Collins S, Raimbault S, Champigny O, Levi-Meyrueis C, Bouillard F, Seldin M, Surwit R, Ricquier D, Warden C. Uncoupling protein 2: a novel gene linked to obesity and hyperinsulinemia. *Nat Genet.* 1997;15:269–272.
39. Gong DW, He Y, Karas M, Reitman M. Uncoupling protein-3 is a mediator of thermogenesis regulated by thyroid hormone, beta3-adrenergic agonists, and leptin. *J Biol Chem.* 1997;272:24129–24132.
40. Busquets S, Sanchis D, Alvarez B, Ricquier D, Lopez-Soriano FJ, Argiles JM. In the rat, tumor necrosis factor alpha administration results in an increase in both UCP2 and UCP3 mRNAs in skeletal muscle: a possible mechanism for cytokine-induced thermogenesis? *FEBS Lett.* 1998;440:348–350.
41. Bing C, Russell ST, Beckett EE, Collins P, Taylor S, Barraclough R, Tisdale MJ, Williams G. Expression of uncoupling proteins-1, -2 and -3 mRNA is induced by an adenocarcinoma-derived lipid-mobilizing factor. *Br J Cancer.* 2002;86:612–618.
42. Strasser F, Bruera ED. Update on anorexia and cachexia. *Hematol Oncol Clin North Am.* 2002;16: 589–617.
43. Tisdale MJ. Metabolic abnormalities in cachexia and anorexia. *Nutrition.* 2000;16:1013–1014.
44. Guirao X. Impact of the inflammatory reaction on intermediary metabolism and nutrition status. *Nutrition.* 2002;18:949–952.
45. Bosaeus I, Daneryd P, Svanberg E, Lundholm K. Dietary intake and resting energy expenditure in relation to weight loss in unselected cancer patients. *Int J Cancer.* 2001;93:380–383.
46. Zylicz Z, Schwantje O, Wagener DJ, Folgering HT. Metabolic response to enteral food in different phases of cancer cachexia in rats. *Oncology.* 1990; 47:87–91.
47. Dills WL Jr. Nutritional and physiological consequences of tumour glycolysis. *Parasitology.* 1993; 107(suppl)177–186.
48. Eden D, Edstrom S, Bennegard K, Schersten T, Lundholm K. Glucose flux in relation to energy expenditure in malnourished patients with and without cancer during periods of fasting and feeding. *Cancer Res.* 1984;44:1718–1724.
49. Burt ME, Aoki TT, Gorschboth CM, Brennan MF. Peripheral tissue metabolism in cancer-bearing man. *Ann Surg.* 1983;198:685–691.
50. Rohdenburg G, Bernhard A, Krehniel O. Sugar tolerance in cancer. *JAMA.* 1919;72:1528–1530.
51. Yoshikawa T, Noguchi Y, Doi C, Makino T, Nomura K. Insulin resistance in patients with cancer: relationships with tumor site, tumor stage, body-weight loss, acute-phase response, and energy expenditure. *Nutrition.* 2001;17:590–593.

52. Kaibara A, Moshyedi A, Auffenberg T, Abouhamze A, Copeland EM III, Kalra S, Moldawer LL. Leptin produces anorexia and weight loss without inducing an acute phase response or protein wasting. *Am J Physiol.* 1998;274(6 pt 2):R1518-R1525.
53. Fried SK, Zechner R. Cachectin/tumor necrosis factor decreases human adipose tissue lipoprotein lipase mRNA levels, synthesis, and activity. *J Lipid Res.* 1989;30:1917–1923.
54. Fiorenza AM, Branchi A, Sommariva D. Serum lipoprotein profile in patients with cancer. A comparison with non-cancer subjects. *Int J Clin Lab Res.* 2000;30:141–145.
55. Beck SA, Mulligan HD, Tisdale MJ. Lipolytic factors associated with murine and human cancer cachexia. *J Natl Cancer Inst.* 1990;82:1922–1926.
56. Wigmore SJ, McMahon AJ, Sturgeon CM, Fearon KC. Acute-phase protein response, survival and tumour recurrence in patients with colorectal cancer. *Br J Surg.* 2001;88:255–260.
57. Argiles JM, Busquets S, Lopez-Soriano FJ. Metabolic interrelationships between liver and skeletal muscle in pathological states. *Life Sci.* 2001;69:1345–1361.
58. Garlick PJ, McNurlan MA. Protein metabolism in the cancer patient. *Biochimie.* 1994;76:713–717.
59. Llovera M, Garcia-Martinez C, Agell N, Marzabal M, Lopez-Soriano FJ, Argiles JM. Ubiquitin gene expression is increased in skeletal muscle of tumour-bearing rats. *FEBS Lett.* 1994;338:311–318.
60. Goodman MN. Tumor necrosis factor induces skeletal muscle protein breakdown in rats. *Am J Physiol.* 1991;260(5 pt 1):E727-E730.
61. Langen KJ, Braun U, Rota Kops E, Herzog H, Kuwert T, Nebeling B, Feinendegen LE. The influence of plasma glucose levels on fluorine-18-fluorodeoxyglucose uptake in bronchial carcinomas. *J Nucl Med.* 1993;34:355–359.
62. Franchi F, Rossi-Fanelli F, Seminara P, Cascino A, Barone C, Scucchi L. Cell kinetics of gastrointestinal tumors after different nutritional regimens. A preliminary report. *J Clin Gastroenterol.* 1991;13:313–315.
63. Rothkopf M. Fuel utilization in neoplastic disease: implications for the use of nutritional support in cancer patients. *Nutrition.* 1990;6(suppl 4):S14-S16.
64. Heys SD, Gough DB, Khan L, Eremin O. Nutritional pharmacology and malignant disease: a therapeutic modality in patients with cancer. *Br J Surg.* 1996; 83:608–619.
65. Barber MD, Ross JA, Voss AC, Tisdale MJ, Fearon KC. The effect of an oral nutritional supplement enriched with fish oil on weight-loss in patients with pancreatic cancer. *Br J Cancer.* 1999;81:80–86.
66. Nebeling LC, Lerner E. Implementing a ketogenic diet based on medium-chain triglyceride oil in pediatric patients with cancer. *J Am Diet Assoc.* 1995;95: 693–697.
67. Daly J, Shinkwin M. Nutrition and the cancer patient. In: Murphy G, Lawrence W, Lenhard R, eds. *American Cancer Society Textbook of Clinical Oncology.* 2nd ed. Atlanta, Ga: American Cancer Society; 1995:580–596.
68. Nebeling LC, Miraldi F, Shurin SB, Lerner E. Effects of a ketogenic diet on tumor metabolism and nutritional status in pediatric oncology patients: two case reports. *J Am Coll Nutr.* 1995;14:202–208.
69. Tisdale MJ. Inhibition of lipolysis and muscle protein degradation by EPA in cancer cachexia. *Nutrition.* 1996;12(suppl 1):S31-S33.
70. Fearon KC, Von Meyenfeldt MF, Moses AG, Van Geenen R, Roy A, Gouma DJ, Giacosa A, Van Gossum A, Bauer J, Barber MD, Aaronson NK, Voss AC, Tisdale MJ. Effect of a protein and energy dense N-3 fatty acid enriched oral supplement on loss of weight and lean tissue in cancer cachexia: a randomised double blind trial. *Gut.* 2003;52:1479–1486.
71. McMillan DC, Preston T, Watson WS, Simpson JM, Fearon KC, Shenkin A, Burns HJ, McArdle CS. Relationship between weight loss, reduction of body cell mass and inflammatory response in patients with cancer. *Br J Surg.* 1994;81:1011–1014.
72. Klimberg VS, Nwokedi E, Hutchins LF, Pappas AA, Lang NP, Broadwater JR, Read RC, Westbrook KC. Glutamine facilitates chemotherapy while reducing toxicity. *JPEN J Parenter Enteral Nutr.* 1992;16(suppl 1, pt 6):S83-S87.
73. Argiles JM, Meijsing SH, Pallares-Trujillo J, Guirao X, Lopez-Soriano FJ. Cancer cachexia: a therapeutic approach. *Med Res Rev.* 2001;21:83–101.
74. Laviano A, Renvyle T, Yang ZJ. From laboratory to bedside: new strategies in the treatment of malnutrition in cancer patients. *Nutrition.* 1996;12:112–122.

Chapter 4

Diet, Cancer Risk, and Cancer Prevention

CONNIE MOBLEY, PHD, RD

INTRODUCTION

A small percentage of cancer cases can be explained by genetics. For most people, however, dietary choices and physical activity are second only to tobacco use in determining their cancer risk (1). This chapter examines the process of carcinogenesis and the relationship between diet and cancer risk. Lifestyle factors, including alcohol consumption, body weight, and physical activity, are reviewed. Because approximately 50% of all cancers could be prevented with the adoption of healthy lifestyles (2), this chapter also explores the relationship of diet to cancer prevention.

DIET AND CANCER RISK

Data suggest that the risk of developing cancer is significantly associated with lifestyle factors (3,4), including diet. According to Doll and Peto (5), approximately one-third of the 500,000 cancer deaths that occur annually in the United States are related to dietary factors. Dietary intake and nutritional status can alter not only the total risk of getting any cancer, but also the risk of specific types of cancer and the age at which they might develop.

Cancer is an assortment of diseases that occur when abnormal cells exhibit uncontrollable growth. In carcinogenesis, a procarcinogen fails to be detoxified or excreted and is converted to a carcinogen that alters genetic material. Figure 4.1 illustrates how bioactive dietary factors can act to prevent promotion and progression of mutant cells to latent tumor cells.

Dietary Fat Intake

The relationship between levels of fat intake and cancer risk has received extensive attention, but the findings are not conclusive. For example, a pooled analysis of cohort studies determined that the intake of meat and dairy products (foods that are generally high in total fat, saturated fat, and dietary cholesterol) has not been consistently or significantly associated with breast cancer risk (6), although dietary patterns characterized by high fiber and low fat intakes have been associated with a lower risk of postmenopausal breast cancer (7). Likewise, positive associations have been found between high-fat diets or intake of specific fatty food types (eg, meat, dairy) and prostate cancer (8). Researchers suggest that these often conflicting findings are because many food groups and nutrients, especially plant foods, may confound associations between relative fat intake and disease risk (9). Historically, ecological studies have identified associations between total fat intake and lung, colon, endometrial, and ovarian cancers (9–11). Studies continue to explore the role of dietary fat as a cancer promoter, the role of fatty acid oxidation, and the relationship of fat intake to changes in genetic material. Studies in progress are focusing on the following

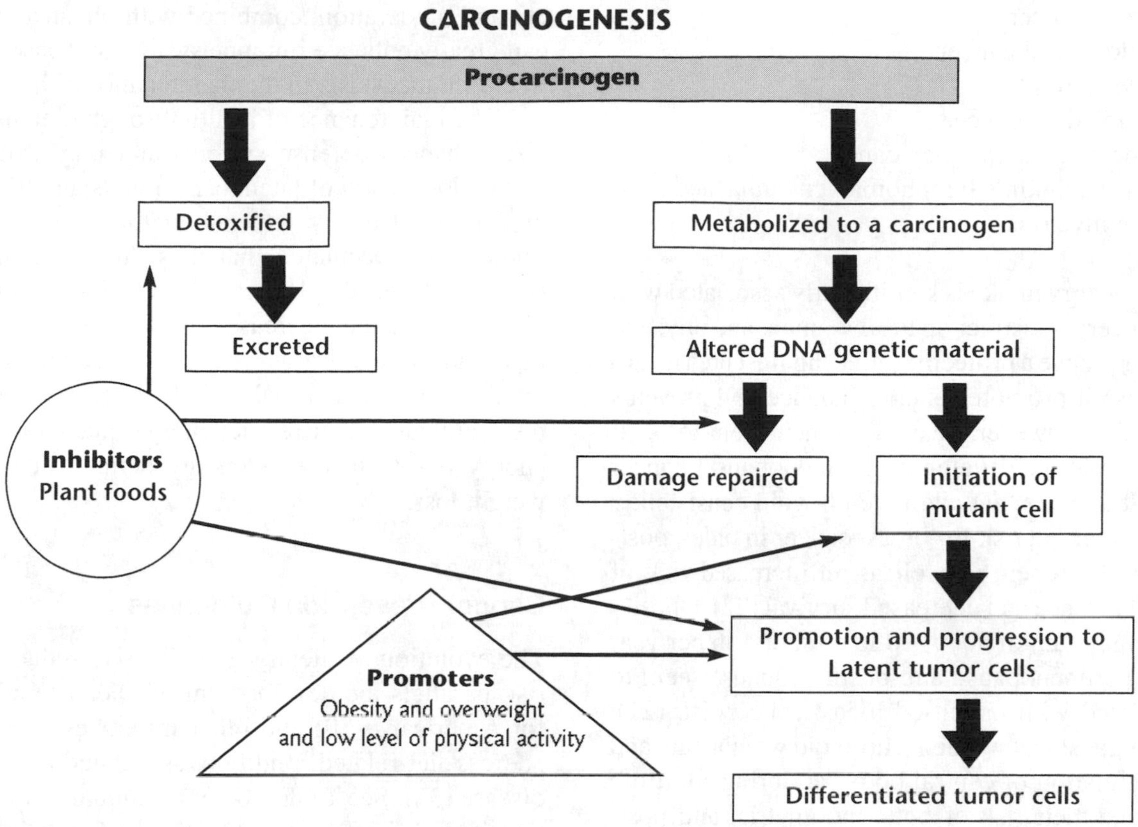

Figure 4.1. Dietary factors that can promote or inhibit carcinogenesis.

issues related to dietary fat intake and the cancer process (10–12):

- Total fat intake related to total energy intake, obesity, percentage body fat, body fat distribution, and sex-hormone levels
- Dietary fat intake related to the intake of fat-soluble carcinogens, especially animal fat
- Types of dietary fat (saturated, n-6-polyunsaturated, n-3-fats) and the mechanisms of cancer progression
- The role of short-chain fatty acids in the carcinogenic process

Alcohol Intake

The risk of developing squamous cell carcinoma of the head and neck has consistently been related to alcohol consumption, smoking, and tobacco use (13–15). Possible relationships between moderate alcohol intake and cancers of the colon, stomach, pancreas, liver, and breast have also been identified (9). Alcoholic beverages may be contaminated with such carcinogens as *N*-Nitroso compounds (micotoxins, urethane), inorganic arsenic, and asbestos; alcohol can also act as a solvent for other carcinogens. Additionally, people who consume excessive alcohol may displace micronutrients, such as folate and vitamins C and E, which have been associated with decreased cancer risk (4). However, moderate alcohol intake (1 to 2 servings per day) may decrease risk of other chronic diseases, such as cardiovascular disease (16).

CANCER RISK AND BODY WEIGHT AND PHYSICAL ACTIVITY

Obesity and associated inactivity may be major determinants of site-specific cancers. At a body mass index (BMI) of 40 or greater, which is indicative of obesity, there is a 52% higher risk of all cancers in men and a 62% higher risk in women (17). Overweight and obesity increase the risk for the following (17–19):

- Esophageal cancer
- Colon and rectum cancer

- Breast cancer
- Endometrial cancer
- Liver cancer
- Gallbladder cancer
- Pancreatic and kidney cancer
- Non-Hodgkin's lymphoma, leukemia, and multiple myeloma

Total energy intake is significantly associated with breast cancer in postmenopausal women, and physical activity may have a protective effect against breast cancer because it promotes energy balance and prevents weight gain. However, heavier women seem to be at decreased risk for developing premenopausal cancer (20,21). It appears that adult weight gain consistently predicts increased risk for breast cancer in older, postmenopausal women, as well as an increased risk of cancer recurrence and decreased survival (22). Obesity and a weight gain of about 10 lb total or 1 lb per year between perimenopause and postmenopause seem to be associated with increased breast cancer risk (21). Studies suggest that women who avoid weight gain and the accumulation of central body fat during adult life may reduce their risk of both endometrial and postmenopausal breast cancer (23).

Central obesity and waist circumference are strong predictors of colon cancer (24). Physical inactivity has been causally linked to the incidence of colon cancer (25). Higher serum estrogen levels in postmenopausal obese women, secondary to a high fat intake, were significantly decreased with a 1-year program of sustained, moderately intense physical activity (26). Steroid hormones or insulin/insulin-like growth factors or free radical generation, body composition, immune modulation, and direct effects on tumors may also be influenced by physical activity (27).

The World Health Organization has identified decreased physical activity (associated with colorectal cancer) and the increasing incidence of overweight and obesity (associated with colorectal, endometrial, esophageal, breast, and kidney cancers) as lifestyle risk factors most convincingly supported by existing evidence (28).

DIET AND CANCER PREVENTION

Achieving a balance among all dietary factors, while meeting nutrient needs, is paramount to cancer prevention. Food choices based on the principles of variety and moderation, combined with physical activity, can greatly enhance immune system response and the role of homeostasis in the maintenance of health.

The maintenance of health through diet and exercise enhances defense systems and may extend the incubation period of latent cancer cells and the ability of cells to detoxify and inhibit the cancer process. Some have speculated that it is the association between increased physical activity and improved dietary intake that decreases risk for cancer (18). Animal studies have shown that energy deficits enhance repair of genetic material (29). The effect occurs when these animals either restrict energy intake or increase energy output to create energy deficits that lead to weight loss.

Cancer Prevention Guidelines

The evolution of dietary guidelines to reduce cancer risk parallels the development of Dietary Guidelines for Americans (30) and other initiatives designed to address diet-related conditions associated with chronic disease (31). See Table 4.1 for a summary of information included in the USDA Dietary Guidelines (30), 1996 National Cancer Institute (NCI) Dietary Guidelines (32), the 2002 American Cancer Society (ACS) Nutrition Guidelines (33), the Dietary Recommendations of the American Institute for Cancer Research (9), and the World Health Organization recommendations (28). Although these guidelines are subject to periodic changes in response to evolving science, they can provide direction to dietetics practitioners engaged in cancer prevention strategies.

To help individuals to decrease cancer risk and promote cancer control through positive dietary behavior changes, health care professionals need to follow a few simple rules and use the simplest, most familiar tools:

- Base dietary recommendations on the USDA Dietary Guidelines.
- Focus on only one message at a time. Provide guidance and information to meet the specific needs and desires of the client. Remind client that behavioral change is a multistep process that takes extended time to accomplish.
- Encourage other health care providers to reinforce nutrition messages.

Table 4.1 Dietary Guidelines and Goals and Recommendations for Cancer Prevention

Organization (reference)	*Dietary Choices and Meal Patterns*	*Healthful Body Weight and Physical Activity*	*Alcohol*	*Other*
USDA, US Dept. of Health and Human Services (30)	• Make smart choices from every food group. • Get the most nutrition from your calories. • Choose a variety of fruits and vegetables every day. • Consume 3 cups of fat-free or low-fat milk or equivalent milk products every day. • Consume 3 or more whole-grain products every day. • Choose lean protein. • Look for foods low in saturated and *trans* fats.	• Find your balance between food and physical activity. • Engage in regular physical activity and reduce sedentary activities to promote health, psychological well-being, and healthy body weight. • Participate in moderate-intensity physical activity for 30 – 60 minutes a day, most days of the week, to maintain a healthy body weight.	• If you drink alcoholic beverages, do so in moderation.	• Choose and prepare foods and beverages with little salt and/or added sugars. • Consume less than 2,300 mg sodium daily. • Choose and prepare foods with little salt. At the same time, consume potassium-rich foods, such as fruits and vegetables.
American Cancer Society (33)	• Eat a variety of healthful foods, with an emphasis on plant sources. • Eat 5 or more servings of a variety of vegetables and fruits each day. • Choose whole grains in preference to processed (refined) grains and sugars. • Limit consumption of red meats, especially those high in fat and processed.	• Adopt a physically active lifestyle. • Maintain a healthful weight throughout life. • Choose foods that help you maintain a healthful weight.	• If you drink alcoholic beverages, limit consumption.	
National Cancer Institute (32)	• Include a variety of fruits and vegetables in the daily diet.	• Avoid obesity.	• Consume alcoholic beverages in moderation, if at all.	

(continued)

Table 4.1 Dietary Guidelines and Goals and Recommendations for Cancer Prevention (*continued*)

Organization (reference)	*Dietary Choices and Meal Patterns*	*Healthful Body Weight and Physical Activity*	*Alcohol*	*Other*
American Institute for Cancer Research (9)	• Choose plant-based diet rich in variety of vegetables, fruits, pulses (legumes), and minimally processed, starchy staple foods. • Eat 15–30 ounces or > 5 servings of vegetables and fruits daily. • Eat 20–30 ounces or > 7 servings of cereals, legumes, nuts, tubers, and plantains daily. • If eaten at all, red meat should provide < 10% total energy. • Total fat/oils should provide 15% to no more than 30% total energy.	• Avoid being over- or underweight, and limit weight gain during adulthood to < 11 pounds. • If activity is low or moderate, walk briskly daily for 1 hour and vigorously exercise for 1 hour weekly.	• Alcohol not recommended.	• Limit salt from all sources to < 6 g/day for adults. • Store and preserve food properly. • Do not eat charred food. • Limit refined sugar to < 10% total energy daily. • For those who follow these goals, dietary supplements are probably unnecessary and possibly unhelpful for reducing cancer risk.
World Health Organization (28)	• Include at least 400 g/day of fruits and vegetables in the diet. • Moderate consumption of preserved meat.	• Maintain desirable BMI, avoid weight gain during adult life, and maintain regular physical activity. • Maintain BMI between 18.5 and 24.9. • 60 minutes/day of moderately intense physical activity.	• Alcohol not recommended. • If consumed, limit to 2 servings/day.	• Moderate consumption of salt and salt-preserved foods. • Minimize exposure to aflatoxins in foods. • Avoid consumption of foods at very hot (scalding) temperatures.

Food Groups to Encourage

Epidemiological data show a probable association between consumption of plant-based foods and reduced risk of cancers of the lung, colon, esophagus, and rectum (34). Published recommendations of the American Cancer Society and the American Institute for Cancer Research for reducing cancer risk encourage Americans to consume a plant-based diet, including the daily consumption of whole grain foods and at least 5 servings of vegetables and fruits (9,33). After adjusting data for ethnic group and energy intake, an increased consumption of vegetables (particularly dark-green vegetables) can reduce cancer risk 20% to 50% (35). In Western nations, an inadequate intake of suggested servings of fruits and vegetables is associated with 1 in 10 of diagnosed cancers (36). See Table 4.2 (4,17–28,34–39) for possible associations between dietary factors and site-specific cancers.

Plant-based foods contain essential nutrients that support optimum tissue and organ responses, as well

Table 4.2 Strength of Evidence of Associations Between Nutrition-Related Factors and Cancers

Hypothesis (References)	*Lung*	*Rectum/Colon*	*Breast*	*Prostate*	*Head and Neck*	*Endometrial*
Diet rich in plant-based foods decreases risk (34-39)	Probable	Probable	Possible	Possible	Probable	Possible
Moderate physical activity decreases risk (20,21,25-27)	Lacking	Convincing	Convincing	Weak	Weak	Probable
Obesity increases risk (17-24,28)	Lacking	Convincing	Convincing	Convincing	Probable	Convincing
Alcohol increases risk (4)	Lacking	Possible	Probable	Lacking	Convincing	Weak

as antioxidants, dietary fiber, and phytochemicals (see Table 4.3). They act to inhibit cancer by functioning as (38)

- Inhibitors of neoplastic transformation by inhibiting hormone-dependent steps in tumor formation and protecting genetic material from carcinogenic agents
- Suppressers of free radical production
- Bulking agents to dilute carcinogens and decrease gastrointestinal transit time
- Stimulators of physiologically active anticancer enzymes

The amount of these plant-based nutrients, including antioxidants, fiber, and phytochemicals, as well as the frequency of ingestion required to prevent the development or promotion of cancer is currently unclear (39).

Carcinogens in the Food Supply

The food supply includes hundreds of procarcinogens (cancer promoters), anticarcinogens (anticancer promoters), and cancer inhibitors (40). Therefore, it is impossible to eat a carcinogenic-free diet. Aflatoxins in peanuts, safrol in some plant oils, tannins in grains and grapes, and benzo(a)pyrene formed by smoking meat and fish are just some examples of naturally occurring carcinogens (41). Potential carcinogens also exist as natural metabolites of plant foods, such as celery, parsley, figs, mustard, pepper, and citrus oils. These metabolites may be part of the plants' natural defense systems. Laboratory data indicate that these natural metabolites are a potential cancer risk only when they are consumed in highly concentrated amounts that are well beyond typical levels of dietary consumption. Naturally found compounds in plants exceed by a factor of at least 10,000 the limits set by the federal government for intake of synthetic carcinogens (such as pesticides and other additives); however, if foods with natural metabolites are properly handled and stored, there is no evidence to suggest adverse health effects (9,41). Some additives, such as BHA and BHT, may even have a protective effect against cancer.

Concern about either naturally occurring or synthetic carcinogens in the food supply can be addressed by

- Choosing in-season, locally grown produce
- Rinsing fruits and vegetables and removing outer leaves before eating
- Practicing food storage and preparation techniques to preserve optimum nutritional value (proper food storage temperatures can delay growth of potent fungal carcinogens)
- Marinating protein foods to decrease total cooking time
- Using cooking methods that avoid contact of foods and food drippings with flames
- Using lower cooking temperatures to reduce production of heterocyclic amines when protein foods are broiled or grilled

Table 4.3 Common Plant-Based Foods, Anticancer Constituents, and Their Roles in Cancer Prevention

Foods	*Phytochemicals*	*Vitamins*	*Fiber*	*Antioxidant Activity*	*Stimulates Anticancer Enzymes*	*Acts as Cancer Inhibitor*
Garlic, onion (Allium vegetables)	Organosulfur compounds		Soluble, insoluble	X		X
Broccoli, cauliflower, cabbage, and other cruciferous vegetables (Brassica vegetables)	Indoles, sulforaphane, isothiocynate	Folate, vitamins A and C	Insoluble			X
Citrus fruit	Terpenes, coumarins, flavonoids	Vitamin C, folate	Soluble	X	X	X
Strawberries, grapes, apples, berries, and nuts	Ellagic acid	Vitamins E and C, beta carotene	Soluble	X	X	X
Carrots, yams, cantaloupe, butternut squash		Beta carotene	Soluble, insoluble	X	X	X
Soybeans, beans, peas, lentils	Genistein, other isoflavones, saponins, phytosterols		Soluble			X
Hot peppers	Capsaicin	Vitamin C		X		X
Flaxseed, whole wheat, barley, brown rice	Lignans		Soluble, insoluble	X		X
Tomatoes, red grapefruit	Lycopene	Vitamin C	Soluble	X		
Green tea, grapes	Polyphenols					X

REFERENCES

1. Mokdad AH, Marks JS, Stroup DF, Gerberding JI. Actual causes of death in the United States, 2000. *JAMA.* 2004;291:1238–1245.
2. Colditz GA, DeJong W, Hunter DJ, Trichopoulos D, Willett WC. Harvard report on cancer prevention. *Cancer Causes Control.* 1996;7(suppl):S1-S55.
3. Herdman R, Lichtenfeld L, eds. *Fulfilling the Potential of Cancer Prevention and Early Detection.* Washington, DC: National Academy Press; 2004.
4. Stein CJ, Colditz GA. Modifiable risk factors for cancer. *Br J Cancer.* 2004;90:299–303.
5. Doll R, Peto R. The causes of cancer: quantitative estimates of avoidable risks of cancer in the United States today. *J Natl Cancer Inst.* 1981;66:1191–1308.
6. Missmer SA, Smith-Warner SA, Spiegelman D, Yaun SS, Adami HO, Beeson WL, van den Brandt PA, Fraser GE, Freudenheim JL, Goldbohm RA, Graham S, Kushi LH, Miller AB, Potter JD, Rohan TE, Speizer FE, Toniolo P, Willett WC, Wolk A, Zeleniuch-Jacquotte A, Hunter DJ. Meat and dairy food con-

sumption and breast cancer: a pooled analysis of cohort studies. *Int J Epidemiol.* 2002;31:78–85.

7. Mattisson I, Wirfalt E, Johansson U, Gullberg B, Olsson H, Berglund G. Intakes of plant foods, fibre and fat and risk of breast cancer—a prospective study in the Malmo Diet and Cancer cohort. *Br J Cancer.* 2004;90:122–127.
8. Fleshner N, Bagnell PS, Klotz L, Venkateswaran V. Dietary fat and prostate cancer. *J Urol.* 2004;171 (suppl):S19-S24.
9. World Cancer Research Fund in Association With American Institute for Cancer Research. *Food, Nutrition and the Prevention of Cancer: A Global Perspective.* Washington, DC: American Institute for Cancer Research; 1997.
10. Kuller LH. Dietary fat and chronic diseases: epidemiologic overview. *J Am Diet Assoc.* 1997;97(suppl 7):S9-S15.
11. Weisburger JH. Dietary fat and risk of chronic disease: mechanistic insights from experimental studies. *J Am Diet Assoc.* 1997;97(suppl 7):S16-S23.
12. Greenwald P, Sherwood K, McDonald SS. Fat, caloric intake, and obesity: lifestyle risk factors for breast cancer. *J Am Diet Assoc.* 1997;97(suppl 7):S24-S30.
13. Jaber MA, Porter SR, Gilthorpe MS, Bedi R, Scully C. Risk factors for oral epithelial dysplasia—the role of smoke and alcohol. *Oral Oncol.* 1999;35:151–156.
14. Zaridze DG, Blettner M, Trapeznikov NN, Kuvshinov JD, Matiakin EG, Poljakov BP, Poddubni BK, Parshikova SM, Rottenberg VI, Chamrakulov TS. Survey of a population with a high incidence of oral and oesophageal cancer. *Int J Cancer.* 1985; 36:153–158.
15. Mashberg A, Garfinkel L, Harris S. Alcohol as a primary risk factor in oral squamous carcinoma. *CA Ca J Clin.* 1981;31:146–155.
16. Burger M, Bronstrup A, Pietrzik K. Derivation of tolerable upper alcohol intake levels in Germany: a systematic review of risks and benefits of moderate alcohol consumption. *Prev Med.* 2004;39:111–127.
17. Calle EE, Rodriguez C, Walker-Thurmond K, Thun MJ. Overweight, obesity, and mortality from cancer in a prospectively studied cohort of U.S. adults. *N Engl J Med.* 2003;348:1625–1638.
18. Key TJ, Schatzkin A, Willett WC, Allen NE, Spencer EA, Travis RC. Diet, nutrition and the prevention of cancer. *Public Health Nutr.* 2004;7:187–200.
19. Pan SY, Johnson KC, Ugnat AM, Wen SW, Mao Y, Canadian Cancer Registries Epidemiology Research Group. Association of obesity and cancer risk in Canada. *Am J Epidemiol.* 2004;159:259–268.
20. Carmichael AR, Bates T. Obesity and breast cancer: a review of the literature. *Breast.* 2004;13:85–92.
21. Hunter DJ, Willett WC. Nutrition and breast cancer. *Cancer Causes Control.* 1996;7:56–68.
22. Ziegler RG. Anthropometry and breast cancer. *J Nutr.* 1997;127(suppl 5):S924-S928.
23. Ballard-Barbash R, Swanson CA. Body weight: estimation of risk for breast and endometrial cancers. *Am J Clin Nutr.* 1996;63(suppl 3):S437-S441.
24. Moore LL, Bradlee ML, Singer MR, Splansky GL, Proctor MH, Ellison RC, Kreger BE. BMI and waist circumference as predictors of lifetime colon cancer risk in Framingham Study adults. *Int J Obes Relat Metab Disord.* 2004;28:559–567.
25. Slattery ML. Physical activity and colorectal cancer. *Sports Med.* 2004;34:239–252.
26. McTiernan A, Tworoger SS, Ulrich CM, Yasui Y, Irwin ML, Rajan KB, Sorensen B, Rudolph RE, Bowen D, Stanczyk FZ, Potter JD, Schwartz RS. Effect of exercise on serum estrogens in postmenopausal women: a 12-month randomized clinical trial. *Cancer Res.* 2004; 64:2923–2928.
27. Westerlind KC. Physical activity and cancer prevention—mechanisms. *Med Sci Sports Exerc.* 2003;35: 1834–1840.
28. WHO/FAO Expert Consultation Panel. *Diet, Nutrition and the Prevention of Chronic Diseases.* WHO Technical Report Series 916. Geneva, Switzerland; 2002.
29. Kritchevsky D. The effect of over- and undernutrition on cancer. *Eur J Cancer Prev.* 1995;4:445–451.
30. US Depts of Agriculture and Health and Human Services. *Nutrition and Your Health: Dietary Guidelines for Americans.* Available at: http://wwww.healthierus .gov/dietaryguidelines. Accessed June 29, 2005.
31. US Department of Health and Human Services. *Healthy People 2010: Understanding and Improving Health.* 2nd ed. Washington, DC: US Government Printing Office; 2000.
32. National Cancer Institute. *Action Guide for Healthy Eating.* Bethesda, Md: National Institutes of Health; 1996. NIH publication 96–3877.
33. Byers T, Nestle M, McTiernan A, Doyle C, Currie-Williams A, Gansler T, Thun M. American Cancer Society 2001 Nutrition and Physical Activity Guidelines Advisory Committee. American Cancer Society guidelines on nutrition and physical activity for cancer prevention: reducing the risk of cancer with healthy food choices and physical activity. *Cancer J Clin.* 2002;52:92–119.
34. Steinmetz KA, Potter JD. Vegetables, fruit, and cancer.

I. Epidemiology. *Cancer Causes Control.* 1991;2: 325–357.

35. Satia-Abouta J, Galanko JA, Martin CF, Ammerman A, Sandler RS. Food groups and colon cancer risk in African-Americans and Caucasians. *Int J Cancer.* 2004;109:728–736.
36. World Health Organization. *IARC Handbook on Cancer Prevention: Fruits and Vegetables.* Volume 8. Geneva, Switzerland; 2004.
37. Riboli E, Norat T. Epidemiologic evidence of the protective effect of fruit and vegetables on cancer risk. *Am J Clin Nutr.* 2003;78(suppl 3):S559-S569.
38. Steinmetz KA, Potter JD. Vegetables, fruit, and cancer. II. Mechanisms. *Cancer Causes Control.* 1991;2: 427–442.
39. Key TJ, Allen NE, Spencer EA, Travis RC. The effect of diet on risk of cancer. *Lancet.* 2002;360:861–868.
40. Ames BN, Gold LS, Willett WC. The causes and prevention of cancer. *Proc Natl Acad Sci USA.* 1995; 92:5258–5265.
41. Sugimura T, Wakabayashi K. Carcinogens in foods. In: Shils ME, Olson JA, Skile M, Ross AC, eds. *Modern Nutrition in Health and Disease.* 9th ed. Philadelphia, Pa: Lea and Fibiger; 1999:1255–1261.

Section 2

Medical Nutrition Therapy in Oncology

Chapter 5

The Nutrition Care Process and Medical Nutrition Therapy

LAURA ELLIOTT, MPH, RD

INTRODUCTION

Nutrition care that is provided in an organized and standardized manner allows for more predictable, effective outcomes. According to Lacey and Pritchett (1), standardizing nutrition care "effectively promotes the dietetics professional as the unique provider of nutrition care when it is consistently used as a systematic method to think critically and make decisions to provide safe and effective nutrition care." This chapter reviews the American Dietetic Association's accomplishments in the standardization of nutrition care, including the Nutrition Care Process (NCP) and medical nutrition therapy (MNT) protocols. This chapter also reviews ADA's development of standards of practice, standards of professional performance, and standardized language.

NUTRITION CARE PROCESS

In 2002, the ADA Nutrition Care Model workgroup developed the NCP in response to the need for a standardized process for critical thinking, decision making, and provision of safe and effective nutrition care (1). The NCP provides a consistent structure and framework to provide nutrition care for both individuals and groups from inpatient to community settings of care. The following are the steps in the NCP (1):

1. *Nutrition assessment*—collecting timely and pertinent information, using valid and reliable methods for data collection, and comparing gathered data to evidence-based standards, norms, and ideals
2. *Nutrition diagnosis*—identifying nutrition problems accurately and consistently, focusing on the primary problems associated with diseases and conditions
3. *Nutrition intervention*—planning, implementing, and documenting evidenced-based interventions that target actual or potential causes of the identified nutrition problems
4. *Nutrition monitoring and evaluation*—collecting and reviewing interval data to evaluate how chosen interventions have altered the signs and symptoms associated with nutrition problems (eg, determining whether the expected outcomes of interventions are achieved and, if not, refining or changing interventions to produce the expected outcomes)

Although the steps in NCP build on one another, they are not necessarily linear. The NCP may involve revisiting previous steps to reassess, revise diagnoses, modify interventions, and evaluate additional outcomes (1).

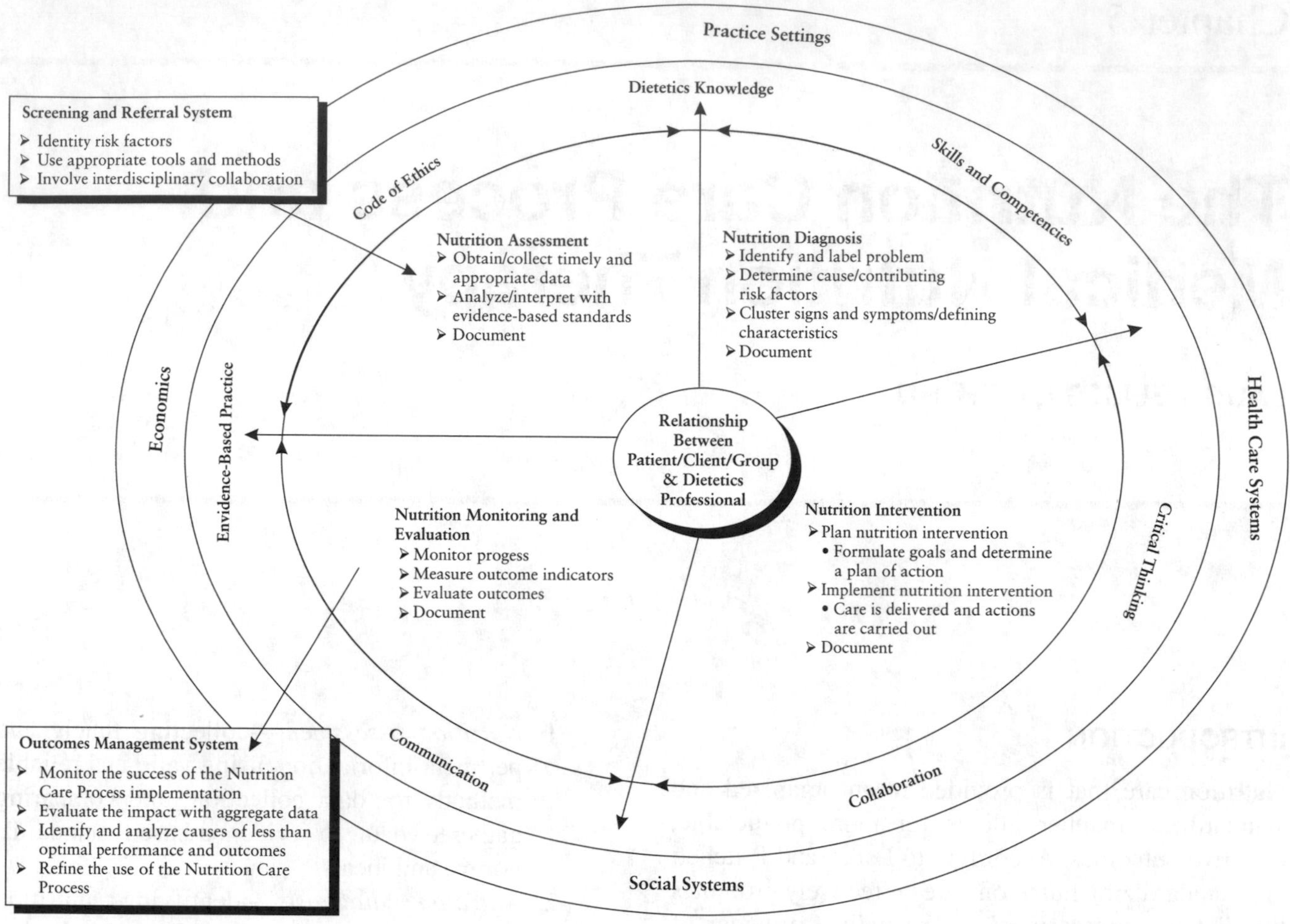

Figure 5.1. American Dietetic Association Nutrition Care Process and Model. Reprinted from Lacey K, Pritchett E. Nutrition care process and model: ADA adopts road map to quality care and outcomes. *J Am Diet Assoc.* 2003;103:1061–1072, with permission from the American Dietetic Association.

Nutrition Care Model

The NCP is represented by the Nutrition Care Model (Figure 5.1) (1). Dietetics professionals should note the following:

- The core is the vital relationship between the patient and the dietetics professional.
- The relationship between patient and the dietetics professional is surrounded by the four steps of the NCP.
- The outer rings represent the strengths and abilities that the dietetics professional brings to the process and the environmental factors and support systems that influence the process.

MEDICAL NUTRITION THERAPY

MNT fits into the framework of nutrition care as the clinical application of the NCP. With a consistent and systematic structure and method by which to think critically and make decisions (1), more consistent practice and outcomes will occur. MNT helps establish the link between quality and nutrition practice and enables the growth of dietetics from experience-based practices to evidence-based practices (2).

MNT is defined by the ADA as a planned series of activities developed through a consultative process that incorporates current professional knowledge and available research and clearly defines the level, content, and frequency of nutrition care appropriate for a disease or condition (2). The MNT protocols were developed to enable practitioners to apply care consistently and to document outcomes in order to meet the challenge of maintaining quality of care while containing costs (3).

Benefits of MNT Protocols

MNT increases effectiveness of care by promoting consistency and by providing clear measurements of quality and effectiveness of care (1). In this era of cost effectiveness, insurers are seeking ways to manage the allocation of health care benefits. It is necessary to show substantial cost savings to the insurer to be included as a covered service. Because of growing evidence of the effectiveness of MNT, the Institute of Medicine recommended in 1999 that MNT provided by registered dietitians (RDs) be included as a benefit to Medicare recipients for all diagnoses upon physician referral (4). Effective January 2002, Medicare reimburses outpatient MNT for beneficiaries with diabetes or nondialysis kidney disease (5).

The MNT protocols also guide future outcomes research. Evaluating nutrition outcomes requires a clear understanding of both the objectives that determine the selection of outcome criteria and the parties that define the objectives. Many studies of cancer treatments, for example, have focused solely on survival rates, regardless of the quality of life experienced by subjects (6). Quality of life may be a more appropriate outcome to measure when evaluating nutrition intervention during cancer treatment. Future research will determine benchmarks for measuring quality of care and effectiveness of MNT, especially with the cancer population.

Oncology Protocols

The oncology protocols are currently under revision by members of the Oncology Nutrition Dietetics Practice Group and the Quality Management and Outcomes Research team of the ADA. The revised protocols will combine the original medical and radiation oncology protocols (7) into one oncology MNT protocol. This most recent work on the protocol reflects ADA's "Priorities for Research" proposal that emphasizes evidence-based practice (8). The basis of the protocols includes current research and existing nationally developed practice guidelines, consensus reports, published MNT protocols, and expert opinion.

The protocols will include explicit statements of the quality and strength of evidence supporting the recommendations. Plans are under way to strengthen the content of the protocols by further validating the protocols (once they are published) in practice. The revised, evidence-based oncology MNT protocols are due to be published in 2006.

STANDARDS OF PRACTICE IN NUTRITION CARE

The Standards of Practice in Nutrition Care reflect the Commission on Accreditation for Dietetics Education (CADE) core educational competencies and the evolving nature of dietetics practice (9). They describe competent practice based on the NCP and Nutrition Care Model and include the following (9):

1. The RD obtains adequate information to identify nutrition-related problems.
2. The RD identifies and describes an actual occurrence of, risk of, or potential for developing a nutrition problem that the RD is responsible for treating independently.
3. The RD identifies and implements appropriate, purposefully planned actions designed with the intent of changing a nutrition-related behavior, risk factor, environmental condition, or aspect of health status for an individual, a target group, or the community at large.
4. The RD monitors and evaluates outcome(s) directly related to the nutrition diagnosis and the goals established in the intervention plan to determine the degree to which progress is being made and goals or desired outcomes of nutrition care are being met.

STANDARDS OF PRACTICE OF RDS IN ONCOLOGY NUTRITION CARE

The Oncology Dietetics Practice Group (ONDPG) of the ADA is in the process of developing the Standards of Practice of Registered Dietitians in Oncology Nutrition Care. These standards will document the fundamental skills required for specialty practice in oncology nutrition and for identifying quality continuing education programs and materials, conducting needed outcomes research, and pursuing certification in oncology nutrition. These Oncology Standards of

Practice will contain the evaluation tools and interventions unique to the oncology population.

STANDARDS OF PROFESSIONAL PERFORMANCE

ADA continues to refine the dietetics profession by developing Standards of Professional Performance (9,10). The Standards of Professional Performance for Dietetics Professionals (formerly called the Standards of Professional Practice) describe a competent level of professional behavior and include the following:

1. Provision of services—The dietetics practitioner provides quality service based on customer expectations and needs.
2. Application of research—The dietetics practitioner effectively applies, participates in, or generates research to enhance practice.
3. Communication and application of knowledge—The dietetics practitioner effectively applies knowledge and communicates with others.
4. Utilization and management of resources—The dietetics practitioner uses resources effectively and efficiently in practice.
5. Quality in practice—The dietetics practitioner systematically evaluates the quality and effectiveness of practice and revises practice as needed to incorporate the results of evaluation.
6. Continued competence and professional accountability—The dietetics practitioner engages in lifelong self-development to improve knowledge and enhance professional competence.

STANDARDIZED LANGUAGE

Using standardized language allows for effective identification of health problems and consistent communication of treatment strategies and evaluation of care (10). Communicating in this way provides a foundation for measuring outcomes and for generating qualitative and quantitative data that can be analyzed and interpreted; hence, a structure with which to validate nutrition care is thereby provided. The ADA task force is developing language to be used much as the International Classification of Diseases (ICD) is used by the medical profession (11); the Current Procedural Terminology (CPT) (12) and systemized Nomenclature of Medicine (SNOMED) (13) codes are used to describe procedures and services; and Nursing Intervention Classification and Nursing Outcomes Classification are used by nurses to document, reflect, and study nursing care (14,15).

REFERENCES

1. Lacey K, Pritchett E. Nutrition Care Process and Model: ADA adopts road map to quality care and outcomes management. *J Am Diet Assoc.* 2003;103:1061–1072.
2. Splett P. *Developing and Validating Evidence-Based Guides for Practice: A Tool Kit for Dietetics Professionals.* Chicago, Ill: American Dietetic Association; 1999.
3. Michalczyk D. Sustaining demand for medical nutrition therapy services: are you meeting the requirements? *J Am Diet Assoc.* 2003;103:1134–1135.
4. Chima CS, Pollack HA. Position of the American Dietetic Association: nutrition services in managed care. *J Am Diet Assoc.* 2002;102:1471–1478.
5. Luthringer S, Kulakowski K. Medical nutritional therapy protocols. In: McCallum P, Polisena C, eds. *The Clinical Guide to Oncology Nutrition.* Chicago, Ill: American Dietetic Association; 2000:24–44.
6. American Dietetic Association. Improving Health and Outcomes of Medicare Beneficiaries. Available at: http://www.eatright.org/Public/GovernmentAffairs/9811351.cfm. Accessed September 14, 2005.
7. American Dietetic Association and Morrison Health Care. *Medical Nutrition Therapy Across the Continuum of Care.* Chicago, Ill: America Dietetic Association; 1998.
8. Vaughan LA, Manning CK. Meeting the challenges of dietetics practice with evidence-based decisions. *J Am Diet Assoc.* 2004;104:282–284.
9. Kieselhorst KJ, Skates J, Pritchett E. American Dietetic Association: Standards of practice in nutrition care and updated standards of professional performance. *J Am Diet Assoc.* 2005;105:641–645.
10. Hakel-Smith N, Lewis NM. A standardized nutrition care process and language are essential components of a conceptual model to guide and document nutrition care and patient outcomes. *J Am Diet Assoc.* 2004;104:1878–1884.
11. World Health Organization. International Classification of Diseases. Available at: http://www.who.int/classifications/icd/en. Accessed April 25, 2005.

12. American Medical Association. Current Procedural Terminology. Available at: http://www.ama-assn.org/ama/pub/category/3113.html. Accessed April 25, 2005.
13. College of American Pathologists. Systematized Nomenclature of Medicine (SNOMED). Available at: http://www.snomed.org. Accessed April 25, 2005.
14. Moorehead S, Johnson M, Maas M, eds. *Nursing Outcomes Classification (NOC)*. 3rd ed. St. Louis, Mo: Mosby; 2004.
15. McCloskey Dochterman J, Bulechek GM, eds. *Iowa Intervention Project: Nursing Interventions Classification (NIC)*. St. Louis, Mo: Mosby; 2004.

Chapter 6

Nutrition Screening and Assessment in Oncology*

PAULA DAVIS MCCALLUM, MS, RD

INTRODUCTION

Proactive nutrition screening and intervention are the cornerstones of success in managing cancer-related cachexia, malnutrition, and nutrition impact symptoms associated with cancer and its treatment (1–3). This chapter defines nutrition screening and assessment and examines tools that have practical applications in oncology settings. This chapter also examines symptom and activity scales that can assist oncology health care professionals in determining individuals' symptoms and abilities. Evaluation of these factors is an important part of the overall nutrition assessment process.

SCREENING AND ASSESSMENT DEFINED

The terms nutrition *screening* and *assessment* are often used interchangeably. As described by Lacey and Pritchett (4), nutrition screening is the identification of an individual's nutrition, health, functional, and behavioral status. Nutrition screening initiates nutrition assessment, which is the first step of the Nutrition Care Process (NCP) and is defined as the collection of timely and pertinent information, the use of valid and reliable methods for data collection, and the comparison of gathered data to evidence-based standards, norms, and ideals. For more information on the NCP, see Chapter 5.

In the oncology setting, health care professionals consider nutrition screening to be the identification of cancer-related malnutrition and cachexia and/or associated nutrition impact symptoms. Because the etiology of cancer-related malnutrition and cachexia is multifactorial (5), and because many of these factors are manageable, especially when identified and treated early in the course of the disease, it is, therefore, essential that nutrition issues be addressed at diagnosis and throughout the course of cancer care.

SCREENING AND ASSESSMENT TOOLS

A number of nutrition screening and assessment tools have evolved over the years. Not all are specific to the oncology population, but the tools listed in the following sections may have some practical applications in oncology settings.

Traditional Nutrition Assessment

Traditional nutrition assessment uses historical, biochemical, and anthropometric data (6). Historical data include pertinent medical history, diet history, and

*With the exception of Figures 6.1 and 6.2, the content of this chapter is adapted with permission from Nutrition Dimension, Inc. Copyright Nutrition Dimension, Inc.

weight history. Biochemical data can include a variety of information, such as visceral protein indexes (albumin, transferrin, pre-albumin, retinol binding protein), total lymphocyte count, hemoglobin, hematocrit, nitrogen balance studies, delayed hypersensitivity skin testing, lipid profiles, and blood glucose level. Indexes of visceral protein are often used in nutrition assessments, although institutions vary as to which indexes are used. Anthropometric data include measurements of weight and height, as well as midarm circumference, triceps skinfold, midarm muscle circumference, and body mass index (BMI).

Although the aforementioned data are objective, a good clinician always uses subjective judgment in completing an assessment. For example, it is not uncommon for an individual diagnosed with cancer to receive large fluid volumes along with chemotherapy. Therefore, decreased albumin may be indicative of hemodilution rather than malnutrition. All these parameters must be evaluated within the context of an individual's history.

The benefits of traditional nutrition assessment are that it relies on multiple parameters, that good clinical judgment can provide an excellent assessment of nutritional status, and that institution-specific protocols may be designed to include triage, which many oncology health care professionals define as the appropriate referral for nutrition intervention and intervention guidelines.

The drawbacks are that laboratory values may be costly or difficult to obtain in some health care settings and that this type of assessment relies on good clinical judgment to evaluate the parameters within the context of the patient's history. Also, traditional nutrition assessment may not include triage guidelines, and protocols using traditional assessments may or may not be validated. Furthermore, skinfold measurements are of limited value in elderly, dehydrated, or edematous individuals, because tissue is more easily compressed in dehydrated individuals and less easily compressed in edematous individuals, giving a false measurement of body fat (7). Finally, delayed hypersensitivity skin tests are not recommended in patients who are immunocompromised (8).

Mini Nutritional Assessment (MNA)

The Mini Nutritional Assessment (MNA) (9) was developed as a quick and efficient tool to screen for malnutrition in the elderly (9,10). Although this tool has been used in individuals diagnosed with cancer, it has not been validated specifically for use in oncology. The MNA considers anthropometric measurements, including BMI, but it does not include laboratory values. There are a number of questions that relate to dietary intake, but none that consider nutritional impact symptoms. The MNA includes both a screening and an assessment component, and both of these are scored, indicating level of risk. There are no intervention guidelines, however.

MNA has several advantages: it is based on multiple parameters (10,11); it is validated for use in the elderly; and it is quick and efficient to use. However, it does not include nutrition impact symptoms specific to cancer, and it is not validated for use in the oncology population.

Prognostic Nutritional Index

The Prognostic Nutritional Index (PNI) measures the risk that a patient has of developing a complication, such as sepsis or death related to malnutrition (6,12). The formula for determining PNI is as follows:

$$PNI\ \% = 158 - 16.6A - 0.78TSF - 0.2TFN - 5.8DH$$

Where: A indicates albumin (g/dL); TSF, triceps skinfold (mm); TFN, transferrin (mg/dL); DH, delayed hypersensitivity skin testing reaction to a recall antigen (usually mumps Candida or streptokinase-streptodornase), with scoring as follows: nonreactive = 0; < 5 mm induration = 1; > 5 mm induration = 2.

Interpretation of the PNI (6,12) is as follows:

- < 40: low risk
- 40–49.99: intermediate risk
- ≥ 50: high risk

Benefits of the PNI are the inclusion of multiple criteria for risk evaluation (11) and its utility for predicting nutrition-related morbidity. Additionally, it is successful in identifying malnourished surgical patients and has been validated in that population (13–16).

However, as previously mentioned, skin testing in individuals with questionable immune function is not reliable, and there are limitations to using albumin values to assess protein malnutrition in this population. Additionally, anthropometrics such as skinfold measurements, midarm circumference, and midarm muscle circumference may not be reliable indicators of nutritional status if the individual is dehydrated or if there is tissue turgor. Furthermore, the PNI does not consider nutrition impact symptoms or changes in weight, and it does not include triage guidelines.

Prognostic Inflammatory and Nutritional Index

The Prognostic Inflammatory and Nutritional Index (PINI) assesses inflammatory markers, which have been associated with cytokine production, weight loss, and cachexia (17–20), as well as albumin and transthyretin (formerly known as pre-albumin or thyroxine-binding pre-albumin). Measurement and comparison of serum proteins can help discriminate between metabolic stress and nutritional deprivation. PINI has been useful in predicting mortality and "chronic institutionalization" (17). The formula for calculating PINI (12) is as follows:

$$\text{PINI} = \frac{(\alpha\text{1-acid glycoprotein} \times \text{C-reactive protein})}{(\text{Albumin} \times \text{Transthyretin})}$$

Where: α1-acid glycoprotein, C-reactive protein, and transthyretin are measured in mg/L; albumin is measured in g/L. Reference ranges for each value are as follows: Transthyretin: 100–400 mg/L; Albumin: 35–50 g/L; Alpha-1 acid glycoprotein: 550–1400 mg/L; C-reactive protein: 0.2–6.1 mg/L.

PINI values may be interpreted as follows:

- < 1: Well-nourished, without infection
- 1–10: Low risk
- 11–20: Medium risk
- 21–30: High risk

Nelson and Walsh (21) found that individuals with advanced cancer had unusually high PINI values, presumably because these subjects had very high C-reactive protein values. Further research is needed to determine whether inflammatory markers are predictive of weight loss and whether they can be used in nutrition screening for early nutrition intervention, particularly with specialty formulas containing production with anti-inflammatory agents like eicosapentaenoic acid (EPA). Inclusion of indexes of both acute and more chronic insult to visceral protein is an attractive feature of the PINI, although liver disease and dilutional/concentration effects can confound interpretation of PINI. Additionally, PINI does not assess weight changes or nutrition impact symptoms, and it does not offer any triage guidelines.

Subjective Global Assessment

The Subjective Global Assessment (SGA) was originally developed by Jeejeebhoy and colleagues in the 1980s (22). The SGA has been used in a number of patient populations (22–26) and has been shown to have superior sensitivity and specificity over more traditional measures of nutrition assessment, such as albumin. The SGA is comprised of history (weight loss, dietary intake, gastrointestinal symptoms, and functional capacity), metabolic demands of the underlying disease, and a nutrition-related physical exam (6). The examination considers loss of subcutaneous fat and presence of muscle wasting, edema, and/or ascites (22).

The rating of nutritional status is subjective and derived from the sum of the parameters, with A = well-nourished, B = moderately malnourished or at risk, and C = severely malnourished. SGA is efficient and cost-effective, and it has been validated in a variety of patient populations. Furthermore, it identifies patients who might otherwise fall between the cracks: those at risk of malnutrition or those whose status borders on malnutrition. The drawbacks to using this tool include professional resistance to performing the nutrition-related physical examination, because some health care professionals are unaware of the benefits of SGA and some do not know how to use it. In addition, there is an incomplete list of nutritional impact symptoms specific to cancer, and it does not include a triage component.

Scored Patient-Generated Subjective Global Assessment

In the mid-1990s, Ottery (27) adapted the SGA to more specifically meet the needs of the oncology population: the gastrointestinal symptom section was increased to include the common nutrition impact symptoms found in cancer (28). Furthermore, the history section of the tool became "patient generated" to streamline the process and involve the patient and family more (29). As time went on, a scoring and triage component (30) was added, and the tool evolved

Box 6.1
Pros and Cons of the Scored PG-SGA

Pros

- Allows patient/family participation
- Streamlines data collection
- More complete list of nutrition impact symptoms
- Parameters are weighted/scored based on nutrition impact
- Easier to use; tables and worksheets included on reverse of form
- Identifies treatable nutrition impact symptoms
- Score can be used to track outcomes
- Validated in oncology setting
- Triage guidelines included

Cons

- Professional resistance to performing physical exam
- Perception of additional workload
- Patients may resist completing more "paperwork"
- Patient-generated section relies on patient literacy

Source: Data are from references 17, 29, 30, 32–35.

into the one in use today (Figures 6.1 and 6.2). Further details about the Scored PG-SGA are located in the Patient-Generated Subjective Global Assessment Training Video and Companion Literature (7), available through the American Dietetic Association.

The scored PG-SGA has been validated for use in oncology patients (30). Isenring and coworkers (31) have also found that the Scored PG-SGA correlates closely with quality of life and can be used to predict the magnitude of change in quality of life of patients undergoing ambulatory radiation therapy. The pros and cons of the Scored PG-SGA are summarized in Box 6.1 (17,29,30,32–35).

The Scored PG-SGA includes calculations of percent change in body weight and a nutrition-related physical exam, both of which are time-consuming, albeit minimally, for the trained clinician. Therefore, adaptations and abridged versions of the Scored PG-SGA have been appearing in individual institutions to facilitate its use. Validation of any adaptation of the Scored PG-SGA, however, must be completed to create scientific basis for its use.

SYMPTOM AND ACTIVITY SCALES

Symptom and activity scales help health care professionals assess individuals' symptoms and abilities. Symptom and activity scales are important pieces of the nutrition assessment process for evaluating psychosocial, socioeconomic, functional, and behavioral factors related to food access, selection, preparation, physical activity, and understanding of health condition. Examples of scales include Common Toxicity Criteria for Adverse Events, Version 3.0 (CTCAE) (36), Karnofsky Performance Scale (KPS) Index (37), Edmonton Symptom Assessment System (ESAS) (38), Activities of Daily Living (ADL) (39), and PedsQL Measurement Model (40). Registered dietitians (RDs) working in the oncology setting should be familiar with the tools discussed in the following sections.

Common Toxicity Criteria

Created by the National Cancer Institute (NCI) in 1988, Common Toxicity Criteria (CTC) is an outcome measure that compares the acute toxicities of different treatments. The latest version of CTCAE (version 3.0) (36) is a widely used tool that grades adverse events from 1 to 5 (see Chapter 8).

Karnofsky Performance Scale Index

The Karnofsky Performance Scale Index (KPS) (37) classifies individuals according to their functional impairment. Health care professionals can use this scale to compare the efficacy of different therapies and to assess an individual's prognosis. Lower scores (less than 40) are associated with rapid disease progression and poor survival rates (1).

Edmonton Symptom Assessment System

The Edmonton Symptom Assessment System (ESAS) (38) was designed as a quick twice-daily assessment of common symptoms associated with advanced cancer. This validated tool consists of nine visual analog scales for pain, activity, nausea, depression, anxiety, drowsiness, appetite, shortness of breath, and sense of well-being. Patients, independently or with assistance,

Patient ID Information

Scored Patient-Generated Subjective Global Assessment (PG-SGA)

History (Boxes 1-4 are designed to be completed by the patient.)

1. Weight *(See Worksheet 1)*

In summary of my current and recent weight:

I currently weigh about _______ pounds
I am about _________ feet _________ tall

One month ago I weighed about _________ pounds
Six months ago I weighed about _________ pounds

During the past two weeks my weight has:
☐ decreased (1) ☐ not changed (0) ☐ increased (0)

Box 1 ☐

2. Food Intake: As compared to my normal intake, I would rate my food intake during the past month as:

- ☐ unchanged (0)
- ☐ more than usual (0)
- ☐ less than usual (1)

I am now taking:

- ☐ *normal food* but less than normal amount (1)
- ☐ little solid food (2)
- ☐ only liquids (3)
- ☐ only nutritonal supplements (3)
- ☐ very little of anything (4)
- ☐ only tube feedings or only nutrition by vein (0)

Box 2 ☐

3. Symptoms: I have had the following problems that have kept me from eating enough during the past two weeks (check all that apply):

- ☐ no problems eating (0)
- ☐ no appetite, just did not feel like eating (3)
- ☐ nausea (1)
- ☐ vomiting (3)
- ☐ constipation (1)
- ☐ diarrhea (3)
- ☐ mouth sores (2)
- ☐ dry mouth (1)
- ☐ things taste funny or have no taste (1)
- ☐ smells bother me (1)
- ☐ problems swallowing (2)
- ☐ feel full quickly (1)
- ☐ pain; where? (3) _________
- ☐ fatigue (1)
- ☐ other** (1) ____________________

** Examples: depression, money, or dental problems

Box 3 ☐

4. Activities and Function: Over the past month, I would generally rate my activity as:

- ☐ normal with no limitations (0)
- ☐ not my normal self, but able to be up and about with fairly normal activities (1)
- ☐ not feeling up to most things, but in bed or chair less than half the day (2)
- ☐ able to do little activity and spend most of the day in bed or chair (3)
- ☐ pretty much bedridden, rarely out of bed (3)

Box 4 ☐

Additive Score of the Boxes 1-4 ☐ A

The remainder of this form will be completed by your doctor, nurse, dietitian, or therapist. Thank you.

Scored Patient-Generated Subjective Global Assessment (PG-SGA)

Additive Score of the Boxes 1-4 (See Side 1) ☐ A

Worksheet 1 - Scoring Weight (Wt) Loss

To determine score, use 1 month weight data if available. Use 6 month data only if there is no 1 month weight data. Use points below to score weight change and add one extra point if patient has lost weight during the past 2

Wt loss in 1 month	Points	Wt loss in 6 months
10% or greater	4	20% or greater
5-9.9%	3	10 -19.9%
3-4.9%	2	6 - 9.9%
2-2.9%	1	2 - 5.9%
0-1.9%	0	0 - 1.9%

Numerical score from Worksheet 1 ☐

5. Worksheet 2 - Disease and its relation to nutritional requirements

All relevant diagnoses (specify) ____________________

One point each:

☐ Cancer ☐ AIDS ☐ Pulmonary or cardiac cachexia ☐ Presence of decubitus, open wound, or fistula
☐ Presence of trauma ☐ Age greater than 65 years ☐ Chronic renal insufficiency

Numerical score from Worksheet 2 ☐ B

6. Work Sheet 3 - Metabolic Demand

Score for metabolic stress is determined by a number of variables known to increase protein & calorie needs. The score is additive so that a patient who has a fever of > 102 degrees (3 points) and is on 10 mg of prednisone chronically (2 points) would have an additive score for this section of 5 points.

Stress	none (0)	low (1)	moderate (2)	high (3)
Fever	no fever	>99 and <101	≥101 and <102	≥102
Fever duration	no fever	<72 hrs	72 hrs	> 72 hrs
Corticosteroids	no corticosteroids	low dose (<10mg prednisone equivalents/day)	moderate dose (≥10 and <30mg prednisone equivalents/day)	high dose steroid (≥30mg prednisone equivalents/day)

Numerical score from Worksheet 3 ☐ C

7. Worksheet 4 - Physical Exam

Physical exam includes a subjective evaluation of 3 aspects of body composition: fat, muscle, & fluid status. Since this is subjective, each aspect of the exam is rated for degree of deficit. Muscle deficit impacts point score more than fat deficit. Definition of categories: 0 = no deficit, 1+ = mild deficit, 2+ = moderate

Muscle Status:				
temples (temporalis muscle)	0	1+	2+	3+
clavicles (pectoralis & deltoids)	0	1+	2+	3+
shoulders (deltoids)	0	1+	2+	3+
interosseous muscles	0	1+	2+	3+
Scapula (latissimus dorsi, trapezius, deltoids)	0	1+	2+	3+
thigh (quadriceps)	0	1+	2+	3+
calf (gastrocnemius)	0	1+	2+	3+
Global muscle status rating	**0**	**1+**	**2+**	**3+**
Fat Stores:				
orbital fat pads	0	1+	2+	3+
triceps skin fold	0	1+	2+	3+
fat overlying lower ribs	0	1+	2+	3+
Global fat deficit rating	**0**	**1+**	**2+**	**3+**

Fluid Status:				
ankle edema	0	1+	2+	3+
sacral edema	0	1+	2+	3+
ascites	0	1+	2+	3+
Global fluid status rating	**0**	**1+**	**2+**	**3+**

Numerical score from Worksheet 4 ☐ D

Total PG-SGA score ☐

(Total numerical score of A+B+C+D above)

(See triage recommendations below)

Clinician Signature ____________________ RD RN PA MD DO Other ___ Date _______

Nutritional Triage Recommendations: Additive score is used to define specific nutritional interventions including patient & family education, symptom management including pharmacologic intervention, and appropriate nutrient intervention (food, nutritional supplements, enteral, or parenteral triage). First line nutrition intervention includes optimal symptom management.

- **0-1** No intervention required at this time. Re-assessment on routine and regular basis during treatment.
- **2-3** Patient & family education by dietitian, nurse, or other clinician with pharmacologic intervention as indicated by symptom survey (Box 3) and lab values as appropriate.
- **4-8** Requires intervention by dietitian, in conjunction with nurse or physician as indicated by symptoms survey (Box 3).
- **≥9** Indicates a critical need for improved symptom management and/or nutrient intervention options.

Figure 6.1. Scored Patient-Generated Subjective Global Assessment (PG-SGA). Reprinted with permission from Faith Ottery.

Worksheets for PG-SGA Scoring

Boxes 1-4 of the PG-SGA are designed to be completed by the patient. The PG-SGA numerical score is determined using 1) the parenthetical points noted in boxes 1-4 and 2) the worksheets below for items not marked with parenthetical points. Scores for boxes 1 and 3 are additive within each box and scores for boxes 2 and 4 are based on the highest scored item checked off by the patient.

Worksheet 1 - Scoring Weight (Wt) Loss

To determine score, use 1 month weight data if available. Use 6 month data only if there is no 1 month weight data. Use points below to score weight change and add one extra point if patient has lost weight during the past 2 weeks. Enter total point score in Box 1 of the PG-SGA.

Wt loss in 1 month	Points	Wt loss in 6 months
10% or greater	4	20% or greater
5-9.9%	3	10 -19.9%
3-4.9%	2	6 - 9.9%
2-2.9%	1	2 - 5.9%
0-1.9%	0	0 - 1.9%

Score for Worksheet 1 ☐
Record in Box 1

Worksheet 2 - Scoring Criteria for Condition

Score is derived by adding 1 point for each of the conditions listed below that pertain to the patient.

Category	Points
Cancer	1
AIDS	1
Pulmonary or cardiac cachexia	1
Presence of decubitus, open wound, or fistula	1
Presence of trauma	1
Age greater than 65 years	1

Score for Worksheet 2 = ☐
Record in Box B

Worksheet 3 - Scoring Metabolic Stress

Score for metabolic stress is determined by a number of variables known to increase protein & calorie needs. The score is additive so that a patient who has a fever of > 102 degrees (3 points) and is on 10 mg of prednisone chronically (2 points) would have an additive score for this section of 5 points.

Stress	none (0)	low (1)	moderate (2)	high (3)
Fever	no fever	>99 and <101	≥101 and <102	≥102
Fever duration	no fever	<72 hrs	72 hrs	> 72 hrs
Corticosteroids	no corticosteroids	low dose (<10mg prednisone equivalents/day)	moderate dose (≥10 and <30mg prednisone equivalents/day)	high dose steroids (≥30mg prednisone equivalents/day)

Score for Worksheet 3 = ☐
Record in Box C

Worksheet 4 - Physical Examination

Physical exam includes a subjective evaluation of 3 aspects of body composition: fat, muscle, & fluid status. Since this is subjective, each aspect of the exam is rated for degree of deficit. Muscle deficit impacts point score more than fat deficit. Definition of categories: 0 = no deficit, 1+ = mild deficit, 2+ = moderate deficit, 3+ = severe deficit. Rating of deficit in these categories are *not* additive but are used to clinically assess the degree of deficit (or presence of excess fluid).

Fat Stores:				
orbital fat pads	0	1+	2+	3+
triceps skin fold	0	1+	2+	3+
fat overlying lower ribs	0	1+	2+	3+
Global fat deficit rating	**0**	**1+**	**2+**	**3+**
Muscle Status:				
temples (temporalis muscle)	0	1+	2+	3+
clavicles (pectoralis & deltoids)	0	1+	2+	3+
shoulders (deltoids)	0	1+	2+	3+
interosseous muscles	0	1+	2+	3+
scapula (latissimus dorsi, trapezius, deltoids)	0	1+	2+	3+
thigh (quadriceps)	0	1+	2+	3+
calf (gastrocnemius)	0	1+	2+	3+
Global muscle status rating	**0**	**1+**	**2+**	**3+**

Fluid Status:				
ankle edema	0	1+	2+	3+
sacral edema	0	1+	2+	3+
ascites	0	1+	2+	3+
Global fluid status rating	**0**	**1+**	**2+**	**3+**

Point score for the physical exam is determined by the overall subjective rating of total body deficit.

No deficit	score = 0 points
Mild deficit	score = 1 point
Moderate deficit	score = 2 points
Severe deficit	score = 3 points

Score for Worksheet 4 = ☐
Record in Box D

Worksheet 5 - PG-SGA Global Assessment Categories

	Stage A	**Stage B**	**Stage C**
Category	Well-nourished	Moderately malnourished or suspected malnutrition	Severely malnourished
Weight	No wt loss **OR** Recent non-fluid wt gain	~5% wt loss within 1 month (or 10% in 6 months) **OR** No wt stabilization or wt gain (i.e., continued wt loss)	> 5% wt loss in 1 month (or >10% in 6 months) **OR** No wt stabilization or wt gain (i.e., continued wt loss)
Nutrient Intake	No deficit **OR** Significant recent improvement	Definite decrease in intake	Severe deficit in intake
Nutrition Impact Symptoms	None **OR** Significant recent improvement allowing adequate intake	Presence of nutrition impact symptoms (Box 3 of PG-SGA)	Presence of nutrition impact symptoms (Box 3 of PG-SGA)
Functioning	No deficit **OR** Significant recent improvement	Moderate functional deficit **OR** Recent deterioration	Severe functional deficit **OR** recent significant deterioration
Physical Exam	No deficit **OR** Chronic deficit but with recent clinical improvement	Evidence of mild to moderate loss of SQ fat &/or muscle mass &/or muscle tone on palpation	Obvious signs of malnutrition (e.g., severe loss of SQ tissues, possible edema)

Global PG-SGA rating (A, B, or C) = ☐

Figure 6.2. Worksheets for PG-SGA Scoring. Reprinted with permission from Faith Ottery.

rate their symptoms by marking a 100-mm line. The point at which the mark is made can be measured with a ruler and quantified. Although the ESAS is not a nutrition screening tool, it does address symptoms, including a few nutrition impact symptoms, in a very simple and concise manner.

Additional Tools

Additional tools include the Activities of Daily Living (ADL) tool (39) and PedsQL Measurement Model (40). The ADL assesses routine activities (eating, bathing, dressing, toileting, transferring [walking], and continence) that people generally do every day without assistance. An individual's ability to perform ADLs is important for determining what type of long-term care (eg, nursing-home care or home care) and coverage the individual needs (eg, Medicare, Medicaid, or long-term care insurance).

The PedsQL Measurement Model is a modular approach to measuring health-related quality of life (HRQOL) in healthy children and adolescents and in those with acute or chronic health conditions. The PedsQL Measurement Model integrates generic core scales and disease-specific modules into one measurement system.

USING SCREENING AND ASSESSMENT TOOLS

In order to be effective and to not merely add more responsibilities to an already over-burdened nursing staff, screening tools must be easy-to-use and cost-effective, must contain an action plan, and must be validated (41). Triage of subsequent nutrition intervention must also be consistent and cost-effective (42).

Despite the myriad of screening and assessment methods available, there is less-than-optimal implementation of consistent screening, triage, and assessment tools that are evidence based. Champetier and colleagues (43) provide guidelines for "good clinical practice," including three types of nutrition consultation, which are diagnostic, preventive, and therapeutic. They recommend nutrition consultation for persons with cancer, those at risk of malnutrition, those without malnutrition but in need of counseling (ie, for management of treatment-related side effects), and those at risk of developing treatment-related side effects. A further recommendation includes completing a nutrition assessment upon initial contact and providing individualized advice both verbally and in written format. The assessment and intervention should be shared with the multidisciplinary team, as well as with patients and their care givers. Finally, outcomes of nutrition intervention, including weight, nutrition impact symptoms, and individual satisfaction, should be measured and documented, consistent with the Nutrition Care Process (see Chapter 5).

REFERENCES

1. Ottery FD. Supportive nutrition to prevent cachexia and improve quality of life. *Semin Oncol.* 1995;22(2 suppl 3):98–111.
2. Lees J. Incidence of weight loss in head and neck cancer patients on commencing radiotherapy treatment at a regional oncology centre. *Eur J Cancer Care (Engl).* 1999;8:133–136.
3. Ferguson ML, Bauer J, Gallagher B, Capra S, Christie DR, Mason BR. Validation of a malnutrition screening tool for patients receiving radiotherapy. *Australas Radiol.* 1999;43:325–327.
4. Lacey K, Pritchett E. Nutrition care process and model: ADA adopts road map to quality care and outcomes. *J Am Diet Assoc.* 2003;103:1061–1072.
5. Rubin H. Cancer cachexia: its correlations and causes. *Proc Natl Acad Sci USA.* 2003;100:5384–5389.
6. Landt K. Preoperative Nutrition. Available at: http://med2.mercer.edu/ncvd/modules/modules/perioperative_nutrition/section4.htm. Accessed March 31, 2005.
7. McCallum PD, Polisena CG. *Patient-Generated Subjective Global Assessment Training Video.* Chicago, Ill: American Dietetic Association; 2001.
8. Shopbell JM, Hopkins B, Shronts EP. Nutrition screening and assessment. In: Gottschlich MM, Fuhrman MP, Hammond KA, Holcombe BJ, Seidner DL, eds. *The Science and Practice of Nutrition Support: A Case-Based Core Curriculum.* Dubuque, Iowa: Kendall/Hunt; 2001:107–140.
9. Nestlé Nutrition. User's Guide to Completing the Mini Nutritional Assessment MNA(r). Available at: http://www.mna-elderly.com/clinical-practice.htm. Accessed March 31, 2005.
10. Vellas B, Guigoz Y, Baumgartner M, Garry PJ, Lauque S, Albarede JL. Relationships between nutritional markers and the mini-nutritional assessment in 155 older persons. *J Am Geriatr Soc.* 2000;48:1300–1309.
11. Schneider SM, Hebuterne X. Use of nutritional scores to predict clinical outcomes in chronic diseases. *Nutr Rev.* 2000;58(2 Pt 1):31–38.

12. The Medical Algorithms Project. Prognostic Nutrition Index. Available at: http://www.medal.org/ch12.html. Accessed March 14, 2004.
13. Nozoe T, Kimura Y, Ishida M, Saeki H, Korenaga D, Sugimachi K. Correlation of pre-operative nutritional complications in surgical treatment for oesophageal carcinoma. *Eur J Surg Oncol.* 2002;28:396–400.
14. Onodera T, Goseki N, Kosaki G. Prognostic nutritional index in gastrointestinal surgery of malnourished cancer patients. *Nippon Geka Gakkai Zasshi.* 1984;85:1001–1005.
15. Buzby GP, Mullen JL, Matthews DC, Hobbs CL, Rosato EF. Prognostic nutritional index in gastrointestinal surgery. *Am J Surg.* 1980;139:160–167.
16. Viera MJ, Gama-Rodrigues JJ, Habr-Gama A, Faintuch J, Waitzberg DL, Pinnotti HW. Preoperative assessment in cases of adult megacolon suffering from malnutrition. *Nutrition.* 1996;12:491–495.
17. Bonnefoy M, Ayzac L, Ingenbleek Y, Kostka T, Boisson RC, Bienvenu J. Usefulness of the prognostic inflammatory and nutritional index (PINI) in hospitalized elderly patients. *Int J Vitam Nutr Res.* 1998;68:189–195.
18. Mahmoud FA, Rivera NI. The role of C-reactive protein as a prognostic indicator in advanced cancer. *Curr Oncol Rep.* 2002;4:250–255.
19. Martin F, Santolaria F, Batista N, Milena A, Gonzalez-Reimers E, Brito MJ, Oramas J. Cytokine levels (IL-6 and IFN-gamma), acute phase response and nutritional status as prognostic factors in lung cancer. *Cytokine.* 1999;11:80–86.
20. Walsh D, Mahmoud F, Barna B. Assessment of nutritional status and prognosis in advanced cancer: interleukin-6, C-reactive protein, and the prognostic and inflammatory nutritional index. *Support Care Cancer.* 2003;11:60–62.
21. Nelson KA, Walsh D. The cancer anorexia-cachexia syndrome: a survey of the Prognostic Inflammatory and Nutritional Index (PINI) in advanced disease. *J Pain Symptom Manage.* 2002;24:424–428.
22. Detsky AS, McLaughlin JR, Baker JP Johnston N, Whittaker S, Mendelson RA, Jeejeebhoy KN. What is subjective global assessment of nutritional status? *JPEN J Parenter Enteral Nutr.* 1987;11:8–13.
23. Enia G, Sicuso C, Alati G, Zoccali C. Subjective global assessment of nutrition in dialysis patients. *Nephrol Dial Transplant.* 1993;8:1094–1098.
24. Hasse J, Strong S, Gorman MA, Liepa G. Subjective global assessment: alternative nutrition-assessment technique for liver-transplant candidates. *Nutrition.* 1993;9:339–343.
25. McLeod RS, Taylor BR, O'Connor BL, Greenberg GR, Jeejeebhoy KN, Royall D, Langer B. Quality of life, nutritional status, and gastrointestinal profile following Whipple procedure. *Am J Surg.* 1995;169:179–185.
26. Barbos-Silva MC, de Barros AJ. Subjective global assessment: Part 2. Review of its adaptations and utilization in different clinical specialties. *Arq Gastroenterol.* 2002;39:248–252.
27. Ottery FD. Cancer cachexia: prevention, early diagnosis, and management [published correction appears in *Cancer Pract.* 1994;2:263]. *Cancer Pract.* 1994;2:123–131.
28. Ottery FD. Definition of standardized nutritional assessment and interventional pathways in oncology. *Nutrition.* 1996;12(suppl 1):S15-S19.
29. Persson C, Sjoden PO, Glimelius B. The Swedish version of the patient-generated subjective global assessment of nutritional status: gastrointestinal vs urological cancers. *Clin Nutr.* 1999;18:71–77.
30. Bauer J, Capra S, Ferguson M. Use of the scored Patient-Generated Subjective Global Assessment (PG-SGA) as a nutrition assessment tool in subjects with cancer. *Eur J Clin Nutr.* 2002;56:779–785.
31. Isenring E, Bauer J, Capra S. The scored Patient-generated Subjective Global Assessment (PG-SGA) and its association with quality of life in ambulatory patients receiving radiotherapy. *Eur J Clin Nutr.* 2003;57:305–309.
32. Ferguson ML, Bauer J, Gallagher B, Capra S, Christie DR, Mason BR. Validation of a malnutrition screening tool for patients receiving radiotherapy. *Australas Radiol.* 1999;43:325–327.
33. Capra S, Ferguson M, Ried K. Cancer: impact of nutrition intervention outcome-nutrition issues for patients. *Nutrition.* 2001;17:769–772.
34. Sacks GS, Dearman K, Replogle WH, Cora VL, Meeks M, Canada T. Use of subjective global assessment to identify nutrition-associated complications and death in geriatric long-term care facility residents. *J Am Coll Nutr.* 2000;19:570–577.
35. Thoresen L, Fjeldstad I, Krogstad K, Kaasa S, Falkmer UG. Nutritional status of patients with advanced cancer: the value of using the subjective global assessment of nutritional status as a screening tool. *Palliat Med.* 2002;16:33–42.
36. National Cancer Institute. Common Terminology Criteria for Adverse Events (CTCAE) v3.0. Available at: http://www.fda.gov/cder/cancer/toxicityframe.htm. Accessed September 15, 2005.
37. Hospice Patients Alliance. Karnofsky Performance

Scale Index. Available at: http://www.hospicepatients.org/karnofsky.html. Accessed April 25, 2005.

38. Bruera E, Kuehn N, Miller MJ, Selmser P, Macmillan K. The Edmonton Symptoms Assessment System (ESAS): a simple method for the assessment of palliative care patients. *J Palliat Care.* 1991;7:6–9.

39. Centers for Disease Control. National Center for Health Statistics. Instrumental Activities of Daily Living (IADL). Available at: http://www.cdc.gov/nchs/datawh/nchsdefs/iadl. Accessed April 25, 2005.

40. PedsQL Measurement Model. Available at: http://www.pedsql.org/about_pedsql.html. Accessed April 25, 2005.

41. Arrowsmith H. A critical evaluation of the use of nutrition screening tools by nurses. *Br J Nurs.* 1999–2000; 8:1483–1490.

42. Brown JK, Radke KJ. Nutritional assessment, intervention, and evaluation of weight loss in patients with non-small cell lung cancer. *Oncol Nurs Forum.* 1998;25:547–553.

43. Champetier S, Bataillard A, Lallemand Y, Montae C, Bachmann P, Blanc-Vincent MP, Bonneteau C, Claude M, Combret D, Cometto F, Dayot F, Duguet A, Duval N, Finch C, Freby-Lehner A, Garabige V, Massoud C, Meuric J, Poiree B, Puel S, Rossignol G, Roux-Bournay P, Simon M, Tran M. Good clinical practice in the dietetic management of cancer patients. *Bull Cancer.* 2000;87:917–926.

Chapter 7

Energy, Macronutrient, Micronutrient, and Fluid Requirements

JEAN D. HURST, MS, RD, CNSD, AND ANITA L. GALLAGHER, MS, RD, CNSD

INTRODUCTION

The presence of cancer, coupled with administration of antineoplastic therapy, frequently leads to alterations in nutritional status (1). Protein-energy malnutrition is the most common secondary diagnosis in individuals with cancer (2,3). The most effective intervention leading to improved nutritional status is to increase energy and protein intake (4). However, the disease process itself, along with the adverse effects of its treatment modalities (eg, surgery, chemotherapy, or radiation therapy), may make it difficult for individuals to consume adequate macronutrients and micronutrients and to maintain adequate fluid intake (2,5).

This chapter examines the energy, macronutrient (protein, carbohydrate, and fat), micronutrient, and fluid requirements of individuals undergoing cancer treatment. The specific macro- and micronutrient needs of individuals will differ, based on nutritional status at time of diagnosis, site of malignancy, tumor burden, type of tumor, treatment modality (6), and patient age, gender, and physical activity level. Individualization of nutrient recommendations is essential (7). Because macronutrient and micronutrient needs will change over the course of treatment and with progression of disease, regular reassessment of nutritional status, with modifications made to the nutritional care plan, as indicated, is also essential (8).

ENERGY REQUIREMENTS

Energy requirements for individuals undergoing cancer treatment have been the subject of numerous studies. Changes in energy metabolism have been documented in tumor-bearing individuals (9). At one time, it was believed that everyone with cancer was hypermetabolic. However, Knox (10) reported that in 200 hospitalized cancer patients, 33% were hypometabolic, 41% were normometabolic, and 26% were hypermetabolic. The study concluded that energy metabolism varies significantly among cancer patients. Other researchers have also concluded that the site of cancer or tumor type does not predictably increase energy needs or resting energy expenditure (REE) (11–13).

When determining energy requirements, best practice dictates that estimates should be individualized and based on clinical judgment. Other factors should include planned antineoplastic therapy, anticipated side effects, current nutritional status, tumor burden, and body weight and composition changes.

Estimating Energy Requirements

Registered dietitians (RDs) can estimate energy requirements for individuals diagnosed with cancer by using established predictive equations and methods. The best-known equation, the Harris Benedict equa-

Box 7.1
Estimating Energy Needs in Adults

Harris Benedict Equation (14)

Men: REE = 66 + 13.7W + 5H – 6.8A

Women: REE = 655 + 9.6W + 1.7H – 4.7A

Where: REE = resting energy expenditure (kcal/d); W = weight (kg); H = height (cm); A = age (years).

Validation Studies: Original studies conducted on healthy volunteers. Note that for obese individuals (BMI > 29.9), formula may overestimate REE by 5% to 15% if actual weight is used (15–17).

Mifflin-St Jeor (18)

Men: REE = 10W + 6.25H – 5A + 5

Women: REE = 10W + 6.25H – 5A – 161

Where: REE = resting energy expenditure (kcal/d); W = weight (kg); H = height (cm); A = age (years).

Validation Studies: Equation developed from a sample of obese and nonobese healthy individuals. Some research has indicated that this equation may provide a more accurate estimation of REE than the Harris-Benedict formula in both obese and nonobese individuals and, therefore, this equation deserves consideration (17).

Ireton-Jones (for hospitalized patients) (19,20)

Ventilator-dependent patients: EEE = 1784 – 11A + 5W + 244S + 239T + 804B

Spontaneously breathing patients: EEE = 629 – 11A + 25W – 609O

Where: EEE = estimated energy expenditure (kcal/d); A = age (y); W = weight (kg); S = sex (male = 1, female = 2); T = diagnosis of trauma (present = 1, absent = 0); B = diagnosis of burn (present = 1, absent = 0); O = obesity > 30% above ideal body weight from 1959 Metropolitan Life Insurance Tables (present = 1, absent = 0).

Validation Studies: Equation developed from a sample of hospitalized patients including critically ill patients and patients with burns (19). Recent research has reported that this equation underestimates energy requirements (21).

Source: Data are from references 14–21.

tion (14), estimates basal energy requirements (REE) for men and women. However, studies have shown that this equation, when compared with indirect calorimetry, overestimates energy needs in healthy individuals, and that there is wide variation in accuracy for critically ill patients (15,16). Box 7.1 (14–21) presents this formula, along with other standardized equations, including Mifflin-St. Jeor and Ireton-Jones.

Activity and Stress/Injury Factors for Harris Benedict and Mifflin-St. Jeor Equations

To calculate an individual's total energy expenditure, the REE value obtained from the Harris Benedict or Mifflin St. Jeor formula is multiplied by stress and activity factors (Table 7.1) (9,22–25). These factors are estimations and can vary based on the individual's current health, body weight, planned therapy, respiratory

Table 7.1 Activity and Stress/Injury Factors*

Activity Factors	
Patient Type	*Factor*
Patients on ventilator support	1–1.1
Bedridden patients	1.2
Ambulatory patients	1.3
Injury Factors	
Condition Present	*Factor*
Mild starvation	0.85–1.0
Cancer, based on severity of illness	1.1–1.45
Cancer, weight maintenance	1.15–1.3
Cancer, nutritional repletion, weight gain	1.5
Ventilator support, catabolic	1.5
Sepsis	1.5

*For use with the Harris Benedict or Mifflin-St. Jeor formula. Multiply the resting energy expenditure calculated with either formula by the activity factor and, if appropriate, the injury factor.

Source: Data are from references 9 and 22–25.

status, and physical activity. Clinical judgment should be used.

Energy Estimates Based on Body Weight

RDs in clinical practice may quickly estimate energy requirements from formulas that suggest that a certain number of kilocalories are required per kilogram of body weight (8,23,26,27). These methods are useful as initial estimates of energy requirements and should be adjusted as individuals' nutritional status and activity levels change. Although these methods are commonly used, they lack evidence-based validation. See Table 7.2 (8,23,27). Actual (current) body weight is used for nonobese patients. For obese individuals (BMI > 29.9), ideal body weight (IBW) should be used because adjusted weight for obesity has not been validated (28).

Indirect Calorimetry

In the hospital setting, indirect calorimetry is used to measure REE in critically ill patients. This energy assessment method may be useful for the following hospitalized patient populations (29–31):

- Severely malnourished individuals
- Morbidly obese individuals
- Critically ill patients with complex medical problems
- Mechanically ventilated patients experiencing difficulties with weaning

A number of devices are available to perform these measurements. Recently, a handheld device and analyzer software were approved by the US Food and Drug Administration for use by health professionals to measure the resting metabolic rate (32). However, at this time in the clinical setting, a portable metabolic cart is the most widely used. Testing is conducted by a trained respiratory therapist.

Measurements can be performed on both ventilator-supported and spontaneously breathing patients. By measuring volume of oxygen consumed (VO_2) and volume of carbon dioxide produced (VCO_2), the respiratory quotient (RQ) can be calculated. Interpretation of RQ values can then be reviewed to determine substrate utilization (15,29). The REE can be derived by inserting the measured values for VO_2 and VCO_2 into the modified Weir formula (Box 7.2) (29,31). The complete Weir formula can be used when the patient's urine from a 24-hour urinary urea nitrogen collection is available during the testing period. This Weir formula helps to correct the REE for the incomplete oxidation of protein. There is less than a 2% difference in the value of the REE obtained when this adjustment for protein oxidation is not made (29).

Table 7.2 Estimated Energy Needs Based on Body Weight*

Condition Present	*Energy Needs, kcal/kg*
Cancer, nutritional repletion, weight gain	30–35
Cancer, nonambulatory, inactive	25–30
Cancer, hypermetabolic, stressed	35
Sepsis	25–30
Stem cell transplant	30–35

*These formulas lack evidence-based validation.

Source: Data are from references 8, 23, and 27.

Box 7.2

Indirect Calorimetry: Guidelines for Interpretation

Weir Formula

(This formula is used if 24-hour nitrogen is collected on the same day as the test.)

$$REE = [(3.9VO_2 + 1.1VCO_2) \times 1.44] - 2.17UN$$

Modified Weir Formula

$$REE = (3.9VO_2 + 1.1VCO_2) \times 1.44$$

Where: REE = resting energy expenditure (kcal/d); VO_2 = oxygen consumption (mL/min); VCO_2 = carbon dioxide production (mL/min); UN = urinary nitrogen (g/d).

Respiratory Quotient (RQ)

$$RQ = VCO_2/VO_2$$

Physiological range of RQ: 0.67–1.3

RQ	*Interpretation*
0.7	Fat oxidation
0.8	Protein oxidation
0.83	Starvation
0.85	Mixed substrate oxidation
1.0	Glucose oxidation
> 1.0	Lipogenesis, overfeeding

REE values should be multiplied by the following stress factors:

- Nonstressed patient requiring maintenance, minimal stress, not malnourished: 1.0
- Stressed patient requiring maintenance, not malnourished: 1.2
- Stressed patient, catabolic, malnourished: 1.3

Source: Data are from references 29 and 31

The REE value is then adjusted for activity as indicated in Box 7.2 (29,31).Changes in nutrition support can then be made based on the results of the values obtained.

Energy Needs and Obesity

Because it is important to avoid overfeeding obese patients, many studies have compared values obtained from indirect calorimetry with those estimated by predictive equations and kcal/kg methods. Box 7.3 (17,18,33–35) reviews some proposed methods for predicting energy requirements for obese patients.

MACRONUTRIENT REQUIREMENTS

Protein

The presence of cancer in the host induces alterations in protein and amino acid metabolism (2). Most

Box 7.3

Estimating Daily Energy Needs for Obese Patients

Option 1: For acutely ill obese patients (BMI: 30–50)
Use the Harris-Benedict formula using average weight (kg) multiplied by an injury factor of 1.3 (no activity factor is used). (Average body weight equals the sum of desired body weight and 50% of excess body weight.)

Validation study: The formula more closely predicted measured energy needs by indirect calorimetry than did the Ireton-Jones formula for obese and hospitalized patients (33).

Option 2: For acutely ill obese patients (BMI: 30–50)
Using actual body weight, estimate 21 kcal per kg body weight.

Validation study: This estimate may be helpful to evaluate the values obtained from other predictive formulas (33).

Option 3: For obese patients (BMI: 30–73)
Use the Ireton-Jones equation for obesity. Results are comparable to measured energy expenditure (MEE) derived from indirect calorimetry (35).

Hospitalized patients: MEE = 606S + 9ABW – 12A + 400V + 1444

Nonhospitalized patients: MEE = 294S + 11ABW + 791

Where: S = sex (male = 1, female = 0); V = ventilator (ventilator support = 1, spontaneous breathing = 0); ABW = actual body weight (kg); A = age (years).

Validation study: These formulas were derived using a regression analysis correlating the measured variables in each equation. Use of actual body weight (instead of ideal body weight) is recommended (32).

Option 4:
Use the Mifflin-St Jeor formula.

Males: REE = 10W + 6.25H – 5A + 5

Females: REE = 10W + 6.25H – 5A – 161

Where: W = weight (kg); H = height (cm); A = age (years).

Validation Studies: The equation was developed from a sample of obese and nonobese healthy individuals. Some research has indicated that this equation may provide a more accurate estimation of REE than the Harris Benedict formula in both obese and nonobese individuals, and, therefore, this equation deserves consideration (17).

Source: Data are from references 17, 18, and 33–35.

patients have been found to be in negative nitrogen balance, a condition that worsens as the malignancy progresses (8). In cancer cachexia, muscle mass is decreased, and there is an increase in muscle proteolysis and an increase in muscle amino acid release (36). Hepatic protein synthesis and amino acid transport are also increased, resulting in a state of negative nitrogen balance (2). In malnourished patients, protein metabolism is thought to be similar to that found in the presence of trauma or infection (1,24). The alterations in host protein metabolism can be summarized as follows (8):

- Increased whole-body protein turnover
- Increased muscle wasting
- Decreased serum protein levels
- Increased liver protein synthesis
- Decreased muscle protein synthesis
- Negative nitrogen balance

Protein requirements are difficult to determine (7,9). Nitrogen balance is affected by many variables, including the stress of treatment modalities such as chemotherapy and radiation (7). Chemotherapy patients with advanced cancer have been shown to exhibit an increase in protein catabolism with resulting negative nitrogen balance (5). Protein should be supplied in amounts sufficient to provide for adequate synthesis while reducing degradation. Adequate nonprotein calories need to be provided to spare protein. If energy intake is inadequate, depletion of the body will occur as the tumor preferentially metabolizes available protein (37). Withholding protein in an attempt to slow tumor growth may only result in decline of individuals' nutritional status and further compromise immune function (7,9).

Measuring Body Composition

The alterations that occur in protein metabolism frequently cause loss of lean muscle tissue (8). Several indirect methods are available to estimate body composition. Anthropometric measurements to evaluate skeletal mass can be done using skin calipers to measure mid-arm circumference (MAC) and mid-arm muscle circumference (MAMC). Skinfold and circumference measurements are used to assess an individual's protein energy status by "pinching" subcutaneous fat at specified body sites with special calipers and measuring specific body locations (38). Errors in practitioner measurement technique, changes in patient's hydration status, and the failure of these measurements to identify small changes in body composition limit the usefulness of this technique in the clinical setting (3,39).

A noninvasive and inexpensive technique for measurement of body fat and fat-free mass is bioelectrical impedance (BIA). This method involves passing a low-voltage electrical current through the body. Body resistance to the current is measured, and fat-free mass is estimated using regression equations. Accuracy of the method can be affected by the patient's hydration status and presence of fever, obesity, and/or electrolyte imbalances. Another problem with accuracy of this method is the lack of good reference standards for interpretation of results of measurements (39).

Data obtained from MAC, MAMC, and BIA represent only estimates of body composition. Muscle atrophy may occur due to prolonged inactivity, not just as a result of malnutrition. Edema may also influence measurements (40). Therefore, use of anthropometry to determine muscle mass with cancer patients is not generally thought to be worthwhile, unless they are being followed long-term or are participating in a research protocol (8,40).

Nitrogen Balance

Protein status can be evaluated in the hospitalized or ambulatory setting using nitrogen balance studies. One method involves measurement of urinary urea nitrogen (UUN). As protein is catabolized, urea is formed in the liver. The urea is subsequently excreted by the kidney. A 24-hour urine collection can be done and evaluated for UUN (in grams). For the same 24-hour period, total protein intake (grams) must be accurately calculated (41). The following formula may then be used to calculate nitrogen balance (6):

Nitrogen Balance = (Protein Intake/6.25) – (UUN + 4)

An accurate calculation of protein intake and a complete urine collection are required for reliable test results. The individual should also be in a steady state and have normal renal function. A factor of "4" is added to the UUN (as above) to account for nonurea nitrogen losses, such as those in the stool and skin. Results will be less reliable when liver disease is present and urea synthesis is affected (41). A positive nitrogen balance of 4 to 6 g/day is desirable. When nitrogen balance is positive, this suggests sufficient protein is being provided (41). If the urinary nitrogen balance is negative, consideration should be given to increasing protein intake. Weekly nitrogen balance studies may help to identify trends in protein status and allows for timely recommendations for changes in the nutrition care plan (6).

When collected urine is not available, protein needs can be quickly estimated, although less

Table 7.3 Estimating Daily Protein Needs in Adult Cancer Patients

Medical Condition	*Estimated Protein Needs, g/kg*
Normal maintenance	0.8–1.0
Nonstressed cancer patient	1.0–1.2
Hypercatabolism	1.2–1.6
Severe stress	1.5–2.5
Requiring nutrition support	1.6–2.0
Stem cell transplant	1.5–2.0
Renal disease	
Acute renal failure	0.5–0.6 (unstressed patient) 1.0 (with stress and hemodialysis)
Predialysis	0.6–0.8
Hemodialysis	1.2–1.5
Peritoneal dialysis	1.2–1.5
Nephrotic syndrome	0.8–1.0
Hepatic disease	
Hepatic failure	1.0–1.5
Hepatitis	0.8–1.0*
End-stage liver disease with encephalopathy	0.6–0.8*
Cirrhosis without encephalopathy	1.0–1.2*

*Dry weight.

Source: Data are from references 3, 6, 8, 9, 27, 37, and 42–46.

accurately, by using the grams of protein per kilogram of body weight formulas outlined in Table 7.3 (3,6,8,9,27,37,42–46). When calculating protein needs for nutrition support, a kilocalorie-to-nitrogen ratio of 125:1 is recommended (9). If renal and/or hepatic dysfunction is present, appropriate adjustments to estimated protein needs will be necessary.

Carbohydrate and Fat

To conserve lean muscle tissue, adequate nonprotein calories (carbohydrate and fat) need to be provided along with the estimated protein-containing calories. Carbohydrates provide important sources of energy and dietary fiber; they are necessary for vitamin and mineral absorption; and through their pre- and probiotic activity, they play a critical role in the function of the gut (47). Consumption of dietary fat is necessary for the digestion, absorption, and transport of fat-soluble vitamins; it provides essential fatty acids not synthesized by the body; and it contributes to the palatability and to the sensation of satiety from foods eaten (47).

The Recommended Dietary Allowance (RDA) for carbohydrate is 130 g/day for adults between the ages of 19 and 70 years (48). There is no adult RDA for fat. The 2005 Dietary Guidelines (49) recommend that 20% to 35% of daily energy intake come from fat, with the emphasis on dietary fat sources from polyunsaturated and monounsaturated fats (eg, fish, nuts, and vegetable oils), and that 45% to 65% of daily energy come from dietary carbohydrate sources that are rich in fiber, such as fruits, vegetables, and whole grains.

MICRONUTRIENT REQUIREMENTS

Recommended intakes of micronutrients (eg, vitamins and minerals) for healthy individuals have been published by the Institute of Medicine. These Dietary Reference Intakes (DRIs) include RDAs), Adequate Intakes (AIs), Estimated Average Requirements (EARs) for groups, and Tolerable Upper Intake Levels (ULs). DRIs can be accessed by visiting the Institute of Medicine's Food and Nutrition Web site (50–55).

Micronutrients are generally needed in relatively small amounts to support normal metabolic processes (56). Twelve vitamins and seven trace elements are known to be essential. See the DRIs (51–54) for recommended oral intake levels of these essential nutrients in healthy individuals.

Determining trace element status is difficult. When cancer is present, there is a potential for micronutrient deficiencies if oral intake is poor, in the presence of maldigestion and malabsorption, with increased excretion or losses, or when requirements are increased (57). Loss of electrolytes may occur with nausea, vomiting, and/or diarrhea related to administration of chemotherapy and/or radiation therapies (4,57).

The presence of cancer can alter the metabolism of some micronutrients, such as iron, vitamin C, vitamin E, selenium, zinc, and copper (56), by the physiological stress that occurs when tumor growth is rapid and uncontrolled (9).

Table 7.4 Adult Parenteral Multivitamin Guidelines

Vitamin	*FDA Requirement per Unit Dose*
Fat-soluble	
Vitamin A (retinol)	3300 IU (1 mg)
Vitamin D (ergocalciferol or cholecalciferol)	200 IU (5 µg)
Vitamin E (alpha-tocopherol)	10 IU (10 mg)
Vitamin K (phylloquinone)	150 µg
Water-soluble	
Vitamin C (ascorbic acid)	200 mg
Folic acid	600 µg
Vitamin B-1 (thiamin)	6.0 mg
Vitamin B-2 (riboflavin)	3.6 mg
Vitamin B-3 (niacinamide)	40 mg
Vitamin B-6 (pyridoxine)	6.0 mg
Vitamin B-12 (cyanocobalamin)	5.0 µg
Pantothenic acid	15.0 mg
Biotin	60 µg

Source: Data are from references 59 and 60.

Table 7.5 Suggested Daily Parenteral Intake of Essential Trace Elements by Adults

	Dosage	
Element	*Stable Patient*	*Patient With Increased Gastrointestinal Losses**
Zinc	2500–4000 µg	Add 12 mg/L of small bowel losses. Add 17 mg/kg of stool or ileostomy losses
Copper	300–500 µg	500 µg
Chromium	10–15 µg	20 µg
Manganese	60–100 µg	60–100 µg

*Serum levels of these elements should be frequently monitored. Adjust dosage as indicated.

Source: Data are from references 57, 61, and 81.

Vitamin and Mineral Supplementation

When oral intake appears to be adequate and nutritional status is not depleted, vitamin and mineral supplementation may not be indicated. However, when inadequate intake and/or increased losses of micronutrients are suspected, a multivitamin and mineral supplement may be appropriate for individuals diagnosed with cancer (4,8,58). See Table 7.4 (59,60) for adult parenteral multivitamin supplementation guidelines. See Table 7.5 (57,61) for recommended adult parenteral dosages of essential trace elements.

Drug-Nutrient Interactions

When examining a patient's nutritional status, RDs should consider the potential for therapeutic drug and nutrient interactions that could induce vitamin and mineral deficiencies. See Table 7.6 (62–64) for some possible nutrient interactions with antibiotics, gastrointestinal (GI) drugs, and diuretics.

Patients receiving chemotherapy may also be at risk for interactions between nutrients and chemotherapeutic agents. The degree to which micronutrient status may be affected by these potential interactions is not precisely known. Clinicians therefore need to review product literature and be aware of the potential for deficiencies associated with drug usage. Chemotherapeutic agents are discussed in Chapter 8.

Vitamin/Mineral Deficiencies

Clinicians need to be aware of the physical signs and symptoms of vitamin and mineral deficiencies (see Table 7.7) (65–68). In the chemotherapy patient, specific nutrient deficiency is almost always identified based on clinical signs and symptoms and the patient's response to therapy. Serum levels of vitamins may not be reliable in identifying deficiencies (5).

Because assessment of trace element status can be difficult, the patient should be carefully observed for signs and symptoms of deficiencies. See Table 7.8 (66,69,70) for some signs of trace element deficiency symptoms and suggested treatments. Deficiencies in trace elements are more frequently reported than toxicities (57). See the DRIs (51,52) for ULs for elements.

Serum levels of trace elements may increase with renal dysfunction (37). Correction of micronutrient deficiencies through appropriate supplementation is thought to be possible (5).

Table 7.6 Drug-Micronutrient Interactions

Drug	*Possible Micronutrient Interaction(s)*	*Notes*
Antibiotics		
Cefalosporin	• Hypokalemia • Vitamin K deficiency	
Gentamicin	• Magnesium and potassium depletion because of increased excretion	
Pentamidine isoethionate	• Folate deficiency, especially with malabsorption or decreased intake • Hypocalcemia • Hyperkalemia	Used in treatment of pneumocystis carinii pneumonia
Tetracycline	• Decreased Vitamin K synthesis • Increased urinary riboflavin and folate loss with potential for deficiency in long-term use • Forms insoluble complexes with calcium, magnesium, iron, and zinc	Used with infections and bronchitis
Trimethoprim with sulfamethoxazole	• Folate depletion • Folate antagonists (methotrexate, phenobarbital, phenytoin sulfasalazine) enhance possibility of deficiency	Used in treatment of pneumocystis carinii pneumonia
Zidovudine	• Megaloblastic anemia • Folate depletion	Used in treatment of HIV and AIDS infections
Ketoconazole	• Calcium and magnesium supplements and antacids should not be taken within 2 hours because these supplements decrease ketoconazole's absorption if taken together	Used for treatment of fungal infections
Gastrointestinal agents		
Bisacodyl	• Malabsorption of vitamins D and K, calcium, and potassium	Laxative
Bismuth subsalicylate	• With chronic use, folate, iron, and vitamin C supplements may be indicated	Antidiarrheal
Calcium carbonate	• Can inactivate thiamin • Hypercalcemia may occur with chronic, high intake; with vitamin D supplementation; or with renal insufficiency	Used as an antacid and for treatment of hypocalcemia and osteoporosis
Ranitidine	• Reduced vitamin B-12 • Iron deficiency	Used for treatment of ulcers and in management of gastroesophageal reflux disease
Senna	• Excessive use associated with hypokalemia, malabsorption, electrolyte imbalance	Used to treat constipation
Phenolphthalein	• Malabsorption of fat-soluble vitamins D and K, calcium, and potassium possible	Used to treat constipation

(continued)

Table 7.6 Drug-Micronutrient Interactions (*continued*)

Drug	*Possible Micronutrient Interaction(s)*	*Notes*
Gastrointestinal agents		
Magnesium hydroxide with aluminum hydroxide	• Vitamin A, folate, riboflavin, iron, phosphorus, copper absorption may be reduced • May inactivate thiamin • May increase magnesium absorption; monitor phosphorus	Used in treatment of ulcers
Famotidine	• Vitamin B-12 depletion	Used in treatment of ulcers and gastroesophageal reflux disease
Diuretics		
Furosemide, thiazides	• Hypomagnesemia • Hypokalemia • Hyponatremia • Hypercalcemia	
Spironolactone	• Hyperkalemia • Hyponatremia • Decreased serum folate	

Source: Data are from references 62–64.

FLUID REQUIREMENTS

Water is an essential nutrient in humans and accounts for 50% to 80% of body weight, depending on the percent of lean body mass (71). The most current DRI report for fluids indicates that the AI for total water intake for men and women 19 to 70 years is 3.7 and 2.7 liters, respectively (72).

The main determinant of adequate hydration in humans is thirst (71). Underhydration can be a problem in patients with a decreased oral intake or inadequate fluid intake from enteral nutrition (8). Volume depletion can occur with vomiting or diarrhea (73). In contrast, overhydration can occur in patients receiving intravenous (IV) fluids or supplemental oral fluid (37). Medical conditions, such as congestive heart failure, pulmonary disease, renal disease, and endocrine abnormalities, may result in fluid overload (8,37).

Estimating Fluid Needs

The 2004 DRI report (72) does not specify exact fluid requirements. Therefore, clinicians may use the following estimates from the American Dietetic Association's *Manual of Clinical Dietetics* as general guidelines for estimating age-specific fluid requirements (74):

- 16–30 years, active: 40 mL/kg
- 31–55 years: 35 mL/kg
- 56–75 years: 30 mL/kg
- 76 years or older: 25 mL/kg

These recommendations are for maintenance needs and should be adjusted for iatrogenic or disease-related fluid overload or dehydration. Table 7.9 (74) reviews the symptoms and alterations in biochemical values associated with dehydration and overhydration.

For determining fluid needs in adults with normal renal and hepatic function, the RDA method is commonly used by clinicians (75):

Fluid Needs = 1 mL fluid per 1 kcal of estimated energy needs

The Body Surface Area (BSA) method is also used in clinical settings (75):

$$\text{Fluid Needs} = 1500\ \text{mL/m}^2\ \textit{or}\ \text{BSA} \times 1500\ \text{mL}$$

Table 7.7 Physical Signs and Symptoms of Vitamin and Mineral Deficiencies

Micronutrient	*Deficiency Signs and Symptoms*
Vitamins	
Vitamin A	• Night blindness • Bitot's spots • Conjunctival xerosis • Follicular hyperkeratosis • Dry mucus membrane • Dry, scaly skin
Vitamin D	• Rickets (children) • Osteomalacia
Vitamin E	• Muscle weakness • Edema • Irritability
Vitamin K	• Abnormal bleeding
Vitamin C	• Impaired wound healing • Scurvy (bruising, hemorrhage, bleeding gums, loose teeth) • Ecchymoses • Petechiae
Vitamin B-1 (thiamin)	• Beriberi (fatigue, loss of appetite, constipation, depression, neuropathy, angular stomatitis, polyneuritis, edema, cardiac failure) • Impaired memory and cognitive function • Ataxia
Vitamin B-2 (riboflavin)	• Cheilosis • Angular stomatitis • Glossitis • Nasolabial seborrheic dermatitis • Scrotal and vulval dermatitis • Peripheral neuropathy
Vitamin B-3 (niacin)	• Pellagra (dermatitis, diarrhea, dementia) • Angular stomatitis • Glossitis • Cheilosis
Vitamin B-6 (pyridoxine)	• Cheilosis • Angular stomatitis • Glossitis • Irritability • Peripheral neuropathy • Convulsions
Vitamin B-12 (cyanocobalamin)	• Glossitis • Peripheral neuropathy • Dementia

(continued)

Table 7.7 Physical Signs and Symptoms of Vitamin and Mineral Deficiencies (*continued*)

Micronutrient	*Deficiency Signs and Symptoms*
Vitamins	
Folic acid	• Pallor • Glossitis • Diarrhea • Macrocytic anemia
Biotin	• Dermatitis • Glossitis
Pantothenic acid*	• Neuritis of arms, legs • Burning sensation of feet
Minerals	
Calcium	• Osteomalacia • Tetany
Phosphorus	• Weakness • Confusion • Seizures • Rickets • Osteomalacia
Potassium	• Weakness • Paralysis
Sodium	• Weakness • Confusion • Seizures • Diarrhea • Oliguria
Chloride	• Tetany • Hypotension • Hyperexcitability of nerves and muscles • Shallow breathing
Magnesium	• Nausea • Vomiting • Weakness • Lethargy • Muscle tremors • Tetany

*Deficiency is rare.

Source: Data are from references 65–68.

Table 7.8 Trace Element Deficiency Symptoms and Treatment

Element	*Causes of Deficiency*	*Deficiency Symptoms*	Treatment *Oral*	 *Parenteral*
Iron	• Low intake • Decreased absorption (postgastrectomy) • Excessive losses (GI bleed)	• Anemia (microcytic, hypochromic) • Fatigue • Tachycardia • Pallor • Cold intolerance • Immunocompetence • Kolloncychia	Ferrous sulfate, 320 mg twice/day for 6–12 mo	Calculate deficit. May give up to 100 mg iron dextran/day in TPN.
Zinc	• Poor intake • Increased losses (diarrhea) • Decreased absorption (small bowel disease)	• Skin lesions • Diarrhea • Decreased taste, smell acuity • Poor wound healing • Alopecia • Growth retardation • Delayed sexual development • Immunocompetence	20–40 mg/day	2500–4000 µg/day in stable patients. Add an additional 2000 µg/day in hypermetabolic patients.
Copper	• Decreased intake • Decreased absorption • Increased losses (stress, burns, GI suction, biliary fistula)	• Neutropenia • Microcytic, hypochromic anemia • Low serum copper and ceruloplasmin levels • Osteoporosis • Hair and skin depigmentation	2 mg/day (cupric sulfate)	300–500 µg/day. Add an additional 500 µg with gastrointestinal losses.
Chromium		• Glucose intolerance • Fasting hyperglycemia • Peripheral neuropathy • Glucosuria • Hyperlipidemia • Metabolic encephalopathy • Insulin resistance	20–35 µg/day	10–15µg/day. Add an additional 20 µg with gastrointestinal losses.
Manganese		• (Not conclusive) • Dermatitis • Hypocholesterolemia	2.0–5.0 mg/day	0.6–1.0 mg/day
Selenium	• Inadequate intake	• Muscle weakness and pain • Myalgia • Cardiomyopathy	50–200 µg/day (selenium sulfate)	≤ 125 µg/day
Molybdenum	• Excess losses with active Crohn's disease	• Headache • Night blindness • Lethargy • Irritability • Nausea	RDA: 45 µg/day	Not widely added to TPN

Abbreviations: RDA, Recommended Dietary Allowance; TPN, total parenteral nutrition.

Source: Data are from references 66, 69, 70, and 81.

Table 7.9 Symptoms and Changes in Biochemical Values Associated With Dehydration and Overhydration

Condition	*Symptoms*	*Biochemical Changes*
Dehydration	• Thirst • Weight loss • Oliguria • Loss of skin turgor • Dry mouth and lips • Coated wrinkled tongue • Dry or sunken eyes • Lowered body temperature • Tachycardia • Restlessness • Delirium	• Increased serum sodium, albumin, BUN, creatinine
Overhydration	• Increased blood pressure • Decreased pulse rate • Edema	• Decreased serum sodium, potassium, BUN, creatinine

Source: Adapted with permission from American Dietetic Association. Nutrition assessment of adults. In: *Manual of Clinical Dietetics.* 6th ed. Chicago, Ill: American Dietetic Association; 2000:14.

Intravenous Hydration

In individuals undergoing cancer treatment, administration of IV fluid may lead to edema and/or respiratory failure. For those who are unable to maintain adequate oral intake, the need for IV hydration should be determined based on input and output records. Generally, the minimum oral fluid need can be assessed based on the 24-hour urine output, with an additional 500 mL for insensible losses. On the average, 1,000 mL of fluid per day provides for adequate urine output and hydration. For individuals receiving palliative treatment, provision of IV hydration should be based on their wishes, taking into account the potential risks and benefits involved (76). For more information on palliative care, see Chapter 17.

REFEEDING SYNDROME

When individuals with head and neck or gastrointestinal cancer (eg, esophageal or gastric tumors) undergo surgery, radiation therapy, or chemotherapy, they may have malnutrition because of insufficient oral intake. Nutrition support, either enteral or parenteral, may be required. Refeeding syndrome is a potential complication that can occur in these individuals. Rapid administration of calorically dense enteral or parenteral formulas may cause hyperglycemia, which in turn can lead to large shifts in phosphorus, magnesium, and potassium from the extracellular to the intracellular spaces (77,78).

The main systems affected by this syndrome are the gastrointestinal and the cardiopulmonary. A decrease in gastric motility during refeeding may lead to nausea and vomiting. Diarrhea may also occur as a result of decreased absorptive surface area and enzyme production. The cardiopulmonary system can also be affected, because of decreased organ mass as a result of the malnourished state. Further complicating this problem is rapid volume expansion, which places increased demands on the cardiac system. As a result, congestive heart failure, respiratory distress, hypercapnia, azotemia, and pericardial effusion may occur. Overfeeding of calories increases oxygen consumption and can result in respiratory and cardiac failure in the already compromised individual (79).

To prevent refeeding syndrome, serum electrolytes and minerals (eg, sodium, potassium, phosphorus, and magnesium) should be assessed and repleted before nutrition support is started. Fluid volume should be corrected slowly, and individuals should be strictly observed for signs of heart failure. Generally, it is recommended that enteral or parenteral feedings be started at 50% of the patient's energy needs, based on current weight, and gradually increased to the goal rate over 3 days (77,78).

Once nutrition support is initiated, it is judicious to monitor for signs of refeeding syndrome, especially during the first 7 days of feeding. This includes checking serum levels of potassium, phosphorus, and magnesium. Repeated correction of these values may be required at this time. Fluid intake and output should be assessed daily along with weight. Excess fluid retention is indicated by a weight increase of greater than 1 kg in 7 days. Also, any intolerance to enteral feedings should be observed, and changes in rate or product formulation should be made as indicated (78–81).

REFERENCES

1. Shils ME. Nutrition and diet in cancer management. In: Shils MD, Olson JA, Shike M, eds. *Modern Nutrition in Health and Disease.* 9th ed. Philadelphia, Pa: Lippincott Williams and Wilkins; 1994:1317–1347.
2. Smith SJ, Souba WW. Nutrition support. In: DeVita VT, Helman S, Rosenberg SA, eds. *Cancer Principles and Practice of Oncology.* Philadelphia, Pa. Lippincott Williams and Wilkins; 2001:3012–3032.
3. Buzby KM. Overview: screening, assessing and monitoring. In: Bloch AS, ed. *Nutrition Management of the Cancer Patient.* Rockville, Md: Aspen Publishers; 1990:3–23.
4. American Dietetic Association, Dietitians of Canada. Cancer. In: *Manual of Clinical Dietetics.* 6th ed. Chicago, Ill: American Dietetic Association; 2000: 235–252.
5. Dreizen S, McCredie KB, Keating MJ, Andersson BS. Nutritional deficiencies in patients receiving cancer chemotherapy. *Postgrad Med.* 1990;87:163–170.
6. Lopez MJ, Tehrani HY. Nutrition and the cancer patient. In: Lenhard RD, Osteen RT, Gansler T, eds. *Clinical Oncology.* Maiden, Mass: American Cancer Society; 2001:811–822.
7. Burgess J. Cancer therapy. In: Skipper A, ed. *Dietitian's Handbook of Enteral and Parenteral Nutrition.* Rockville, Md: Aspen Publishers;1989:119–135.
8. Bloch AS. Cancer. In: Matarese LE, Gottschlich MM, eds. *Contemporary Nutrition Support Practice: A Clinical Guide.* Philadelphia, Pa: WB Saunders; 1998: 475–495.
9. Dempsey DT, Mullen JL. Macronutrient requirements in the malnourished cancer patient. How much of what and why. *Cancer.* 1985;55(suppl):290–294.
10. Knox LS, Crosby LO, Feurer ID, Buzby GP, Miller CL, Mullen JL. Energy expenditure in malnourished cancer patients. *Ann Surg.*1983;197:152–162.
11. Merrick HW, Long CL, Grecos GP, Dennis RS, Bakemore WS. Energy requirements for cancer patients and the effect of total parenteral nutrition. *JPEN J Parenter Enteral Nutr.*1988;12:8–14.
12. Hansell DT, Davies JW, Burns HJ. The relationship between resting energy expenditure and weight loss in benign and malignant disease. *Ann Surg.* 1986;203: 240–245.
13. Hansell DT, Davies JW, Shenkin A, Burns HJ. The oxidation of body fuel stores. *Ann Surg.* 1986;204: 637–642.
14. Harris JA, Benedict FG. *Biometric Studies of Basal Metabolism in Man.* Washington, DC: Carnegie Institution of Washington; 1919. Publication 270.
15. McClave S, Snider HL. Use of indirect calorimetry in clinical nutrition. *Nutr Clin Pract.* 1992;7:207–221.
16. Frankenfield D. Energy and macrosubstrate requirements. In: Gottschlich MM, Fuhrman MP, Hammond KA, Holcombe BJ, Seidner DL, eds. *The Science and Practice of Nutrition Support: A Case-Based Core Curriculum.* Dubuque, Iowa: Kent/Hunt Publishing; 2001:31–52.
17. Frankenfield DC, Rowe WA, Smith JS, Cooney RN. Validation of several established equations for resting metabolic rate in obese and nonobese people. *J Am Diet Assoc.* 2003;103:1152–1159.
18. Mifflin MD, St Jeor ST, Hill LA, Scott BJ, Daugherty SA, Koh YO. A new predictive equation for resting energy expenditure in healthy individuals. *Am J Clin Nutr.* 1990;51:241–247.
19. Ireton-Jones CS, Turner WW, Liepa GU, Baxter CR. Equations for estimation of energy expenditures in patients with burns with special reference to ventilatory status. *J Burns Care Rehabil.* 1992;13: 330–333.
20. Ireton-Jones CS, Jones JD. Why use predictive equations for energy expenditures of hospitalized patients? *J Am Diet Assoc.* 1997;97(suppl):A-44.
21. Frankenfeld D, Smith S, Cooney RN. Validation of 2 approaches to predicting resting metabolic rate in critically ill patients. *JPEN J Parenter Enteral Nutr.* 2004;28:259–264.
22. Souba WW, Wilmore DW. Diet and nutrition in the care of the patient with surgery, trauma, and sepsis. In: Shils MD, Young VR, eds. *Modern Nutrition in Health and Disease.* 7th ed. Philadelphia, Pa: Lea and Febiger; 1988:1207–1240.

23. Trujillo EB, Robinson MK, Jacobs DO. Critical illness. In: Merritt RJ, Souba WW, eds. *The ASPEN Nutrition Support Practice Manual.* Silver Spring, Md: ASPEN; 1998:18.1–18.14.
24. Schwartz D. Pulmonary failure. In: Matarese LE, Gottschlich MM, eds. *Contemporary Nutrition Support Practice: A Clinical Guide*. Philadelphia, Pa: WB Saunders; 1998:395–409.
25. Peck MD. Sepsis. In: Zaloga GP, ed. *Nutrition in Critical Care*. St. Louis, Mo: Mosby; 1994:599–616.
26. Alberda C, Snowden L, McCargar L, Gramlich L. Energy requirements in critically ill patients. *Nutr Clin Pract.* 2002;17:38–42.
27. Lenssen P, Aker SN. Adult hematopoietic stem cell transplantation. In: Hasse JM, Blue LS, eds. *Comprehensive Guide to Transplant Nutrition*. Chicago, Ill: American Dietetic Association; 2002:123–152.
28. Ireton-Jones C, Turner W. Actual or ideal body weight: which should be used to predict energy expenditure? *J Am Diet Assoc*. 1991;91:193–195.
29. Matarese LE. Indirect calorimetry. *Support Line.* 1997;14:6–12.
30. Porter C, Cohen NH. Indirect calorimetry in critically ill patients: role of the clinical dietitian in interpreting results. *J Am Diet Assoc.* 1996;96:49–57.
31. Ireton-Jones. Indirect calorimetry. In: Skipper A, ed. *Dietitian's Handbook of Enteral and Parenteral Nutrition*. Gaithersburg, Md: Aspen Publishers; 1998: 148–164.
32. HealtheTech Inc. HealtheTech receives FDA clearance, CE marking and Canadian medical device license. *PR Newswire Europe Ltd.* July 16, 2002. Available at: http://www.prnewswire.co.uk/cgi/news/release?id=88191. Accessed November 15, 2005.
33. Glynn CC, Greene GW, Winkler MF, Albina JE. Predictive versus measured energy expenditure using limits-of-agreement analysis in hospitalized, obese patients. *JPEN J Parenter Enteral Nutr.* 1999;23: 147–154.
34. Amato P, Keating KP, Quercia RA, Kabonic J. Formulaic methods of estimating calorie requirements in mechanically ventilated obese patients: a reappraisal. *Nutr Clin Pract*. 1995;10:229–232.
35. Malone A. Anthropometric assessment. In: Charney P, Malone A, eds. *ADA Pocket Guide to Nutrition Assessment.* Chicago, Ill: American Dietetic Association; 2004:142–152.
36. Shaw JH, Humberstone DM, Douglas RG, Korea J. Leucine kinetics in patients with benign disease, non-weight-losing cancer, and cancer cachexia: Studies at the whole-body and tissue level and the response to nutritional support. *Surgery.* 1991;109:37–50.
37. Bloch AS. Cancer. In: Gottschlich MM, Matarese LE, Shronts EP, eds. *Nutrition Support Dietetics Core Curriculum.* 2nd ed. Silver Spring, Md: American Society for Parenteral and Enteral Nutrition; 1993: 213–226.
38. Wang J, Thornton JC, Kolesnik S, Pierson RN. Anthropometry in body composition. An overview. *Ann N Y Acad Sci.* 2000;904:317–326.
39. Shopbell JM, Hopkins B, Shronts EP. Nutrition screening and assessment. In: Gottschlich MM, Furman MP, Hammond KA, Holcombe BJ, Seidner DL, eds. *The Science and Practice of Nutrition Support: A Case-Based Core Curriculum.* Dubuque, Iowa: Kent/Hunt Publishing; 2001:107–140.
40. Geerts SP. Assessment. In: Bloch AS, ed. *Nutrition Management of the Cancer Patient.* Rockville, Md: Aspen Publishers, Inc; 1990:25–36.
41. Grant A, DeHoog S. Biochemical assessment. In: Grant A, DeHoog S, eds. *Nutrition: Assessment Support and Management.* 5th ed. Seattle, Wash: Grant/DeHoog; 1999:157–213.
42. Matarese LE. Renal failure. In: Gottschlich MM, Matarese LE, Shronts EP, eds. *Nutrition Support Dietetics Core Curriculum.* 2nd ed. Silver Spring, Md: American Society for Parenteral and Enteral Nutrition; 1993:327–339.
43. Goldstein DJ, Abrahamian-Gebeshian C. Nutrition support in renal failure. In: Matarese LE, Gottschlich MM, eds. *Contemporary Nutrition Support Practice: A Clinical Guide.* Philadelphia, Pa: WB Saunders; 1998:447–471.
44. Raup SM, Kaproth P. Hepatic failure. In: Matarese LE, Gottschlich MM, eds. *Contemporary Nutrition Support Practice: A Clinical Guide.* Philadelphia, Pa: WB Saunders; 1998:441–446.
45. Shronts EP, Fish J. Hepatic failure. In: Gottschlich MM, Matarese LE, Shronts EP, eds. *Nutrition Support Dietetics: Core Curriculum.* 2nd ed. Silver Spring, Md: American Society for Parenteral and Enteral Nutrition; 1993:311–325.
46. Hamwi GJ. Changing dietary concepts. In: Danowski TS, ed. *Diabetes Mellitus: Diagnosis and Treatment.* New York, NY: American Diabetes Association; 1964:73–78.
47. Ettinger S. Macronutrients: carbohydrates, proteins, and lipids. In: Mahan KL, Escott-Stump S, eds. *Krause's Food, Nutrition, & Diet Therapy*. 11th ed. Philadelphia, Pa: WB Saunders; 2004:37–74.

48. Institute of Medicine. *Dietary Reference Intakes for Energy, Carbohydrate, Fiber, Fat, Fatty Acids, Cholesterol, Protein, and Amino Acids.* Washington, DC: National Academies Press; 2002.
49. US Department of Health and Human Services (HHS) and the Department of Agriculture (USDA). Dietary Guidelines for Americans 2005. Available at: http://www.healthierus.gov/dietaryguidelines. Accessed November 3, 2005.
50. Institute of Medicine. *Recommended Dietary Allowances*. 10th ed. Washington, DC: National Academies Press; 1989.
51. Institute of Medicine. *Dietary Reference Intakes for Vitamin A, Vitamin K, Arsenic, Boron, Chromium, Copper, Iodine, Iron, Manganese, Molybdenum, Nickel, Silicon, Vanadium, and Zinc.* Washington, DC: National Academies Press; 2000.
52. Institute of Medicine. *Dietary Reference Intakes for Calcium, Phosphorus, Magnesium, Vitamin D, and Fluoride.* Washington, DC: National Academies Press; 1997.
53. Institute of Medicine. *Dietary Reference Intakes for Vitamin C, Vitamin E, Selenium, and Carotenoids.* Washington, DC: National Academies Press; 2000.
54. Institute of Medicine. *Dietary Reference Intakes for Thiamin, Riboflavin, Niacin, Vitamin B6, Folate, Vitamin B12, Pantothenic Acid, Biotin, and Choline.* Washington, DC: National Academies Press; 2000.
55. Institute of Medicine. Food and Nutrition Web site. Available at: http://www.iom.edu/topic.asp?id=3708. Accessed April 25, 2005.
56. Huffman FA. Micronutrient requirements of cancer patients. *Cancer.* 1985;55(suppl):295–300.
57. Baumgartner TG. Trace elements in clinical nutrition. *Nutr Clin Pract.* 1993;8:251–263.
58. Brown JK, Byers T, Doyle C, Coumeya KS, Demark-Wahnefried W, Kushi LH, McTieman A, Rock CL, Aziz N, Bloch AS, Eldridge B, Hamilton K, Katzin C, Koonce A, Main J, Mobley C, Morra ME, Pierce MS, Sawyer KA; American Cancer Society. Nutrition and physical activity during and after cancer treatment: an American Cancer Society guide for informed choices. *CA Cancer J Clin.* 2003;53:268–291.
59. Parenteral multivitamin products; drugs for human use; drug efficacy study implementation; amendment. (21 CFR 5.70). *Fed Reg.* 2000;65: 21200–21201.
60. Helphingstine CJ, Bistrian BR. New Food and Drug Administration requirements for inclusion of vitamin K in adult parenteral multivitamins. *JPEN J Parenter Enteral Nutr.* 2003;27:220–224.
61. Guidelines for essential trace element preparations for parenteral use: a statement by an expert panel. AMA Department of Foods and Nutrition. *JAMA.* 1979; 24:2051–2054.
62. Grant A, DeHoog S. Drug and nutrient interactions. In: Grant A, DeHoog S. *Nutrition: Assessment Support and Management.* 5th ed. Seattle, Wash: Grant/DeHoog; 1999:219–277.
63. Karch AM. *2004 Lippincott's Nursing Drug Guide.* Philadelphia, Pa: Lippincott Williams & Williams; 2004.
64. Thomson CA, LaFrance RJ. Pharmacotherapeutics. In: Gottschlich MM, Matarese LE, Shronts EP, eds. *Nutrition Support Dietetics: Core Curriculum*, 2nd ed. Silver Spring, Md: American Society for Parenteral and Enteral Nutrition; 1993:433–456.
65. Mueller DH, Burke F. Vitamin and mineral therapy. In: Morrison G, Hark L, eds. *Medical Nutrition and Disease.* Cambridge, Mass: Blackwell Science; 2003: 39–74.
66. Grant A, DeHoog S. Physical signs in nutrient deficiency and toxicity. In: Grant A, DeHoog S, eds. *Nutrition: Assessment, Support, and Management,* 5th ed. Seattle, Wash: Grant/DeHoog; 1999:149–155.
67. Grant A, DeHoog S. Tests of mineral status. In: Grant A, DeHoog S, eds. *Nutrition: Assessment, Support, and Management,* 5th ed. Seattle, Wash: Grant/DeHoog; 1999:187–193.
68. Cresci G. Nutrition assessment and monitoring. In: Shikora SA, Martindale RG, Schwaitzberg SD, eds. *Nutritional Considerations in the Intensive Care Unit: Science, Rationale and Practice.* Dubuque, Iowa: Kendall/Hunt Publishing; 2002:21–30.
69. Hopkins B. Assessment of nutritional status. In: Gottschlich MM, Matarese LE, Shronts EP, eds. *Nutrition Support Dietetics Core Curriculum,* 2nd ed. Silver Spring, Md: American Society for Parenteral and Enteral Nutrition; 1993:49–57.
70. Braunschweig C. Minerals and trace elements. In: Matarese LE, Gottschlich MM, eds. *Contemporary Nutrition Support Practice: A Clinical Guide.* Philadelphia, Pa: WB Saunders; 1998:163–173.
71. Kleiner SM. Water: an essential but overlooked nutrient. *J Am Diet Assoc.* 1999;99:200–206.
72. Institute of Medicine. *Dietary Reference Intakes: Water, Potassium, Sodium, Chloride, and Sulfate.* Washington, DC: National Academies Press; 2004.
73. Huckleberry Y. Intravenous fluids: which solution and why? *Support Line.* 2001;23:12–16.
74. American Dietetic Association, Dietitians of Canada. Nutrition assessment of adults. In: *Manual of Clinical*

Dietetics. 6th ed. Chicago, Ill: American Dietetic Association; 2000:3–37.

75. Russell M, Malone A. Nutrient requirements. In: Charney P, Malone A, eds. *ADA Pocket Guide to Nutrition Assessment.* Chicago, Ill: American Dietetic Association; 2004:153–188.
76. Steiner N, Bruera E. Methods of hydration in palliative care patients. *J Palliat Care.* 1998;14:6–13.
77. Kein CJ, Stanek GS, Wiles CE III. Overfeeding macronutrients to critically ill adults: metabolic complications. *J Am Diet Assoc.* 1998;98:795–806.
78. Russell M, Cromer M, Grant J. Complications of enteral nutrition therapy. In: Gottschlich MM, Fuhrman MP, Hammond KA, Holcombe BJ, Seidner DL, eds. *The Science and Practice of Nutrition Support: A Case-Based Core Curriculum.* Dubuque, Iowa: Kent/Hunt Publishing; 2001:189–209.
79. Havala T, Shronts E. Managing the complications associated with refeeding. *Nutr Clin Pract.* 1990; 5:23–29.
80. Fuhrman MP. Management of complications of parenteral nutrition. In: Matarese LE, Gottschlich MM, eds. *Contemporary Nutrition Support Practice: A Clinical Guide.* Philadelphia, Pa: WB Saunders; 1998:243–263.
81. Brown RO, Minard G. Parenteral nutrition. In Shils ME, Shike M, Ross AC, Caballero B, Cousins R, eds. *Modern Nutrition in Health and Disease,* 10 ed. Philadelphia, PA: Lippincott Williams & Wilkins, 2006:1567–1597.

Chapter 8

Nutritional Implications of Chemotherapy

BARBARA GRANT, MS, RD, AND JAMES BYRON, RPH, BCOP

INTRODUCTION

Chemotherapy uses chemical agents or medications to interfere with the steps of the cell cycle specifically involved in the synthesis of DNA and the replication of tumor cells (1). This chapter reviews the goals of chemotherapy and the ways in which chemotherapy is used. This chapter also examines the classification of chemotherapeutic agents and the toxicities and side effects of chemotherapy.

GOALS

Chemotherapy has three primary goals (2,3):

1. Cure
   - Obtain a durable response to treatment of a specific cancer
2. Control
   - Extend the length of life when cure is not possible
   - Eradicate microscopic metastasis after tumors are surgically removed
   - Reduce tumor bulk before surgery and/or radiation therapy
3. Palliation
   - Improve comfort when cure or control is not possible
   - Improve quality of life
   - Reduce tumor burden, thereby helping to relieve cancer-related symptoms, such as pain and organ obstruction

CHEMOTHERAPY USES

Chemotherapeutic agents are used for individuals with solid tumors who have been or who are at risk for systemic disease. Chemotherapeutic agents can also be used as the following (1,4–6):

- A primary treatment in hematological cancers, such as lymphomas or leukemias
- Single agents or in combination with other agents to achieve maximum cell kill for each drug within a tolerated range of toxicity, to provide a broader range of activity against different subgroups or a heterogeneous tumor population, and to prevent or retard the development of new resistant cell lines
- An adjuvant treatment to decrease the risk of recurrence after surgery, primarily in breast and colorectal cancer
- A neo-adjuvant treatment (before surgery) to improve the possibility of optimal surgery, most commonly used in breast and rectal cancers
- A myeloablation treatment to obliterate bone marrow in preparation for blood or marrow transplantation

- A radiosensitizer to enhance the response to radiation therapy
- A palliative treatment in individuals with incurable disease
- A chemopreventive treatment to prevent cancer in high-risk individuals

CLASSIFICATION OF CHEMOTHERAPEUTIC AGENTS

The three main classifications of FDA-approved chemotherapeutic agents discussed in this chapter are (*a*) cytotoxic therapies, (*b*) hormonal therapies, and (*c*) biotherapies, which include biological response modifiers and molecularly targeted agents. Chemotherapeutic agents vary in their modes of action, and they are classified as cell cycle- (phase) specific, or cell cycle- (phase) nonspecific. Cell cycle-specific agents have their effect during a specific phase or phases of the cell cycle. Cell cycle-nonspecific agents act on cells whether they are actively dividing in any phase of the cell cycle or in the resting (nonreplicating) state (7).

Cytotoxic agents include alkylating agents, antibiotics, antimetabolites, miscellaneous agents, and plant alkaloids. These agents have specific mechanisms of action and are toxic to malignant cells and normal host cells that have a high replication rate (4).

Hormonal agents are used in the treatment of hormone-sensitive cancers, such as prostate, endometrial, and breast cancer (8). Hormone therapy can alter the body's hormonal environment, causing changes in the cancer cell's normal growth, and the suppression or removal of the stimulus for tumor growth.

Biological therapies alter the host-tumor relationship and include cytokines, such as hematopoietic growth factors, and immune therapies (eg, interleukins and interferon), monoclonal antibodies (eg, rituximab), and targeted molecular therapies (eg, trastuzumab, vaccines, and other substances that stimulate or modulate the body's immune system) (9). Hematopoietic growth factors include colony-stimulating factors that stimulate production of blood cells in the bone marrow to assist with recovery from chemotherapy (10).

Immune therapies enhance the ability of the host to attack the cancer through immunomodulation and immunoregulation of leukocytes (4). Monoclonal antibodies work in a variety of ways to modify the immune response, so that cancer cells are injured or killed (9). Targeted molecular therapies therapeutically act on identified and potential molecular flaws in the cell.

Table 8.1 (6,11) describes the effects of chemotherapeutic agents and their mechanisms of action.

FACTORS TO CONSIDER IN CHEMOTHERAPY REGIMENS

Many factors should be considered when selecting a chemotherapy regimen. These include tumor burden, histology, cancer stage, efficacy of treatment modalities (surgery, radiation therapy, and/or chemotherapy), and the goal or intent of the planned therapy.

Patient-specific factors include age, comorbid disease, psychosocial issues, bone marrow reserve, nutritional status, performance status, educational needs, and general health (4). Concurrent patient problems that can affect treatment decisions include infection, malignant effusions, and metabolic abnormalities such as hypercalcemia (10).

Tumors are most likely to be responsive to chemotherapy when they are small and vascular, rather than later when cell proliferation slows, because of crowding, poor vascularization, and limited nutrients (1). The higher the proliferative rate of a tumor, the more effective the chemotherapy. Ideally, it is best to begin therapy when consideration can be given to debulking the mass. Tumors are generally heterogeneous, and cell clones may show resistance to a particular agent, continuing to grow even during treatment (1). Combining chemotherapy agents that are synergistic and act at different phases of the cell cycle can provide greater cell kill. In addition, combining agents that produce different toxicities allows for the administration of maximal dosages of each agent (4).

DOSAGES AND ADMINISTRATION

Chemotherapy dosages are usually calculated based on body surface area. The dosage should be based on the individual's actual height and weight obtained before each course of therapy (10). The dosage may also be based on renal function, as determined by the serum creatinine and actual or estimated creatinine clearance (4).

Chemotherapy is administered by systemic or regional modes of delivery. In systemic chemotherapy, the goal is to attain a maximum therapeutic cytotoxic effect without extreme toxicity to normal tissue, and the delivery methods are oral, intravenous, subcutaneous, intramuscular, or intraosseous. In regional chemotherapy, the goal is to deliver chemotherapeutic agents directly into blood vessels supplying the tumor or into a cavity in which the tumor is located. Delivery methods for regional chemotherapy are intrathecal, intra-arterial, or intracavitary (4,10).

TOXICITIES AND ADVERSE EFFECTS OF CHEMOTHERAPEUTIC AGENTS

Chemotherapeutic agents are potent and have the potential to cause many adverse events (10). Toxicities and side effects are often a result of damage to rapidly dividing cells. The actions of chemotherapeutic agents can be cytotoxic to normal cells as well as to malignant cells, in particular those cells with a rapid turnover, such as bone marrow, hair follicles, and oral and intestinal mucosa. Adverse effects range from mild to life-threatening. Dosage adjustments or discontinuation of therapy may be indicated, depending on tolerance to the chemotherapy regimen (4).

Classifying Adverse Events

Developed by the National Cancer Institute as a standardized grading system for assessing and reporting treatment-related adverse events, the Common Terminology Criteria for Adverse Events (CTCAE) Version 3.0 (12) uses a classification system of Grades 1 through 5, with specific clinical descriptions of severity for each adverse event experienced:

- Grade 1: Mild adverse event
- Grade 2: Moderate adverse event
- Grade 3: Severe adverse event
- Grade 4: Life-threatening or disabling adverse event
- Grade 5: Death-related adverse event

Myelosuppression

Myelosuppression (the suppression of bone marrow activity) is the most common dose-limiting toxicity of chemotherapy (4). When bone marrow production is interrupted by chemotherapy, leukopenia (a decrease in the number of white blood cells) and neutropenia (a decrease in the number of neutrophils) can occur. Neutropenia is a substantial predisposing factor to infection in cancer patients. The absolute neutrophil count (ANC) is calculated by multiplying the percentage of granulocytes (neutrophils = segments + bands) by the total white blood cell count (WBC). The risk of infection rises as the WBC count falls; the greatest risk occurs when ANCs are less than 500/mm^3 (13). Chemotherapy can also cause a decrease in the number of red blood cells (anemia), and platelets (thrombocytopenia) (14). The nadir is defined as the lowest value of blood counts and usually occurs within 7 to 14 days of chemotherapy administration. When blood

Table 8.1 Classification of Antineoplastic Chemotherapeutic Agents

Drug	*Mechanism of Action*
Alkylating agents	Interfere with replication of DNA and transcription of RNA by cross-linking DNA strands
Antibiotics	Inhibit cell division by binding to DNA and interfering with RNA transcription
Antimetabolites	Interfere with nucleic acid synthesis by substituting drug for purines or pyrimidines necessary for normal cellular function
Hormones	Alter cellular metabolism by changing body hormonal milieu for unfavorable tumor growth
Plant alkaloids	Inhibit mitotic spindle formation and block mitosis
Targeted molecular therapies	Act therapeutically on identified and potential molecular flaws
Biologic response modifiers	Modify host biologic responses to tumor
Platinum coordination complexes	Inhibit DNA synthesis by cross-linking DNA strands
Substituted ureas	Inhibit DNA synthesis and ribonucleotide reductases
Methylhydrazine derivatives	Break the chromosome and separate DNA strands

Source: Data are from references 6 and 11.

counts return to acceptable levels (ANC > 1,000), the next dose of chemotherapy can be administered.

Common Nutrition-Related Side Effects

Adverse effects of chemotherapy include nausea, vomiting, anorexia, mucositis, esophagitis, fatigue, and alterations in bowel habits (constipation, bloating, or diarrhea). Normal gut function may also be affected because of damage to the cells that line the gastrointestinal tract. Resulting changes in digestion and absorption can compromise nutritional status.

Chemotherapy agents can also adversely impact hepatic and renal function. Neutropenia, anemia (ie, iron-deficiency and folate-deficiency anemias) and thrombocytopenia require strict attention to food safety and handling, as well as dietary modifications. The severity of side effects experienced is related to the chemotherapy regimen, the individual's response, supportive medications given, and performance status. Aggressive and thorough management of nutrition related side effects throughout the course of treatment can have a positive effect on nutritional status and well-being (8). Refer to Appendix A for nutrition recommendations for managing treatment-related side effects and to Chapter 7 for estimated energy, protein, and fluid requirements.

As many as 50% of all cancer patients receiving chemotherapy experience some degree of nausea and vomiting (15). Chemotherapy-induced nausea and vomiting are commonly classified as follows:

- Acute: Occurring 24 hours or less after chemotherapy
- Delayed: Occurring 1 to 6 days immediately after chemotherapy
- Anticipatory: Occurring within 1 week before the actual administration of chemotherapy

The risks for chemotherapy-induced nausea and vomiting are related to the agent(s) administered as well as to patient factors (18). Both the chemotherapy medication given and the dosage prescribed determine the emetogenic potential (see Tables 8.2 and 8.3) (6,10,16–19). The time of onset and the duration of nausea and vomiting are highly variable, although agents with the shortest onset generally tend to be the most emetogenic (16). Careful assessment of the emetogenic potential of chemotherapeutic agents is important to accurately provide the most effective antiemetic treatment.

Table 8.2 Emetogenic Potential of Chemotherapeutic Agents

Level	*Individuals Experiencing Emesis*
5 (very high)	> 90%
4 (high)	60%–90%
3 (moderate)	30%–60%
2 (low)	10%–30%
1 (very low)	< 10%

Source: Data are from reference 16.

OTHER SUPPORTIVE THERAPIES

The management of side effects may also include other supportive therapies for patients undergoing chemotherapy treatment. Measures may include the use of biologic therapies or blood products to manage episodes of treatment-induced bone marrow suppression, use of prophylactic antibiotics to minimize the occurrence and severity of treatment-related infections of the urinary and gastrointestinal tracts, and medications such as antidiarrheals and antiemetics to aid in the management of chemotherapy-induced diarrhea and nausea.

CASE STUDY

A 40-year-old premenopausal woman is diagnosed with invasive breast cancer that is estrogen receptor–negative (ER–), and progesterone receptor–negative (PR–), with HER-2/neu – overexpression. The tumor is 1.6 cm and there are three positive axillary nodes. Her treatment plan is considered adjuvant therapy and consists of the following (20):

- Surgery: Total mastectomy with surgical axillary staging
- Chemotherapy: Four cycles of doxorubicin (Adriamycin, Pharmacia & Upjohn, Peapack, NJ 07977) and cyclophosphamide (Cytoxan,

Table 8.3 Nutritional Implications of Chemotherapeutic Agents

Antineoplastic Agent (Trade Name and Manufacturer)	*Myelosuppression*	*Nausea and Vomiting**	*Anorexia*	*Mucositis and Esophagitis*	*Diarrhea*	*Renal Effects*	*Hepatic Effects*	*Other*
Cytotoxics								
asparaginase (Elspar, Merck & Co, West Point, PA 19486)		3	x	x		x	x	Decreased protein synthesis; hypoalbuminemia; pancreatitis; weight loss; hyperglycemia; clotting disorder; risk of acute allergic reaction
bleomycin (Blenoxane, Bristol Myers Squibb, Princeton, NJ 08540)	None to mild	1	x	x				Weight loss; xerostomia; fever; cumulative risk for pulmonary fibrosis
busulfan (Myleran, GlaxoSmithKline, Research Triangle Park, NC 27709; Busulfex, Orphan Medical, Minnetonka, MN 55305)	Mild to moderate	4–5†	x	x			x	May cause weight loss; pulmonary fibrosis
capcitabine (Xeloda, Roche Laboratories, Nutley, NJ 07110)	Moderate	1			x	x		Fatigue; hand and foot syndrome; fever; headache
carboplatin (Paraplatin, Bristol Myers Squibb, Princeton, NJ 08540)	Moderate to severe	4			x	x	x	Ototoxicity; risk for postadministration allergic reaction
carmustine (BCNU, Bristol Myers Squibb, Princeton, NJ 08540)	Moderate to severe (delayed—4 to 6 weeks after administration)	4–5†	x	x		x	x	Pulmonary toxicity; phlebitis

chlorambucil (Leukeran, GlaxoSmithKline, Research Triangle Park, NC 27709)	Mild to moderate	1						Pulmonary fibrosis
cisplatin (CDDP Platinol, Bristol Myers Squibb, Princeton, NJ 08540)	Mild to moderate	4–5†	x		x	x—severe†		Decreased serum Mg, K, Zn; renal tubular necrosis; metallic taste; ototoxicity
cyclophosphamide (Cytoxan, Mead Johnson Oncology, Princeton, NJ 08540)	Moderate to severe	2–3†	x	x				Xerostomia; abdominal pain; pulmonary fibrosis; cystitis
cytarabine (Ara-C, Faulding, Paramus, NJ 07652)	Moderate to severe	3–5†	x	x	x	x	x	Flu-like symptoms; CNS toxicity
dacarbazine (DTIC, DTIC-Dome, Bayer Corporation, West Haven, CT 06516)	Moderate	5	x	x	x			Metallic taste; flu-like symptoms; phlebitis
dactinomycin (Actinomycin-D, ACT, Merck & Co., West Point, PA 19486)	Moderate to severe	5	x	x—severe†	x			Xerostomia; taste alterations; radiation recall; phlebitis
daunorubicin hydrochloride (Daunomycin, Abbott Laboratories, Abbott Park, IL 60064)	Moderate to severe	3- 4†	x	x—severe†	x			Xerostomia; change in taste acuity; cardiotoxicity
docetaxel (Taxotere, Aventis Pharmaceuticals, Bridgewater, NJ 08807)	Severe	2					x	Risk for acute allergic reaction during infusion
doxorubicin hydrochloride (Adriamycin, Pharmacia & Upjohn, Peapack, NJ 07977)	Moderate to severe	2–4†	x	x—severe†	x			Xerostomia; cardiotoxicity; radiation recall; alopecia; hand and foot syndrome

(*continued*)

Table 8.3 Nutritional Implications of Chemotherapeutic Agents (*continued*)

Antineoplastic Agent (Trade Name and Manufacturer)	*Myelosuppression*	*Nausea and Vomiting**	*Anorexia*	*Mucositis and Esophagitis*	*Diarrhea*	*Renal Effects*	*Hepatic Effects*	*Other*
Cytotoxics								
epirubicin hydrochloride (Ellence, Pharmacia & Upjohn, Peapack, NJ 07977)	Moderate to severe	2–4†			x			Hair loss; stomatitis; cardiotoxicity
Etoposide (VePesid, VP-16, Bristol Myers Squibb, Princeton, NJ 08540)	Moderate	2	x	x	x		x	Hypertension; fever
fludarabine phosphatase (Fludara, Berlex Laboratories, Wayne, NJ 07470)	Moderate to severe	1	x	x	x	x		Neurotoxicity
fluorouracil (5-FU, 5-Fluorouracil, Pharmacia & Upjohn, Peapack, NJ 07977)	Moderate	2		x—severe†	x		x	Taste alterations; avoid pyroxidine supplements; cardiotoxicity; hand and foot syndrome; myocardial schemia
gemcitabine hydrochloride (Gemzar, Eli Lilly and Company, Indianapolis, IN 46285)	Mild to moderate	2		x	x	x		Fever; rash; dyspnea
hydroxyurea (Hydrea, Berlex Laboratories, Wayne, NJ 07470)	Moderate	1	x	x	x			
idarubicin (Idamycin, Pharmacia & Upjohn, Peapack, NJ 07977)	Mild to moderate	3		x	x		x	Cardiotoxicity; alopecia

ifosfamide (Ifex, Bristol Myers Squibb, Princeton, NJ 08540)	Moderate to severe	3				x		Confusion; lethargy; cystitis; CNS toxicity
irenotecan (Camptosar, Pharmacia & Upjohn, Kalamazoo, MI 49001)	Moderate to severe	4	x		x—severe†			Fever; abdominal pain; asthenia
mechlorethamine (Nitrogen Mustard, HN2 Mustargen, Merck & Co., West Point, PA 19486)	Severe	5	x		x			Metallic taste; fever; chills; tinnitis; severe vesicant
melphalan (Alkeran, Glaxo-SmithKline, Research Triangle Park, NC 27709)	Moderate	1						Pulmonary fibrosis
mercaptopurine (Purinethol, Glaxo-SmithKline, Research Triangle Park, NC 27709)	Moderate	1	x	x	x	x	x	Biliary stasis; cholestatic jaundice; rash; pancreatitis
methotrexate sodium (Methotrexate sodium, American Pharmaceutical Partners, Los Angeles, CA 90049)	Moderate	2–4†	x	x—severe†	x	x	x	Decreased absorption of B-12, folate, and D-xylose; change in taste acuity; pneumonitis
mitomycin (Mitomycin-C, MTC Mutamycin, Bristol Myers Squibb, Princeton, NJ 08540)	Severe	2	x	x	x	x	x	Hypercalcemia; cumulative stem cell toxicity
mitoxantrone (Novantrone, Amgen, Thousand Oaks, CA 91320)	Mild to moderate	3		x	x		x	Blue discoloration of urine

(continued)

Table 8.3 Nutritional Implications of Chemotherapeutic Agents (*continued*)

Antineoplastic Agent (Trade Name and Manufacturer)	*Myelosuppression*	*Nausea and Vomiting**	*Anorexia*	*Mucositis and Esophagitis*	*Diarrhea*	*Renal Effects*	*Hepatic Effects*	*Other*
Cytotoxics								
oxalaplatin (Eloxatin, Sanofi-Synthelabo, New York, NY 10016)	Mild to moderate	3			x			Peripheral neuropathy; pharyngeal dysesthesia; bowel wall injury
paciltaxel (Taxol, Bristol Myers Squibb, Princeton, NJ 08540)	Moderate to severe	2		x	x		x	Fatigue; neuropathy; risk of acute allergic reaction
procarbazine hydrochloride (Matulane, Sigma-Tau Pharmaceuticals, Gaithersburg, MD 20877)	Moderate to severe	4	x	x	x	x	x	Monoamine oxidase inhibitor; low tyramine diet; decreased serum K, Ca, PO4
temozolamide (Temodarr, Schering-Plough, Kenilworth, NJ 07033)	Moderate to severe	3	x				x	Fatigue
thioguanine (6-Thioguanine, TG Thioguanine, Glaxo-SmithKline, Research Triangle Park, NC 27709)	Severe	1	x	x	x		x	
topotecan hydrochloride (Hycamtin, Glaxo-SmithKline, Research Triangle Park, NC 27709)	Severe	2	x		x			Fever

vinblastine sulfate (Velban, American Pharmaceutical Partners, Los Angeles, CA 90049)	Moderate	3		x	x		x	Constipation; neuropathy
vincristine sulfate (Vinscar, Pharmacia & Upjohn, Peapack, NJ 07977)	Mild	1	x	x	x		x	Peripheral neuropathy; abdominal pain; hyponatremia; alternating diarrhea and constipation
vinorelbine tartate (Navelbine, GlaxoSmithKline, Research Triangle Park, NC 27709)	Moderate to severe	2	x					Constipation; neuropathy
Hormonals								
prednisone‡ dexamethasone‡ (Decadron, Merck & Co, West Point, PA 19486)	Lymphopenia							Hyperphagia; sodium and fluid retention; GI upset; glucose intolerance; potassium wasting; hyperlipidemia; osteoporosis; negative nitrogen balance; CNS symptoms
flutamide§ (Eulexin, Schering-Plough, Kenilworth, NJ 07033)		1				x	x	Hot flashes; decreased libido; impotence
bicalutamide§ (Casodex, AstraZeneca, Pharmaceuticals, Wilmington, DE 19850)		1			x			Hot flashes; gynecomastia; constipation

(continued)

Table 8.3 Nutritional Implications of Chemotherapeutic Agents (*continued*)

Antineoplastic Agent (Trade Name and Manufacturer)	*Myelosuppression*	*Nausea and Vomiting**	*Anorexia*	*Mucositis and Esophagitis*	*Diarrhea*	*Renal Effects*	*Hepatic Effects*	*Other*
tamoxifen citrate[‖] (Novaldex, AstraZeneca, Pharmaceuticals, Wilmington, DE 19850)	Mild	1	x					Bone pain; edema fluid retention; hypercalcemia; hot flashes; menstrual dysfunction
toremifene citrate[‖] (Fareston, Shire US, Newport, KY 41071)	Mild							Hot flashes; menstrual irregularities
anastrozole[¶] (Arimedex, AstraZeneca, Pharmaceuticals, Wilmington, DE 19850)		1						Hot flashes; sexual dysfunction; headaches
letrozole[¶] (Femara, Novartis Pharmaceuticals, East Hanover, NJ 07936)		1						Musculoskeletal pain; hot flashes
megestrol acetate[#] (Megace, Mead Johnson Oncology, Princeton, NJ 08540)		1						Increased appetite; fluid retention; weight gain; hypercalcemia
leuprolide acetate** (Lupron, TAP Pharmaceuticals, Deerfield, IL 60015)		1						Bone pain; hot flashes; decreased libido
goserelin acetate** (Zolodex, AstraZeneca, Pharmaceuticals, Wilmington, DE 19850)								Sexual dysfunction

Biotherapies				
interferon alfa†† (Alfa n-l Lymphoblastiod Wellferon, Schering-Plough, Kenilworth, NJ 07033)	Mild to moderate	3	x	Fatigue; weight loss or weight gain; flu-like symptoms
aldesleukin†† (Interleukin-2, IL-2 Roferon-A, Roche Laboratories, Nutley, NJ 07110)	Moderate	2		Weight loss or weight gain; hypotension; chills; fatigue; capillary leak syndrome
epoetin alfa‡‡ (Erythropoietin, EPO Procrit, Ortho Biotech, Raritan, NJ 08869)				Fever; decreased transferrin and ferritin levels; iron supplementation usually necessary
filgastim‡‡ (Granulocyte Colony Stimulating Factor, GM-CSF Neupogen, Amgen, Thousand Oaks, CA 91320)				Bone pain; flu-like symptoms; fever
pegfilgastin‡‡ (Pegylated Granulocyte Colony Stimulating Factor Neulasta, Amgen, Thousand Oaks, CA 91320)				Bone pain; flu-like symptoms; fever
sargramostin‡‡ (Granulocyte Macrophage Colony Stimulating Factor, GM-CSF Leukine, Immunex, Seattle, WA 98119)	Mild to moderate			Bone pain; flu-like symptoms; fever

(*continued*)

Table 8.3 Nutritional Implications of Chemotherapeutic Agents (*continued*)

Antineoplastic Agent (Trade Name and Manufacturer)	*Myelosuppression*	*Nausea and Vomiting**	*Anorexia*	*Mucositis and Esophagitis*	*Diarrhea*	*Renal Effects*	*Hepatic Effects*	*Other*
Moleculary Targeted Therapies								
bevacizumab (Avastin, Genentech, South San Francisco, CA 94080)						x		Gastrointestinal perforation; impaired wound healing; hemorrhage; hypertension; congestive heart failure
bortezomib (Velcade, Millennium Pharmaceuticals, Cambridge, MA 02139)	Moderate	2	x		x		x	Fluid retention; edema; rash; effusions
cetuximab (Erubitux, Imclone Systems, Inc., Branchburg, NJ 02139)								Rash; risk of acute allergic reaction
gefitinib (Iressa, AstraZeneca, Pharmaceuticals, Wilmington, DE 19850)		2					x	Rash
imatinib (Gleevec, Novartis Pharmaceuticals, East Hanover, NJ 07936)		3	x		x		x	Fatigue; rash; peripheral neuropathy

rituximab (Rituxan, Genentech, South San Francisco, CA 94080)	1		Fever; chills; rash
trastuzumab (Herceptin, Genentech, South San Francisco, CA 94080)	1	x	Fever; chills; rash; risk of acute allergic reaction; CHF

*Refer to Table 8.2 for explanation of classification.
†Dose dependent
‡Glucocorticoid
§Antiandrogen
‖Antiestrogen
¶Aromatase inhibitor
#Aromatase Inhibitor
**Gonadotropin-releasing hormone analog
††Cytokine
‡‡Hematopoeitic agent
Source: Data are from references 6, 10, and 16–19.

Mead Johnson Oncology, Princeton, NJ 08540), followed by 12 cycles of paciltaxel (Taxol, Bristol Myers Squibb, Princeton, NJ 08540) with tratsuzmab (Herceptin, Genentech, South San Fransico, CA 94080)
- Postchemotherapy radiation therapy to the chest wall and to the supraclavicular nodal area

Anticipated side effects may include moderate to severe myelosuppression and nausea/vomiting, fatigue, anorexia, neuropathy, mucositis/esophagitis, and diarrhea. Nutrition care plan management suggestions for this patient are as follows:

- Advise patient to exercise safety in handling food (neutropenic precautions).
- Provide tips for managing nausea and vomiting, improving appetite, maintaining weight, and incorporating nutritionally dense foods into daily eating plan.
- Provide tips for managing treatment-related fatigue. For example, the patient should use easy-to-prepare foods and seek assistance from friends and family in meal planning and preparation.
- Recommend a soft-textured, bland diet to aid in management of sore/tender mouth and throat.
- Consider use of a low-fiber diet to aid in diarrhea management. RDs should note that constipation is common with antiemetic agents, so take this into consideration when prescribing low-fiber diets.
- Encourage the intake of fluids for adequate hydration.
- Encourage the avoidance of high-fat, greasy, or fried foods.
- Encourage open communication with the health care team with regard to any nutrition problems encountered and efficacy of management suggestions.

REFERENCES

1. Kemper M, Stewart Haapoja I, Goodman M. Principles of chemotherapy. In: Gates RA, Fink RM, eds. *Oncology Nursing Secrets.* 2nd ed. Philadelphia, Pa: Hanley and Belfus; 2001:44–52.
2. Dollinger M, Rosenbaum EH, Cable G. What happens in chemotherapy. In: *Everyone's Guide to Chemotherapy.* 3rd ed. Kansas City, Mo: Andrew McMeel Publishing; 1997:57–67.
3. Powell LL, Fishman MA, Mrozek-Orlowski M. *Principles of Cancer Chemotherapy. Guidelines and Recommendations for Practice.* Pittsburgh, Pa: Oncology Nursing Press; 1996.
4. Brown KA, Esper P, Kelleher LO, Brace O'Neill JE, Polovich M, White JM, eds. *Chemotherapy and Biotherapy.* Pittsburgh, Pa: Oncology Nursing Press; 2001.
5. Fink RM, Hinshaw I. Principles of therapy. In: Gates RA, Fink RM, eds. *Oncology Nursing Secrets.* 2nd ed. Philadelphia, Pa: Hanley and Belfus; 2001:21–34.
6. Wilkes G, Ingwersen K, Barton-Burke M. *Oncology Nursing Drug Handbook*. Sudbury, Mass: Jones and Bartlett Publishers; 2003.
7. Tenebaum L. The cell cycle chemotherapy. In: Tenebaum L. *Cancer Chemotherapy and Biotherapy: A Reference Guide.* Philadelphia, Pa: WB Saunders; 1989.
8. Lenhard RE Jr, Osteen RT, Gansler T, eds. *Clinical Oncology*. Atlanta, Ga: Blackwell Science; 2001.
9. Rieger PT. Biotherapy: an overview. In: Rieger PT. *Biotherapy: A Comprehensive Overview.* 2nd ed. Sudbury, Mass: Jones and Bartlett Publishers; 2001:3–37.
10. Baltzer Cleri L, Haywood R. *Oncology Pocket Guide to Chemotherapy*. 5th ed. Philadelphia, Pa: Mosby Medical Communications/Elsevier Science; 2002.
11. Fred Hutchinson Cancer Research Center. *BMT/PBSCT Nutrition Care Criteria Manual*. Seattle, Wash: Fred Hutchinson Cancer Research Center; 1995.
12. National Cancer Institute. Cancer Therapy Evaluation Program. Common Terminology Criteria for Adverse Events v3.0 (CTCAE). Available at: http://ctep.cancer.gov/reporting/ctc.html. Accessed April 8, 2004.
13. Gates R. Infections in immunosuppressed patients. In: Gates RA, Fink RM, eds. *Oncology Nursing Secrets.* 2nd ed. Philadelphia, Pa: Hanley and Belfus; 2001: 459–469.
14. Groenwald SL, Frogge MH, Goodman M, Yarbro CH. *Cancer Symptom Management.* Sudbury, Mass: Jones and Bartlett Publishers; 1996.
15. Wickman R. Nausea and vomiting. In: Gates RA, Fink RM, eds. *Oncology Nursing Secrets.* 2nd ed. Philadelphia, Pa: Hanley & Belfus; 2001:353–364.
16. Hesketh PJ, Kris MG, Grunberg SM, Beck T, Hainsworth JD, Harker G, Aapro MS, Gandara D, Lindley CM. Proposal for classifying the acute emetogenicity of cancer chemotherapy. *J Clin Oncol.* 1997;15:103–109.

17. Ettinger DS. Preventing chemotherapy-induced nausea and vomiting: an update and review of emesis. *Semin Oncol.* 1995;23(suppl 10):S6-S18.
18. American Society of Health-System Pharmacists. *AHFS Drug Information*. Bethesda, Md: American Society of Health-System Pharmacists; 2004.
19. *Drug Facts and Comparisons*. St. Louis, Mo: Wolters Kluwer; 2004.
20. National Comprehensive Cancer Network. Clinical Practice Guidelines in Oncology. Breast Cancer. Available at: http://www.nccn.org. Accessed April 26, 2005.

Chapter 9

Nutritional Implications of Radiation Therapy

SANDRA L. LUTHRINGER, RD

INTRODUCTION

Nutrition support of individuals receiving radiation therapy is vital. Adequate screening and medical nutrition therapy performed proactively can prevent or decrease the nutrition impact symptoms that radiation therapy can cause (1). This chapter explains the action of radiation therapy and examines its potential effects on nutritional status.

ACTION OF RADIATION THERAPY

Radiation therapy uses ionizing radiation to injure or destroy cells in the area being treated. The energy released from the radiation damages the genetic material, making it impossible for the cells to continue to grow (2). All cells, both cancerous and healthy, in the treatment area are affected by the radiation, but the healthy cells recover more quickly. Because tolerance of healthy tissue to radiation therapy is the limiting factor for total dose administration, radiation therapy is delivered in multiple, small doses, allowing for recovery of healthy tissue and maximizing the total dosage that may be administered to the tumor (2).

RADIATION THERAPY USES

Radiation is considered a local treatment because only cells in the area being treated are affected. Radiation may be used to treat localized solid tumors, such as cancers of the breast, brain, colon, larynx, or prostate. It can also be used to treat leukemia and lymphoma.

Radiation therapy may be used in early-stage cancers to cure or to control the disease; it can be used before surgery to shrink the tumor; and it can be used after surgery to prevent the cancer from recurring. Radiation therapy may also be used to treat symptoms such as pain caused by cancer that has metastasized from the original site. In some instances, radiation therapy has been used prophylactically, to treat areas known to develop metastases from other cancers (3). For example, radiation therapy is often delivered to the brain to prevent the spread from some lung cancers. Radiation therapy is often used in combination with other forms of treatments, such as surgery and chemotherapy.

TYPES OF RADIATION THERAPY

External-Beam Radiation Therapy

External-beam radiation therapy is the most common type of treatment given and is noninvasive. In external-beam radiation therapy, rays are directed at the tumor or tumor bed from outside the body. The treatments are generally given daily for 6 to 8 weeks, although in some cases, twice-a-day treatment protocols may be used. As the treatments progress, cell damage increases, frequently causing nutrition-related side effects.

Internal Radiation Therapy

Internal radiation therapy, also called brachytherapy, is a more invasive procedure and is performed by placing the radiation source into the body cavity as close as possible to the cancer cells. Radioactive material, sealed in a thin wire, catheter, or tube, is placed directly into the affected cancerous site. This method concentrates the radiation on the cancer cells and minimizes the radiation damage to the healthy tissue nearby. Nutrition-related side effects do not generally occur (3).

Stereotactic Radiosurgery

Stereotactic radiosurgery is a procedure commonly used to treat brain tumors. It involves precisely delivering high-dose radiation with steep dose gradients to small volumes. These treatments can be delivered via a retrofitted linear accelerator or by a dedicated unit such as a Gamma Knife (Elekta, Stockholm, Sweden) or CyberKnife (Accuray Incorporated, Sunnyvale, CA 94089). These machines use Co-60 sources that emit high-energy gamma rays directed at the tumor to avoid harming other parts of the brain (4). Nutrition-related side effects do not generally occur.

New Approaches

Several new approaches to radiation therapy are being evaluated to determine their effectiveness in treating cancer. Intraoperative irradiation delivers large doses of radiation to the tumor site and surrounding tissue during surgery. Intraoperative irradiation may be used in abdominal or pelvic cancers that have a high recurrence rate (5).

Scientists are also testing radiosensitizers, which may be more likely to damage tumor cells than healthy ones, and radioprotectors, which may protect healthy tissues. It is hoped that these methods will increase the effectiveness of radiation therapy or decrease its side effects (6).

Hyperthermia therapy (the use of heat created by microwaves and ultrasound) may be combined with radiation to make it more effective (7). The delivery of radiation directly to the cancer site by radioimmunotherapy is another new area of research. In radioimmunotherapy, antibodies are attached to radioactive substances and injected into the body. The antibodies actively seek out the cancer cells, which are in turn destroyed by the cytotoxic action of the radiation. The success of this technique will depend on both the identification of the appropriate radioactive substances and the determination of the safe and effective dosage of radiation delivered (6).

NUTRITION IMPACT SYMPTOMS

The side effects of radiation therapy are specific to the area irradiated, total dosage, duration, and whether the radiation is given in combination with another form of treatment, such as chemotherapy. Nutrition impact symptoms seen with radiation therapy are listed in Table 9.1 (8,9). Most side effects are acute, beginning around the second or third week of treatment, and they diminish 2 to 3 weeks after therapy is completed. Some side effects may be chronic (eg, taste and saliva changes due to head and neck irradiation or radiation enteritis from pelvic irradiation) (see Table 9.1).

Individuals receiving radiation therapy to any part of the gastrointestinal (GI) tract are especially susceptible to nutrition-related side effects because the GI tract is composed of rapidly dividing cells. Patients most at risk for experiencing side effects from treatment are those whose cancers involve the aerodigestive tract, including the head and neck, lungs, esophagus, pelvic regions, colorectal area, or pancreas.

MANAGING NUTRITION IMPACT SYMPTOMS

For radiation therapy patients, medical nutrition therapy is directly connected to symptom management. Adequate calories and protein intake can help the patient to maintain strength and prevent body tissues from catabolism. If individuals do not consume adequate calories and protein, stored nutrients are used as an energy source, leading to protein wasting and weight loss (9). If a patient is at risk for developing nutrition-related side effects from treatment, a dietetics professional should see the patient within the first week of treatment. The goal is to provide patients with information to help them manage potential nutrition impact symptoms before they occur, rather than waiting until problems and/or weight loss occurs.

Table 9.1 Common Nutrition Impact Symptoms Associated With Radiation Therapy

Site of Radiation Therapy	*Acute Effects*	*Late Effects**
Central nervous system (brain and spinal cord)	• Nausea, vomiting • Elevated blood glucose due to steroid administration • Fatigue • Loss of appetite	• Headache, lethargy
Head and neck area (tongue, larynx, pharynx, oropharynx, nasopharynx, tonsils, salivary glands)	• Xerostomia • Sore mouth and throat • Dysphagia, odynophagia • Mucositis • Alterations in taste and smell • Fatigue • Loss of appetite	• Mucosal—atrophy, dryness, ulceration • Salivary glands—xerostomia, fibrosis • Osteoradionecrosis • Trismus • Alterations in taste and smell
Thorax (esophagus, lung; also breasts if treatment field involves esophagus)	• Dysphagia, odynophagia • Heartburn • Fatigue • Loss of appetite	• Esophageal—fibrosis, stenosis, necrosis • Cardiac—angina on effort, pericarditis, cardiac enlargement • Pulmonary—dry cough, fibrosis, pneumonitis
Abdomen and pelvis (gastrointestinal system, reproductive organs, prostate, colon, rectum, testicles)	• Nausea, vomiting • Changes in bowel function—diarrhea, cramping, bloating, gas • Changes in urinary function—increased frequency, burning sensation with urination • Acute colitis or enteritis • Lactose intolerance • Fatigue • Loss of appetite	• Diarrhea, malabsorption, maldigestion • Chronic colitis or enteritis • Intestinal—stricture, ulceration, obstruction perforation, fistula • Urinary—hematuria, cystitis

*More than 90 days after treatment.

Source: Data are from references 8 and 9.

Initial Consultation

The initial meeting with the dietetics professional may require 30 to 45 minutes per patient and should include the following:

- Diet history or assessment of the patient's current intake
- Patient's weight history
- Current nutrition-related symptoms
- Determination of baseline nutritional status

Refer to Chapter 6 for the screening and assessment process.

Common side effects should be discussed and specific suggestions given to the patient and/or family, even if the patient currently has no problems. Refer to Appendix A for practical patient suggestions.

Energy and protein requirements should be discussed with each patient and specific goals should be outlined. Nutrient requirements vary with each cancer type, patient's age, gender, and current nutritional status (see Chapter 7).

Follow-up Appointments

Follow-up appointments may require 15 minutes each. The need for follow-up can be determined at the initial assessment and can vary among individuals. Some patients may need to be seen only every 2 to 3 weeks throughout the course of treatment; others, specifically those with cancers of the head or neck, will require weekly visits.

It is usually simple to schedule counseling sessions because individuals undergoing radiation therapy return to the treatment center daily, generally at the same time of day. Radiation treatments are brief, 15 to 20 minutes, and often the patient and/or family members can be available before or immediately after their scheduled treatment time.

Additional Considerations

Medications

Many medications are available to help manage the side effects of radiation treatment (see Chapter 15). Knowledge of frequently prescribed medications, including their schedule and form, is important.

Food Preparation and Availability

Dietetics professionals should encourage patients to keep easy-to-eat foods, such as single portions of canned fruit, yogurt, pudding, or commercially available nutrition supplements, handy at all times, especially on days when they have appointments with their physicians or expect to be away from home for a prolonged period of time.

If the patient lives far from the treatment facility and occupies temporary housing, meeting nutrition needs can be challenging. Appropriate nutrition can be especially difficult for patients staying in a hotel without cooking facilities in their room. Dietetics professionals must adjust the nutrition plan and goals as necessary.

Restrictive Therapeutic Diets

If the patient's oral intake is compromised, dietetics professionals may consider relaxing dietary restrictions. Diabetes meal plans and low-fat and low-cholesterol diets can be liberalized during radiation therapy. The goal is to maintain current weight and nutritional status as much as possible. The patient's health care team may need to provide new target values (ie, blood glucose values) or establish a new desired range for the patient, to help assure the patient that he or she is able to eat as well as possible. Adjustments to medications (such as oral hypoglycemic agents, insulin, or other medications taken for chronic illness) may be necessary during this time.

Supplements

If the patient's diet is lacking in energy, protein, or other nutrients, a variety of nutrition products for supplementation may be considered. Pharmaceutical companies often provide samples so that patients can try the products and various flavors before purchasing them.

Client Education

Each client should receive written material on how to help manage nutrition impact symptoms. Client education texts should be written clearly and simply. Education materials written at a 6th- to 8th-grade reading level can be read by a large number of patients and their caregivers.

The American Dietetic Association and the Oncology Nutrition Dietetic Practice Group have published a set of educational materials, *Management of Nutrition Impact Symptoms in Cancer and Educational Handouts* (10), which is available for purchase from the American Dietetic Association. For a list of client education resources on relieving cancer side effects, see Appendix B.

Enteral Nutrition

Enteral nutrition support must be considered when oral nutrition is not adequate, when oral intake is not possible because of mechanical obstruction, or when nutrition impact symptoms are severe enough to impede oral intake (see Chapter 13). The combination of chemotherapy and radiation therapy can exacerbate the symptoms associated with treatment, especially mucositis (11). Weight loss and wasting can be kept to a minimum if proactive nutrition support is provided before the start of combined chemotherapy and radiation therapy treatments. If combined planned therapies to the esophagus or head and neck indicate that the patient will have difficulty maintaining adequate oral intake, nutrition support may include the placement of a gastrostomy tube (12).

Total Parenteral Nutrition

Total parenteral nutrition (TPN) is rarely used in individuals undergoing radiation therapy because most patients can be fed orally or enterally. However, TPN may be used in chronic radiation enteritis, which can affect approximately 5% of individuals who receive pelvic irradiation (13). For a discussion of parenteral nutrition, see Chapter 14.

EMERGING RESEARCH

During the past several years, researchers have studied ways to reduce side effects from treatments using specific nutrients or medications. Glutamine, zinc sulfate, and amifostine (Ethyol, MedImmune, Gaithersburg, Md 20878) are being examined for their role in minimizing mouth sores, mucositis, diarrhea, altered taste, and xerostomia.

Glutamine

The amino acid glutamine may play a role in minimizing or preventing mouth sores and mucositis, which sometimes occur when receiving radiation therapy to the head and neck area, and it may help to relieve or prevent diarrhea when radiation therapy is administered to the pelvic region (14). In randomized studies, prophylactic glutamine mouthwashes reduced the incidence, severity, and duration of oral mucositis in subjects undergoing radiation therapy and chemotherapy (15,16). These results are encouraging but remain inconclusive; further trials of glutamine supplementation as an adjuvant therapy are indicated (17).

Zinc Sulfate

Although more studies are needed, some randomized clinical trials have shown that supplementation of zinc sulfate during head and neck irradiation may help expedite the return of taste after the therapy is completed (18). A randomized clinical trial in Italy found that oral supplementation of zinc sulfate tablets (45 mg) reversed the loss of taste that is often associated with this form of treatment (19).

Amifostine

Some nutrition impact symptoms caused by radiation therapy can be serious and irreversible. For example, xerostomia can have a pronounced effect on a patient's quality of life. Treatments for this problem have been limited, but clinical trials (20-22) have demonstrated that amifostine infusions significantly reduced the incidence of both chronic and acute xerostomia in subjects undergoing postoperative irradiation for head and neck cancers. Although the benefits of amifostine have been well demonstrated, subjects treated with the drug do report more adverse effects, such as nausea, vomiting, and hypotension, than subjects who do not use the drug (23). Studies are underway to determine whether amifostine has a role in reducing the incidence and severity of side effects caused by radiation therapy to the pelvic region (24).

REFERENCES

1. Rivadeneira DE, Evoy D, Fahey TJ, Lieberman MD, Daly JM. Nutritional support of the cancer patient. *CA Cancer J Clin.* 1998;48:69–80.
2. National Cancer Institute. *Radiation Therapy and You: A Guide to Self-Help During Cancer Treatment.* Available at: http://nci.nih.gov/cancertopics/radiation-therapy-and-you. Accessed April 26, 2005.
3. American Cancer Society. Goals of Radiation Therapy. Available at: http://www.cancer.org/docroot/ETO/Content/eto_1_4x_Goals_of_Radiation_Therapy.asp. Accessed December 21, 2005.
4. Khan FM. *The Physics of Radiation Therapy.* 3rd ed. Philadelphia, Pa: Lippincott Williams & Wilkins; 2003:507–520.
5. Hu KS, Harrison LB. Results and complications of surgery combined with intraoperative radiation therapy for the treatment of locally advanced or recurrent cancers in the pelvis. *Semin Surg Oncol.* 2000;18:269–278.
6. National Cancer Institute Information. Radiotherapy, Cancer Facts. Available at: http://cis.nci.nih.gov/fact/7_1.htm. Accessed April 26, 2005.
7. Algan O, Fosmire H, Hynynen K, Dalkin B, Cui H, Drach G, Stea B, Cassady JR. External beam radiotherapy and hyperthermia in the treatment of patients with locally advanced prostate carcinoma—results of long term follow-up. *Cancer.* 2002;89:399–403.
8. Ottery FD. Supportive nutritional therapy in cancer. *Semin Oncol.* 1995;22(suppl 6):3–44.
9. National Cancer Institute. *Nutrition in Cancer Care (PDQ).* Available at: http://www.cancer.gov/cancerinfo/pdq/supportivecare/nutrition/healthprofessional. Accessed April 26, 2005.
10. Eldridge B, Hamilton KK, eds. *Management of Nutrition Impact Symptoms in Cancer and Educational Handouts.* 2nd ed. Chicago, Ill: American Dietetic Association; 2004.
11. Marcy PY, Magne N, Bensadoun RJ, Bleuse A, Falewee MN, Voit M, Bruneton JN. Systematic percutaneous fluoroscopic gastrostomy for concomitant radiochemotherapy of advanced head and neck cancer:

optimization of therapy. *Support Care Cancer.* 2000;8: 410–413.

12. Schweinfurth JM, Boger GN, Feustel PJ. Preoperative risk assessment for gastrostomy tube placement in head and neck cancer patients. *Head Neck.* 2001;23: 376–382.
13. Scolapio JS, Ukleja A, Burnes JU, Kelly DG. Outcome of patients with radiation enteritis treated with home parenteral nutrition. *Am J Gastroenterol.* 2002;97: 662–666.
14. Savarese DM, Savy G, Vahdat L, Wischmeyer PE, Corey B. Prevention of chemotherapy and radiation toxicity with glutamine. *Cancer Treat Rev.* 2003;29: 501–513.
15. Anderson PM, Schroeder G, Skubitz KM. Oral glutamine reduces the duration and severity of stomatitis after cytotoxic cancer chemotherapy. *Cancer.* 1998; 83:1433–1439.
16. Huang EY, Leung SW, Wang CJ, Chen HC, Sun LM, Fang FM, Yeh SA, Hsu HC, Hsiung CY. Oral glutamine to alleviate radiation-induced oral mucositis: a pilot randomized trial. *Int J Radiat Oncol Biol Phys.* 2000;34:300–303.
17. Decker GM. Glutamine: indicated in cancer care? *Clin J Oncol Nurs.* 2002;6:112–115.
18. Ertekin MV, Koc M, Karslioglu I, Sezen O. Zinc sulfate in the prevention of radiation-induced oropharyngeal mucositis: a prospective, placebo-controlled, randomized study. *Int J Radiat Oncol Biol Phys.* 2004; 58:167–174.
19. Ripamonti C, Zecca E, Brunelli C, Fulfaro F, Villa S, Balzarini A, Bombardieri E, De Conno F. A randomized, controlled clinical trial to evaluate the effects of zinc sulfate on cancer patients with taste alterations caused by head and neck irradiation. *Cancer.* 1998;82: 1938–1945.
20. Rosenthal DI, Chambers MS, Weber RS, Eisbruch A. A phase II study to assess the efficacy of amifostine for submandibular/sublingual salivary sparing during the treatment of head and neck cancer with intensity modulated radiation therapy for parotid salivary sparing. *Semin Oncol.* 2004;31(6 Suppl 18):25–28.
21. Vacha P, Fehlauer F, Mahlmann B, Marx M, Hinke A, Sommer K, Richter E, Feyerabend T. Randomized phase III trial of postoperative radiochemotherapy +/- amifostine in head and neck cancer. Is there evidence for radioprotection? *Strahlenther Onkol.* 2003;179: 385–389.
22. Anne PR. Phase II trial of subcutaneous amifostine in patients undergoing radiation therapy for head and neck cancer (erratum in *Semin Oncol.* 2003;30:417). *Semin Oncol.* 2002;29(6 Suppl 19):80–83.
23. Brizel DM, Wasserman T, Henke M, Strnad V, Rudat V, Monnier A, Eschwege F, Zhang J, Russell L, Oster W, Sauer R. Phase III randomized trial of amifostine as a radioprotector in head and neck cancer. *J Clin Oncol.* 2000;18:3339–3345.
24. Athanassiou H, Antonadou D, Coliarakis N, Kouveli A, Synodinou M, Paraskevaidis M, Sarris G, Georgakopoulos GR, Panousaki K, Karageorgis P, Throuvalas N. Protective effect of amifostine during fractionated radiotherapy in patients with pelvic carcinomas: results of a randomized trial. *Int J Radiat Oncol Biol Phys.* 2003;56:1154–1160.

Chapter 10

Nutritional Implications of Surgical Oncology

SHEELA THOMAS, MS, RD, CNSD

INTRODUCTION

Surgery is the primary treatment modality for many cancers and can affect the body by mechanical and physiological alterations. The immediate metabolic response to surgery in cancer patients is similar to those who have surgery for benign disease. Commonly experienced side effects of surgery include fatigue, increased calorie and protein needs for wound healing, and temporary alterations in appetite and bowel function caused by anesthesia and analgesia (1). This chapter discusses general nutrition guidelines for all oncological surgery patients, with emphasis on surgical interventions in head and neck cancers and gastrointestinal cancers, as well as nutrition guidelines for commonly experienced postsurgical complications. Surgery to the areodigestive system can affect normal peristalsis, digestion, and absorption, resulting in altered nutritional status. Prompt nutrition assessment and close monitoring pre- and postsurgery is vital to all surgical patients.

MEDICAL NUTRITION THERAPY FOR INDIVIDUALS UNDERGOING SURGERY

Regardless of the site of cancer diagnosis, malnourished individuals undergoing surgery have compromised wound healing and increased morbidity and mortality (2). Individuals who are well nourished have been shown to tolerate surgical interventions with fewer complications than individuals who are malnourished (3). The intent of nutrition support should be to minimize weight loss and to prevent nutrient deficiencies, and nutritional support should continue until the planned anticancer therapy has been completed and healing has occurred (2).

Preoperative Enteral Nutrition Support

The American Dietetic Association's *ADA Pocket Guide to Enteral Nutrition* (4) indicates that the following criteria should be met before initiating preoperative nutrition support:

1. The individual is severely malnourished.
2. There is a demonstrated improvement in clinical outcome as a result of the nutrition support for the surgical procedure.
3. Surgery is either elective or can be safely delayed for 7 to 10 days.

Refer to Chapter 13 for further guidelines on providing enteral nutrition support.

Immune-Enhancing Nutrition Support

In patients undergoing gastrointestinal tract surgery, the use of immune-enhancing nutrition support (eg, enteral formulas supplemented with arginine, n-3 fatty acids, and glutamine) has been shown to reduce postoperative morbidity, as evidenced by fewer infections and decreased length of stay, as well as to reduce the cost of patient care (5–7). Use of immune-enhancing formulas is indicated orally for 5 to 7 days before surgery and for a minimum of 5 days enterally after surgery, to reduce postoperative complications (5).

Parenteral Nutrition

Results of randomized clinical trials have shown no significant benefit in the use of total parenteral nutrition (TPN) in well-nourished or mildly malnourished individuals with cancer who are being treated with surgery, chemotherapy, and/or radiation therapy (2). Of note, in individuals who are severely malnourished undergoing elective major surgery (eg, substantial bowel resection) or receiving intensive therapy associated with bone marrow transplantation, improved clinical outcomes (eg, decreased postoperative complications, improved nutritional markers, and improved mortality rates) have been shown with the use of TPN (2,8). If enteral nutrition support is not tolerated in 5 to 10 days postsurgery, parenteral nutrition may be indicated, to minimize postsurgical complications and to restore and maintain nutritional status (2). Refer to Chapter 14 for further guidelines on providing parenteral nutrition support to individuals who have had significant bowel resections.

PRIMARY CANCER SITES AND SURGERIES

Breast cancer is the most frequently diagnosed cancer in women, and prostate cancer is the most commonly diagnosed cancer in men (9). Cancers of the lung and bronchus are the second most commonly diagnosed cancers in men and women and the leading cause of cancer deaths in both men and women (9). Depending on the stage of an individual's cancer at diagnosis, anticancer therapy includes surgery, radiation therapy, and chemotherapy, or a combination of these therapies. The surgical treatment of the cancers in Table 10.1 does not affect the alimentary tract, but individuals may have complications that will require nutrition management.

WEIGHT LOSS IN PATIENTS WITH VISCERAL ORGAN TUMORS

In the surgical population, weight loss is often more severe in patients with visceral organ tumors (eg, pancreas or stomach cancer), because of changes to normal digestion and absorption, than in those with nonvisceral organ tumors (eg, breast cancer) (1). A recent weight loss of 10% or more has also been shown to increase the incidence of morbidity and mortality in these patients due to protein-calorie malnutrition (1).

HEAD AND NECK CANCERS

Head and neck cancers include cancers of the oral cavity (lip, tongue, and mandible), pharynx, larynx, salivary glands, and sinus (10). Although most head and neck cancers are squamous cell in origin, head and neck cancers also include more rarely found forms of nonsquamous tumors, such as tumors found in sinus and salivary glands (11).

For individuals with head and neck cancers, the location of the tumor may impede appropriate mastication and swallowing long before a diagnosis is made. These individuals often experience substantial weight loss before diagnosis and are at a very high risk for malnutrition and postoperative complications (12,13). Impaired nutrition intake—combined with poor dietary habits and histories of tobacco and alcohol abuse—contributes to the high incidence of malnutrition in this population (13). Weight loss of 10% or more during the 6 months before diagnosis may lead to a significantly higher rate of complications after surgical removal and reconstruction in these patients and may lead to reduced survival rates (14).

Surgical intervention is often the first course of treatment for head and neck cancer, followed by radiation therapy and chemotherapy. Initial nutrition assessment and intervention is recommended before the individual begins cancer treatment (14).

Postsurgical Nutritional Complications

Because of the tumor's location, surgical reconstruction, chemotherapy, and radiation therapy, individuals often experience adverse nutritional effects from treatment of head and neck cancers (see Table 10.2) (15,16). Aggressive nutrition therapy is essential for these individuals and is often required throughout the course of treatment and recovery from treatment. See Table 10.3 (15–18) for nutrition guidelines for common postsurgical complications. With this population of individuals, clinicians must consider their medical and surgical history, psychosocial factors, age, and tobacco and alcohol use.

Table 10.1 Primary Cancer Sites Requiring Surgery

Site of Cancer/Surgery	*Surgical Complications*	*Nutrition Interventions*
Ovarian: abdominal surgery TAH/BSO	• Bloating, cramps, increase in gas • Inability to meet calorie/protein needs • Bowel alterations • Wound healing • Fatigue	• Avoid gassy foods/beverages. • Eat nutrient-dense foods that are easy to prepare. • Alter fiber intake to reduce gas and promote normal bowel function. • Ensure adequate micronutrient consumption, especially vitamin C and zinc.
Prostate: prostatectomy	• Incontinence • Fatigue • Wound healing	• Ensure adequate hydration. • Eat nutrient-dense foods that are easily prepared. • Ensure adequate micronutrient consumption, especially vitamin C, vitamin A, and zinc.
Breast: mastectomy or lumpectomy Spleen: splenectomy Lymph node dissection	• Fatigue • Wound healing	• Eat nutrient-dense foods that are easily prepared. • Ensure adequate micronutrient consumption, especially vitamin C, vitamin A, and zinc.
Brain: brain surgery	• Steroid medication • Nausea/vomiting • Decreased appetite • Fatigue • Wound healing	• Monitor blood glucose levels and avoid simple carbohydrates as necessary. • See Appendix A for symptom management suggestions. • Eat nutrient-dense foods that are easily prepared. • Ensure adequate micronutrient consumption, especially vitamin C, vitamin A, and zinc.

Meticulous attention to oral hygiene and care is important to help keep the mouth clean and healthy during and after radiation therapy and chemotherapy (19). A visit to the dentist for a thorough dental evaluation and teeth cleaning is advised before undergoing therapy, as well as close dental monitoring and follow-up once therapy has been completed (20).

Enteral Nutrition Support

Enteral nutrition support before and after surgical reconstruction may be necessary to provide adequate nutrition and to alleviate or prevent many postoperative complications. Percutaneous endoscopic gastrostomy (PEG) feeding tubes are often placed before or during surgery, to provide enteral nutrition access (21). Many individuals with head and neck cancer have more advanced-stage disease at the time of diagnosis and require chemotherapy and radiation therapy after surgery. Placing a PEG feeding tube at the time of surgery and before additional antineoplastic therapy can provide access for nutrition support if the combination of side effects from surgery and chemotherapy and radiation therapy make swallowing difficult or unsafe (eg, odynophagia or risk of aspiration) (21). A PEG placement has a low complication rate and is a viable option for individuals undergoing head and neck surgery, reconstruction, and chemotherapy and radiation therapy (22,23). In addition, the placement of a feeding tube before the initiation of radiation and chemotherapy is recommended, to help prevent dehydration and delays in treatment (21).

Table 10.2 Nutritional Complications After Head and Neck Cancer Surgery

Surgery	*Compromised Swallowing and Aspiration Potential*	*Delayed Swallowing (> 10 sec)*	*Dysphagia, Odynophagia, Postoperative Swelling*	*Dental Extraction/ Altered Dentition*	*Dry Mouth, Altered Taste*	*Inability to Meet Energy Needs*
Base of tongue resection	X		X			X
Total glossectomy	X	X	X			X
Partial glossectomy	X		X			
Floor of mouth resection		X	X	X		X
Hypopharyngeal resection	X	X	X			X
Total laryngectomy		X	X			X
Partial laryngectomy	X		X			X
Total maxillectomy	X		X			X
Pharyngolaryngectomy		X	X			X
Oropharyngeal resection	X	X	X	X		X
Nasopharyngeal resection		X	X	X		X
Mandibulectomy			X	X	X	X
Buccal/mucosal resection			X	X	X	
Loss of 7th cranial nerve	X	X				X
Thyroidectomy			X		X	

Source: Data are from references 15 and 16.

Table 10.3 Nutritional Complications and Guidelines After Head and Neck Cancer Surgery

Complication	*Guidelines*
Compromised swallowing and aspiration potential	• Avoid sticky, bulky, or thin fluids and foods that crumble. • Use thickening agent in liquids. • Use pureed thick liquid diet. • Use supplemental tube feeding if intake by mouth is $< 60\%$ of estimated needs.
Delayed swallowing (> 10 sec)	• Mandatory nasogastric tube feeding for first 10-21days • Begin oral diet at 10 days if palatal drop* is present. • Goal is to maintain weight and prevent weight loss while maintaining adequate hydration.
Placement of obturator† or palatal drop prosthesis*	• Full liquid and pureed foods are allowed once packing is removed, 2 to 3 days after surgery.
Dental extractions	• Modify food texture. • Assess long-term dental prognosis and provide appropriate instruction for texture alteration, recipes for home, and mouth and dental care management. • Discuss with dental team appropriate timing of dentures. (Most patients receiving radiation therapy are advised that they will have to wait 1 year before denture fitting, if there are no sores, exposed bony tissue, or signs of recurrence.) • Educate the patient and caregiver on the importance of consuming adequate protein and energy while the oral surgery site is healing, with the goal of weight maintenance.
Dysphagia, odynophagia, postoperative swelling	• Consider moist foods or pureed foods if significant pain and swelling. • Avoid highly spiced, acidic, and abrasive foods. • Use liquid supplements and shakes. • To prevent dehydration, keep track of amount of fluids consumed daily.
Dry mouth/altered taste	• Frequent liquids. • Soft/moist meals. • Avoid dry foods, such as bread, toast, pancakes. • For altered taste, take zinc sulfate lozenges (45 mg zinc sulfate 3 times/day). • Dental and mouth care management. • Frequently rinse mouth, especially before and after eating. • Carry drink bottle at all times. • To ensure adequate hydration needs are being met, keep track of amount of fluids consumed daily.
Inability to meet energy needs before surgery	• Perioperative enteral feedings.‡ • Parenteral nutrition with nonfunctioning GI tract, presence of pharyngocutaneous or chylous fistula.§

*A removable bridge that fits contour of palate; reduces palatal height to enable food mastication and speech in patients with speech and dental impairment.

†Synthetic customized removable device of varying form and function, which may be used in head and neck cancer patients to aid in speech and swallowing.

‡See Chapter 13.

§See Chapter 14.

Source: Data are from references 15–18.

For additional information on enteral nutrition, see Chapter 13.

Monitoring

Individuals with head and neck cancer must be monitored closely throughout treatment and for up to 1 year after treatment. After intensive radiation therapy and chemotherapy, individuals may experience swallowing difficulties (dysphagia and odynophagia) or dry mouth (xerostomia) and may need additional modifications to the consistency and texture of foods and beverages for 1 year or more (24,25). Surgical interventions to the head and neck can also result in lasting alterations in swallowing ability, and individuals may benefit from a referral to a speech pathologist for assessment and evaluation of swallowing function and risk of aspiration (26). To alleviate treatment-related xerostomia, the use of over-the-counter oral moisturizers and saliva substitutes can help to moisten and lubricate the oral cavity (19,20).

GASTROINTESTINAL CANCERS

Gastrointestinal (GI) cancers include esophageal cancer, gastric cancer, pancreatic cancer, liver cancer, carcinoma of the gall bladder, carcinoma of the bile duct, cancer of the small bowel, and colorectal cancer. For most GI cancers, surgery is the primary treatment modality.

Individuals who have had GI surgeries may experience a wide range of nutritional complications (see Table 10.4) (27). Table 10.5 (2,18,28–34) outlines appropriate nutrition interventions for these complications.

ESOPHAGEAL CANCER

Most malignant esophageal tumors are either squamous cell carcinomas or adenocarcinomas (35). Squamous cell carcinomas can develop anywhere along the length of the esophagus, and adenocarcinomas most frequently originate in the lower esophagus (36). Increased risk of esophageal cancer has been associated with tobacco and alcohol abuse (37).

Esophagectomy remains the standard of care of treatment for individuals diagnosed with esophageal cancer, although combined modality therapy using chemotherapy and radiation therapy with or without surgery is currently being evaluated through controlled clinical trials (38). Surgical treatment consists of removing the diseased portion of the esophagus (39,40). Complications of surgical resection of the esophagus include anastomotic leaks, wound infection, laryngeal nerve injury, and bleeding. Endoscopic laser therapy (ELT) is used in noncircumferential lesions in the middle or distal esophagus. The most common complication is esophageal perforation.

Refer to Tables 10.4 and 10.5 for common nutritional complications and appropriate nutrition interventions. Additional complications associated with esophagectomy may include stricture, dysmotility, early satiety, vomiting, and the need for neoadjuvant therapies (eg, chemotherapy and radiation therapy), all of which can affect nutritional status (33). Jejunostomy tube feedings are often used for at least 10 to 14 days after surgery and is tapered when an individual's intake by mouth is at least 75% of the estimated nutrition needed. Gastrostomy tubes may not be indicated if the distal esophagus and the gastroesophageal junction (lower esophageal sphincter) are altered or surgically removed.

Dysphagia occurs in more than 90% of the patients with esophageal cancer (41). Malnutrition and associated weight losses from dysphagia are common (33). Photodynamic therapy (PDT) is a treatment option for dysphagia and is used as a means to palliate obstructing esophageal carcinomas (42). PDT is used in tumors near the cricopharyngeus area that are more than 10 cm long. Skin photosensitivity and fistula formation are the side effects of this treatment. Self-expanding metallic stents are sometimes placed to help with dysphagia associated with end-stage disease. Complications include stent migration, perforation, and occlusion (41).

GASTRIC CANCER

Adenocarcinomas account for 95% of gastric cancers (43). Although the incidence of gastric cancer below the gastric cardia has decreased significantly over the last century, there has been a significant increase in the incidence of proximal gastric and gastroesophageal junction adenocarcinomas since the mid 1980s (44). Some of the factors associated with the increased risk of developing gastric cancer are high salt and nitrate consumption, poor food preparation and lack of refrigeration, and cigarette smoking, as well as *Helicobacter pylori* infection (45). Dietary factors believed to lower the risk of gastric cancer are diets rich in vitamins A

Table 10.4 Nutritional Complications After Gastrointestinal Surgery

Type of Surgery	*Gastro-paresis*	*Fat Mal-absorption*	*Hyper-glycemia*	*Hyper-triglyceri-demia*	*Encepha-lopathy*	*Fluid-Electrolyte Imbalance*	*Anasto-motic Leak*	*Chyle Leak*	*Dumping Syndrome*	*Vitamin Malabsorption*	*Mineral Malabsorption*
Esophagastric	X					X	X	X	X		
Gastric	X	X	X						X	B-12, D	Iron, calcium
Pancreas	X	X	X			X	X	X	X	A, D, E, K, B-12	Iron, calcium, zinc
Hepatocellular			X	X	X	X		X		A, D, E, K, B-12, folic acid	Magnesium, zinc
Gall bladder	X	X	X			X		X		B-12, A, D, E, K	Iron, calcium, zinc
Bile duct	X	X	X			X		X		B-12, A, D, E, K	Iron, calcium, zinc
Small bowel	X	X	X			X		X		B-12, A, D, E, K	Iron, calcium, zinc
Colon or rectum						X				B-12	Sodium, potassium, magnesium, calcium

Source: Data are from reference 27.

Table 10.5 Nutrition Suggestions for Complications of Gastrointestinal Surgery

Complications	*Management Suggestions*
Gastroparesis, gastric stasis, gastric reflux	*For individuals with tube feedings:* • Continue tube feeding until patient is able to meet more than 70% to 75% of assessed nutrition requirements by oral intake alone. • Feeding JT can be placed during surgery. Tube feeding is initiated postoperatively and advanced as tolerated. Feeding pump with frequent water flushes is recommended. • Formula selection depends on type of surgery, development of complications, and intolerance. For esophageal and gastric cancer, a polymeric high-protein formula can be used. For pancreas, duodenal, bile duct, and gall bladder surgeries, a low-fat, high-MCT formula may be used, because of possible fat malabsorption. MCT absorption occurs directly into the portal circulation without hydrolysis with pancreatic lipase. Tube feeding regimen should achieve optimal glucose control. May use ½ tsp Viokase powder* per 240 mL tube feeding for steatorrhea.
	In the absence of tube feedings: • A GT can be placed to drain stomach contents. With improvement in gastric motility, GT can be clamped. An oral diet can then be initiated and advanced, as tolerated, from clear liquids to six regular, small feedings. Patient is discharged on a regular diet of six small meals. High-fiber foods should be avoided. • Patient should not eat 2-3 hours before bedtime. • Foods that are high in fat or hard to digest should be avoided. • Patient should keep head and shoulders elevated above stomach. • Patient should avoid tight clothing around the waist.
Fat malabsorption (steatorrhea)	• Pancreatic enzymes: Pancreatic lipase is needed for the hydrolysis of most dietary fat. Oral pancreatic enzyme replacement can partially correct pancreatic insufficiency, so dietary restriction of fat may not always be necessary. Enzymes need to be used with meals and snacks. • Low-fat diet: Fat malabsorption due to decreased secretion of bile salts is treated with a low-fat diet and use of MCT oil.
Hyperglycemia	• Antihyperglycemics: Hyperglycemia should be controlled by an oral hypoglycemic agent and/or insulin. • Patient should avoid added sweets and concentrated sweets.
Hypertriglyceridemia	*For individuals on TPN:* • Avoid overfeeding with TPN. 25–35 kcal/kg body weight is recommended. • Do not administer IV lipids if triglycerides are > 400 mg/dL. • If triglycerides are > 400 mg/dL for ≥ 2 weeks, provide 1 g IV lipid per kg body weight twice weekly over 24 hours (to prevent the onset of EFA deficiency).
Hepatic encephalopathy	• Provide adequate energy and protein to facilitate hepatic cell nutrition without excess production of ammonia from endogenous and exogenous protein catabolism. • Protein: For acute hepatic encephalopathy, begin with 0.5 g protein/kg/day and increase to 1–1.5 g protein/kg/day. Protein intake should be calculated using the patient's ideal body weight. • Energy: Daily energy intake is commonly calculated at 30–35 kcal/kg/day.

(*continued*)

Table 10.5 Nutrition Suggestions for Complications of Gastrointestinal Surgery *(continued)*

Complications	*Management Suggestions*
Fluid and electrolyte balance	• Ensure adequate intake of fluids and electrolytes as monitoring indicates. • Fluid intake should be increased if the patient has fluid losses secondary to nasogastric or gastrostomy output or vomiting and diarrhea. • A fluid restriction is indicated in the presence of dilutional hyponatremia; with fluid limited to 1,000-1,500 mL/day. Sodium is often restricted to further aid in diuresis. • Electrolyte requirements are often increased if the patient is experiencing diarrhea secondary to intestinal resection. Closely monitor electrolytes needs: sodium, potassium, magnesium, calcium, and zinc.
Anastomotic leak/breakdown	• Full nutrition support via JT or TPN (if no enteral access is available distal to the leak) is recommended.
Chyle leak (if thoracic duct or lymph accidentally nicked during surgery)	• Patient should take minimal to no fat by mouth or enterally. • Enteral feeding formula should have minimal fat and/or be high in MCT oil. • Consider MCT supplementation. (MCT oil is an absorbable form of fat, which bypasses lymphatic absorption and goes directly to portal circulation). • Patient may require TPN.
Dumping syndrome	• Avoid hyperosmolar feedings (limit concentrated carbohydrates) to help with both early and late dumping. • Patient should consume foods that are high in protein and complex carbohydrates. • Small, more frequent meals and snacks throughout the day are recommended. • Patient should take liquids 30–60 minutes before and after meals. If early satiety is affecting food intake, suggest drinking fluids after meals. Patients with gas should avoid carbonated beverages. • Limit very cold or very hot foods. • Foods high in pectin (apples, bananas, oatmeal, rice, potatoes) or 1 tsp pectin 3 times a day may help reduce transit time. • Patient should minimize activities and lie down after a meal; this may reduce the transit time of food. • Encourage patient to eat slowly in a relaxed atmosphere. • Use of pancreatic enzyme may be helpful in total gastrectomy patients. • Monitor weight and use nocturnal tube feedings into jejunum if needed.
Vitamins	• For a patient experiencing steatorrhea, a supplement containing fat-soluble vitamins is indicated. • Monitor patient for vitamin B-12 and folic acid deficiency. Patients with these deficiencies may be supplemented intramuscularly, orally, or nasally after gastrectomy and pancreaticoduodenectomy. Vitamin B-12 deficiency can be treated with monthly injections of 100 mg. • Vitamin D absorption can be altered after duodenal bypass or gastrectomy; therefore, supplementation is recommended.
Minerals	• Calcium absorption can be altered after duodenal bypass or gastrectomy; therefore, supplementation is recommended. Monitor patient for metabolic bone disease and osteopenia/osteoporosis. • Calcium oxalate stones may develop after colorectal surgery. Encourage increased fluid intake. Restrict high-oxalate foods, if indicated. • Monitor patient for microcytic anemia, and supplement with iron if indicated based on laboratory analysis (eg, serum iron studies). In patients requiring iron supplementation, intake of vitamin C-containing foods should be encouraged to enhance oral iron absorption.

Abbreviations: GT, gastrostomy tube; JT, jejunostomy tube; MCT, medium-chain triglycerides; TPN, total parenteral nutrition.
*Axcan Scandipharm, Birmingham, AL 35242.

Source: Data are from references 2, 18, and 28–34.

and C, and micronutrients such as selenium, zinc, copper, iron, and manganese (46). Individuals diagnosed with gastric cancer often present with early satiety, weight loss, anorexia, and gastric pain (2).

Surgery is the most common treatment for gastric cancer. Surgical intervention, in combination with chemotherapy and radiation therapy, is frequently used preoperatively or postoperatively to improve disease control and survival (43). Surgery is also a common palliative approach. Surgical options include distal subtotal gastrectomy, proximal subtotal gastrectomy, or total gastrectomy. The gastrointestinal tract is maintained by anastomosis of the small intestine to the gastric remnant, distal stomach to the esophagus, and small intestine to the esophagus (with or without jejunal reservoirs).

Refer to Tables 10.4 and 10.5 for common nutritional complications and appropriate nutrition interventions. Dumping syndrome is the most commonly recognized complication postgastrectomy (2). The severity of the syndrome depends on the rate of gastric emptying. Dumping syndrome can be classified as early or late, based on the time elapsed after a meal and the development of symptoms. Early dumping syndrome may occur anywhere from 15 to 60 minutes postprandial and can cause both GI and vasomotor symptoms (29,47). These symptoms may be due to the loss of reservoir function of the stomach, which results in rapid emptying of hyperosmolar contents into the small bowel (29,47). Vasomotor symptoms include fatigue, tachycardia, faintness, diaphoresis, headache, flushing, difficulty concentrating, hunger, and desire to lie down. GI symptoms include abdominal cramps, diarrhea, nausea, vomiting, and early satiety (29,47). Late dumping may occur 1 to 3 hours after a meal and is attributed to reactive hypoglycemia caused by rapid absorption of glucose and resultant hyperinsulinemia response (29,47). Symptoms may be mainly vasomotor in nature.

Other postgastrectomy intolerances and deficiencies include lactose intolerance, fat malabsorption, anemia, metabolic bone disease, and gastric stasis. Exocrine pancreatic enzyme supplementation might reduce fecal fat excretion. The most common nutrient deficiencies associated with this condition include fat-soluble vitamins, vitamin B-12, iron, and calcium (29). Folate deficiency secondary to vitamin B-12 deficiency should also be monitored and treated with oral or intramuscular supplements (29).

PANCREATIC CANCER

Approximately 90% of the pancreatic exocrine cancer originates from pancreatic duct epithelium, and 80% of these are adenocarcinomas. Sixty percent to seventy percent of pancreatic adenocarcinomas arise in the head of the pancreas (1). A very rare type of pancreatic cancer that begins in the cells of islets of Langerhans is called islet cell cancer or endocrine cancer (48).

Eighty percent of individuals diagnosed with pancreatic cancer have lost 15% of preillness weight at the time of diagnosis (49). Malabsorption (resulting from pancreatic enzyme deficiency due to pancreatic duct obstruction) and anorexia result in progressive weight loss. Tumor obstruction in the ampulla of Vater or common bile duct may also cause malabsorption and nutritional deterioration due to bile insufficiency (2,33). Glucose intolerance is also common in individuals diagnosed with pancreatic cancer (50). The combined effects of the anatomic location, endocrine and exocrine hormonal insufficiency, and treatment-related toxicity puts individuals at high risk for developing symptoms that affect their ability to eat and absorb adequate nutrition (51). Severe peripheral muscle wasting, involuntary weight loss, anemia, and anorexia resulting in cancer cachexia are major reasons for the increased morbidity and mortality in these patients.

Although surgery offers the best chance of a cure, approximately 80% of individuals are ineligible for a curative procedure at the time of presentation (52). For those patients who are eligible, surgical intervention is used in the following ways (52):

- For solid tumors without evidence of metastasis
- As palliative treatment in obstructive disease that has failed nonoperative regimens
- For patients after chemoradiation that has responded with shrinkage of tumor and a clear vein

Types of Surgery

The most commonly used surgical procedure to remove the exocrine cancer of the pancreas is the Whipple procedure or a pancreaticoduodenectomy. The standard Whipple procedure is removal of the head of the pancreas, duodenum, distal stomach, and a portion of bile duct (1,48,53). Pylorus-preserving pancreatoduodenectomy (PPPD) is a modification of the standard Whipple procedure, where distal gastrectomy is not performed. This procedure may be used instead of the Whipple procedure, because PPPD provides multiple benefits, including the preservation of the stomach, which decreases the incidence of stomal ulceration and dumping syndrome, improves postoperative nutritional status, and helps control diabetes mellitus (54,55). One of the drawbacks associated with PPPD procedure is that some patients experience a temporary inability to empty the stomach after digestion and this may result in a longer period of hospitalization after surgery (54,55).

Postsurgical Nutritional Complications

For postsurgical nutritional complications, refer to Table 10.4. Nutrition interventions are outlined in Table 10.5. The most common nutritional complications after the Whipple procedure include early satiety, delayed gastric emptying, anastomotic leak, diarrhea, dumping, ulceration, and bile acid reflux gastritis (33). After surgery, patients may require gastric decompression because of delayed gastric emptying. Frequent, small feeding will be helpful in patients with early satiety.

Jejunal Enteral Nutrition Support

Jejunal enteral nutrition support may be necessary until oral intake is adequate. Jejunal feedings for 4 to 6 weeks after surgery is common (34). Use of an enteral formula low in fat and/or with MCT oil may be better tolerated because of pancreatic exocrine deficiency.

Malabsorption

About 25% of patients who undergo a Whipple procedure may also have malabsorption due to deficiency in exocrine pancreatic secretions (56). Oral pancreatic enzyme replacement can partially correct pancreatic insufficiency, so dietary restriction of fat may not always be necessary (18). Supplementation with 30,000 to 40,000 U of lipase, which is needed for the hydrolysis of most dietary fat, will be beneficial with each meal (34). Monitoring of glucose levels is essential, and insulin may be required (2). Conventional dietary restrictions may need to be liberalized to achieve adequate caloric intake (2).

CANCERS OF THE LIVER

Hepatocellular carcinoma is the most common type of primary liver cancer in adults (57). The liver is also the most common site of metastasis. Other types of malignant liver tumors include angiosarcomas, cholangiocarcinomas, and hepatoblastomas in children. Conditions that are associated with predisposing individuals to the development of liver cancer include injury to liver: hepatitis virus B or C infection, cirrhosis, chemical carcinogens (eg, alcohol abuse and aflatoxin), and metabolic diseases such as hemachromatosis (58). Individuals diagnosed with cancers of the liver can present with anorexia, nausea and vomiting, weight loss, steatorrhea, diarrhea, jaundice, ascites, and abnormal liver function tests.

Surgical resection of liver cancer often requires removal of significant liver tissue and is associated with high rates of morbidity and mortality (33). Surgical resection of metastatic liver lesions is beneficial in patients with colorectal cancer and Wilms' tumor. (57).

For postsurgical nutritional complications, refer to Table 10.4. Nutrition interventions are outlined in Table 10.5. Hypophosphatemia is commonly seen after major liver resections and is associated with increased cardiorespiratory complications, infections, and hemorrhages (33,59). The exact mechanism is not understood but may be due partly to regeneration of the liver. Phosphorous levels may be lowest on postoperative day 2, and patients with phosphorus levels ≤ 1.5 mg/dL are at increased risk for more complications and increased length of stay (58).

Other nutrition issues include hepatic encephalopathy and ascites. Treatment for hepatic encephalopathy includes providing adequate calories and protein to facilitate hepatic cell nutrition without excess production of ammonia from endogenous and exogenous protein catabolism. Thirty to thirty-five kcal/kg/day and 1 to 1.5 g/kg of protein using dry weight are adequate (18). In the presence of encephalopathy, protein may be restricted to 0.6 to 0.8 g/kg dry weight. Nutrition therapy for ascites commonly includes a restriction of sodium to 2 to 4 g/day and fluid to 1 to 1.5 L/day (60). The amount of sodium and fluid allowed each day is dependent on the severity of the ascites.

CARCINOMA OF THE GALL BLADDER

Gallbladder cancer is rare in the United States (61), and its incidence is believed to be related to cholelithiasis and exposure to chemical carcinogens (62). Gall bladder tumors can be resected in 15% to 30% of cases (41). Surgical treatment is based on the extent of the disease and is usually treated with cholecystectomy, liver resection, and lymphadenectomy (57). Surgical implications and nutrition interventions are similar to pancreas and hepatocellular cancer (see Table 10.5).

CARCINOMA OF THE BILE DUCT

Cancer of the bile duct (cholangiocarcinoma) is rare, and because of its proximity to the pancreas and liver, surgical intervention usually includes pancreatic and hepatic resections or both (63). Most patients are diagnosed in advanced stages, and, therefore, palliative management to relieve symptoms of biliary obstruction is required (eg, low-fat diet and avoidance of gas-forming foods and beverages) (41,64). The surgical implications and nutrition interventions are similar to those for patients with liver and pancreatic cancer (see Tables 10.4 and 10.5).

CANCER OF THE SMALL BOWEL

Malignant neoplasms of the small bowel include adenocarcinoma, carcinoid, non-Hodgkin's lymphoma, leiomyosarcoma, liposarcoma, myxoliposarcoma, and lymphangiosarcoma (65). Although small-bowel cancer is rare, metastatic lesions from other sites can occur. Metastasis from the colon, pancreas, lungs, breast, malignant melanoma, stomach, liver, ovary, and appendix are the most common (65). Malignancies are most frequently found in the lower duodenum and in the lower ileum. Individuals with malignant tumors have symptoms that can include bowel pain, obstruction, weight loss, bleeding, and perforation (66).

Surgical resection with negative margins is the main form of treatment in most small-bowel neoplasms (65). Side effects depend on the length of the resection and the ability of the small bowel to adapt. The degree of malabsorption increases with the length of resection (67).

Jejunal resections result in hyperplasia of the ileum and assumption of proximate absorptive functions except jejunal enterohormone secretions (67). Terminal ileal resection greater than 100 cm and/or loss of ileocecal valve results in steatorrhea and impaired absorption of fat, fat-soluble vitamins, and Vitamin B-12 (67). It is also necessary to monitor and supplement calcium and zinc (67). Surgical implications and nutrition interventions are similar to pancreaticoduodenectomy (see Tables 10.4 and 10.5).

COLORECTAL CANCER

Cancers of the colon and rectum are the third most common cancers among American men and women (9). Individuals with colorectal cancers can experience symptoms such as changes in bowel habits, rectal bleeding, and pain and cramping in their lower abdomens. Risk factors for the development of colorectal cancer are 50 years of age or older, personal or family history of polyps, and history of inflammatory bowel disease (68). Lifestyle risk factors for colorectal cancer include diets high in saturated fat and red meat, alcohol consumption, poor intake of vegetables and fruits, physical inactivity, and smoking (9).

Surgery is the most common treatment for colon and rectal cancers. A colectomy with resection of paracolonic lymph nodes is performed in cases of neoplastic polyps that show invasion to muscularis mucosae or the vascular system, or when the polyps contain poorly differentiated tumor cells. Resection of the tumor and primary anastomosis is the most common procedure used in cancers of the colon and upper third of the rectum (65). Colostomies are usually not needed in colon cancer and are seen more in rectal cancer resections. If the tumor is within 2 to 3 cm of the anus, and if the sphincter muscles and rectum are resected, permanent colostomies are needed (65). Temporary colostomies may be reversed with a second surgery in 3 to 6 months. If proctocolectomy is indicated, an ileal pouch-anal anastomosis (IPAA) or ileoanal anastomosis is usually performed. These procedures can replace ileostomies as long as the rectal sphincter muscles are intact. The pouch is made from the small bowel above the anus, to collect waste material. This enables normal passage of bowel movements but will be more frequent and watery. If anus and rectal sphincter muscles are removed, a permanent ostomy is indicated. A permanent colostomy is also needed with pelvic exenteration (68).

Ostomies can promote high losses of fluid and electrolytes. These losses are usually related to location of the ostomy and functional ability of the remaining GI tract. Ileostomies cause greater losses of fluid than colostomies, because the colon is bypassed (major site of fluid absorption) (69). Fluid and electrolyte

Box 10.1

Ileostomy Diet Guidelines

1. Eat small, frequent, balanced meals at regular times.
2. Eat slowly, thoroughly chewing food.
3. Avoid foods that caused problems before surgery for 4–6 weeks after surgery, to minimize complications associated with stoma blockage and gas.
4. To reduce ostomy output at night, avoid high-fiber foods at dinnertime and eat main meal at lunchtime.
5. Add new foods to the diet gradually. Try 1–2 tablespoons of a new food to assess tolerance. If a food is not tolerated, write this down and try the food again in another month. Try only one new food at a time. Try each food several times before giving up on it.
6. Introduce milk products slowly and in small amounts. Try cultured yogurt, buttermilk, or cottage cheese first.
7. Drink plenty of caffeine-free fluids, and dilute juices with water or club soda.
8. Avoid high-fiber foods, such as broccoli, brussels sprouts, cabbage, celery, Chinese greens, dried fruits, fruit and vegetable skins, nuts, popcorn, poppy seeds, and sesame seeds, for 4 to 6 weeks after surgery.
9. Try these stool-thickening snack foods: applesauce, bananas, creamy peanut butter, marshmallows, pretzels, white rice, and tapioca.
10. Try these foods that contain soluble fiber, which helps to slow down diarrhea by forming a gel: acorn squash, applesauce, apricots, asparagus tips, bananas, barley, beets, canned fruits, carrots, peeled apples, cornflakes, cornbread, grits, oat bran, peas, boiled rice, rutabaga, potatoes, summer squash, tapioca, turnips, and zucchini.
11. Avoid these foods that may increase output: caffeine, some fruits and juices, especially prune juice and licorice, some dairy foods, rich foods such as gravies and cream sauces, whole grains, wheat bran, nuts and seeds, broccoli, cabbage, cauliflower, brussels sprouts, and spicy foods.
12. Avoid these foods that may increase odors: dried peas and beans, asparagus, broccoli, brussels sprouts, cabbage, cauliflower, eggs, fish, garlic, onions, sauerkraut, spicy foods, strong cheeses, and turnips.
13. Avoid the following foods that may increase gas production: beans, beer, broccoli, brussels sprouts, cabbage, radishes, onions, carbonated drinks, cauliflower, bleu cheese, corn, cucumbers, melons, milk, mushrooms, peas, Roquefort cheese, spinach, turnips, asparagus, sweet potatoes, turkey, prunes, apples, raisins, bananas, foods that are high in fat (eg, deep-fried or greasy foods), and very sweet foods such as frosting or heavy syrups.
14. If bile acid deficiency occurs from major ileal resection, then a low-fat diet with MCT oil supplementation may be needed.

Source: Data are from reference 69.

balance should be monitored closely. Additional fluids, sodium, potassium, magnesium, calcium, and zinc may be required if the ostomy output is high. Output may also be excessive with macronutrient malabsorption (69). Bile salt deficiency is common after an ileal resection. It is often necessary to restrict dietary fat and supplement with MCT oil (69). Colostomies may have little effect on stool output if much of the colon is still functional; ileostomies, on the other hand, can be expected to produce stool with a more liquid consistency (69).

Patients with colostomies at the ascending colon will need to follow an ileostomy diet for 6 to 8 weeks after surgery. This diet eliminates high-fiber foods that increase risk of obstruction, such as nuts, skins, seeds, popcorn, raw fruits, raw vegetables, and dried fruits. For common postsurgical nutritional complications and appropriate interventions, see Tables 10.4 and 10.5. See Box 10.1 (68) for nutrition guidelines for ileostomy care.

Other modalities of anticancer therapy, such as chemotherapy and radiation therapy, are commonly prescribed before or after surgery for individuals who have colorectal cancers that have spread to their lymph nodes or have invaded the bowel wall (68). For individuals with metastatic colorectal cancers, novel new targeted therapies have recently been approved by the Food and Drug Administration (9).

REFERENCES

1. Feig BW, Berger DH, Fuhrman GM, eds. *The MD Anderson Surgical Oncology Handbook.* 2nd ed. Philadelphia, Pa: Lippincott Williams and Wilkins; 1999:478–483.
2. Barrera R. Nutrition support in cancer patients. *JPEN J Parenter Enteral Nutr.* 2002;26(suppl 5):S63-S71.
3. Campos A, Mequid M. A critical appraisal of the usefulness of perioperative nutritional support. *Am J Clin Nutr.* 55;117–130.
4. Thompson C. Initiation, advancement, and transition of enteral feedings. In: Charney P, Malone A, eds. *ADA Pocket Guide to Enteral Nutrition.* Chicago, Ill: American Dietetic Association; 2005;123–154.
5. Sax HC. Effect of immune enhancing formulas (IEF) in general surgery patients. *JPEN J Parenter Enteral Nutr.* 2001;25(suppl 2):S19-S22.
6. Braga M, Gianotti L. Preoperative immunonutrition: cost-benefit analysis. *JPEN J Parenter Enteral Nutr.* 2005;29(suppl 1):S57-S61.
7. Gianotti L, Braga M, Nespoli L, Radaelli G, Beneduce A, Di Carlo V. A randomized controlled trial of preoperative oral supplementation with a specialized diet in patients with gastrointestinal cancer. *Gastroenterology.* 2002;122:1763–1770.
8. Sundaram A, Koutkia P, Apovian CM. Nutritional management of short bowel syndrome in adults. *J Clin Gastroenterol.* 2002:34;207–220.
9. American Cancer Society. *Cancer Facts and Figures 2005.* Atlanta, Ga: American Cancer Society; 2005.
10. Gibson MK, Forastier AA. Multidisciplinary approaches to the management of advanced head and neck tumors: state of the art. *Curr Opin Oncol.* 2004; 16:220–224.
11. Licitra L, Locati LD, Bossi P, Cantu G. Head and neck tumors other than squamous cell carcinoma. *Curr Opin Oncol.* 2004,16.236–241.
12. Van Bokhorst-de van der Schueren MA, van Leeuwen PA, Sauerwein HP, Kuik DJ, Snow GB, Quak JJ. Assessment of malnutrition parameters in head and neck cancer and their relation to postoperative complications. *Head Neck.* 1997;19:419–425.
13. Van Bokhorst-de van der Schueren MA, van Leeuwen PA, Kuik DJ, Klop WM, Sauerwein HP, Snow GB, Quak JJ. The impact of nutritional status on the prognoses of patients with advanced head and neck cancer. *Cancer.* 1999;86:519–527.
14. Hammerlid E, Wirblad B, Sandin C, Mercke C, Edsrom S, Kaasa S, Sullivan M, Westin T. Malnutrition and food intake in relation to quality of life in head and neck cancer patients. *Head Neck.* 1998;20:540–548.
15. McClure S. *Nutritional Management of the Head and Neck Cancer Patient.* Houston, Tex: University of Texas MD Anderson Cancer Center, Department of Clinical Nutrition; 1997.
16. Kyle U. The patient with head and neck cancer. In: Bloch AS, ed. *Nutrition Management of the Cancer Patient.* Rockville, Md: American Society for Parenteral and Enteral Nutrition; 1990:53–64.
17. Ripamonti C, Zecca E, Brunneli C, Fulfaro F, Villa S, Balzarini A, Bombardieri E, Conno FD. A randomized, controlled clinical trial to evaluate the effects of zinc sulfate on cancer patients with taste alterations caused by head and neck irradiation. *Cancer.* 1998;82:1938–1945.
18. ASPEN. *The Science and Practice of Nutrition Support: A Case-Based Core Curriculum.* Dubuque, Iowa: Kendall/Hunt Publishing; 2001.
19. Iwamoto RR. Xerostomia. In: Groenwald SL, Goodman M, Frogge MH, Yarbo CH, eds. *Cancer Symptom Management.* Sudbury, Mass: Jones & Bartlett; 1996: 252–258.
20. Oncology Reference Guide to Oral Health: Prevention and management of oral complication from head and neck therapy, chemotherapy, and blood and marrow transplant. National Oral Health Information Clearinghouse. Available at: http://www.nohic.nidcr.nih.gov. Accessed October 28, 2005.
21. Scolapio JS, Spangler PR, Romano MM, McLaughlin MP, Salassa JR. Prophylactic placement of gastrostomy feeding tubes before radiotherapy in patients with head and neck cancer: is it worthwhile? *J Clin Gastroenterol.* 2001;33:215–217.
22. Schweinfurth JM, Boger GN, Feustel PJ. Preoperative risk assessment for gastrostomy tube placement in head and neck cancer patients. *Head Neck.* 2001;23: 276–382.
23. Chandu A, Smith AC, Douglas M. Percutaneous endoscopic gastrostomy in patients undergoing resection for oral tumors: a retrospective review of complications and outcomes. *J Oral Maxillofac Surg.* 2003;61: 1279–1284.
24. List MA, Siston A, Haraf D, Schumm P, Kies M, Stenson K, Vokes EE. Quality of life and performance in advanced head and neck cancer patients on concomitant chemoradiotherapy: a prospective examination. *J Clin Oncol.* 1999;17:1020–1028.
25. Deleyiannis FW, Weymuller EA Jr, Coltrera MD. Quality of life of disease-free survivors of advanced

(stage III or IV) oropharyngeal cancer. *Head Neck.* 1997;19:466–473.

26. Barbour LA. Dysphagia. In: Groenwald SL, Goodman M, Frogge MH, Yarbo CH, eds. *Cancer Symptom Management*. Sudbury, Mass: Jones & Bartlett; 1996:197–218.
27. Bloch AS. Nutrition implications in esophageal and gastric cancer. In: Bloch AS, ed. *Nutrition Management of the Cancer Patient.* Rockville, Md: American Society for Parenteral and Enteral Nutrition; 1990: 73–83.
28. Vokes EE, Weichseibaum RR, Lippman SM, Hong WK. Head and neck cancer. *N Engl J Med.* 1993;328: 184–194.
29. American Dietetic Association, Dietitians of Canada. Gastric surgery. In: *Manual of Clinical Dietetics.* 6th ed. Chicago, Ill: American Dietetic Association; 2000:397–400.
30. University of Pittsburgh Medical Center. Dumping syndrome diet. Available at: http://patienteducation.upmc.com/Pdf/DumpingSynDiet.pdf. Accessed April 26, 2005.
31. Grant JP, Chapman G, Russell MK. Malabsorption associated with surgical procedures and its treatment. *Nutr Clin Pract.* 1996;11:43–52.
32. Nelson JK, Moxness KE, Jensen MD, Gastineau CF. *Mayo Clinic Diet Manual: A Handbook of Nutrition Practice.* 7th ed. St Louis, Mo: Mosby; 1994.
33. Wong PW, Enriquez A, Barrera R. Nutrition support in critically ill patients with cancer. *Crit Care Clin.* 2001;17:743–767.
34. Baradi H, Walsh RM, Henderson JM, Vogt D, Popovich M. Postoperative jejunal feeding and outcome of pancreaticoduodenectomy. *J Gastrointest Surg.* 2004;8:428–433.
35. Blot WJ, McLaughlin JK. The changing epidemiology of esophageal cancer. *Semin Oncol.* 1999:26–28.
36. American Cancer Society Web site. Detailed guide: esophagus cancer. Available at: http://www.cancer.org/docroot/cri/content/cri_2_4_1x_what_is_esophagus_cancer_12.asp?sitearea=cri. Accessed April 18, 2005.
37. Blot WJ. Alcohol and cancer. *Cancer Res.* 1992;52 (suppl):2119S-2123S.
38. O'Reilly S, Forastierre AA. Is surgery necessary with multimodality treatment of esophageal cancer? *Ann Oncol.* 1995;6:519–521.
39. Ellis FH Jr. Esophagogastrectomy for carcinoma: technical considerations based on anatomic location of lesion. *Surg Clin North Am.* 1980;60:265–279.
40. Ellis HF Jr, Shahlan DM. Tumors of the esophagus. In: Glenn WWL, Baue AE, Geha AS, Hammon GL, Laks H, eds. *Thoracic and Cardiovascular Surgery.* 4th ed. Norwalk, Conn: Appleton & Lange; 1983:566.
41. Sial SH, Catalano MF. Gastrointestinal tract cancer in the elderly. *Gastroenterol Clin North Am.* 2001;30: 565–590.
42. Ell C, Gossner L. Photodynamic therapy. *Rec Results Cancer Res.* 2000:155;175–181.
43. Layke JC, Lopez PP. Gastric cancer: diagnosis and treatment options. *Am Fam Physician.* 2004;69: 1133–1140.
44. Salvon-Harmon JC, Cady B, Nikulasson S, Khettry U, Stone MD, Lavin P. Shifting proportions of gastric adenocarcinomas. *Arch Surg.* 1994:129;181–189.
45. Nomura A, Grove JS, Stemmermann FN, Severson RK. A prospective study of stomach cancer and its relation to diet, cigarettes, and alcohol consumption. *Cancer Res.* 1990;50:627–631.
46. Dorgan JF, Schatzkin A. Antioxidant micronutrients in cancer prevention. *Hematol Oncol Clin North Am.* 1991;5:43–68.
47. Padda S. Dumping syndrome. Available at: http://www.emedicine.com/med/topic589.htm. Accessed April 13, 2004.
48. American Cancer Society. Detailed guide: pancreatic cancer. Available at: http://www.cancer.org/docroot/home/index.asp. Accessed April 26, 2005.
49. Staging of cancer of the pancreas. Cancer of the Pancreas Task Force. *Cancer.* 1981;47(suppl 6):S1631-S1639.
50. Permert J, Ihse I, Jorfeldt L, von Schenck H, Arnqvist HJ, Larsson J. Pancreatic cancer is associated with impaired glucose metabolism. *Eur J Surg.* 1993:159; 101–107.
51. Ottery F. Supportive nutritional management of the patient with pancreatic cancer. *Oncology (Huntingt).* 1996;10(suppl 9):S26-S32.
52. Cooperman AM, Fader A, Cushin B, Golier F, Feld M, Kasmin F, Cohen S, Mahadevia P, Shah K. Surgery and cancer of the pancreas: will common sense become common practice? *Hematol Oncol Clin North Am.* 2002;16:81–94.
53. Murphy GP, Lawrence W Jr, Lenhard RE Jr, eds. *American Cancer Society Textbooks of Clinical Oncology.* Atlanta, Ga: American Cancer Society; 1995: 282–303.
54. Lin YJ, Lin PW. Prospective randomized comparison between pylorus-preserving and standard pancreaticoduodenectomy. *Br J Surg.* 1999;86:603–607.
55. Ohtsuka T, Yamaguchi K, Chijiiwa K, Tanaka M. Postoperative pancreatic exocrine function influences body

weight maintenance after pylorus-preserving pancreatoduodenectomy. *Am J Surg.* 2001;182:524–529.

56. Ellison NM, Chevlen E, Still CD, Dubagunta S. Supportive care of patients with pancreatic adenocarcinoma: symptom control and nutrition. *Hematol Oncol Clin North Am.* 2002;16:105–121.
57. American Cancer Society. All about liver cancer. Available at: http://www.cancer.org/docroot/CRI/CRI_2x.asp?sitearea=&dt=25. Accessed April 26, 2005.
58. Rustgi V. Epidemiology of hepatocellular carcinoma. *Gastroenterol Clin North Am.* 1987:16;545–551.
59. Smyrniotis V, Kostopanagiotou G, Katsarelias D, Theodoraki K, Hondros K, Kouskouni E. Changes of serum phosphorus levels in hepatic resections and implications on patients' outcomes. *Int Surg.* 2003;88:100–104.
60. Escott-Stump S. Ascites. In: Escott-Stump S, ed. *Nutrition and Diagnosis-Related Care*. 5th ed. Philadelphia, Pa: Lippincott Williams & Williams; 2002:342–343.
61. American Cancer Society Web site. Detailed guide: gallbladder cancer. Available at: http://www.cancer.org/docroot/CRI/CRI_2_3x.asp?dt=68. Accessed November 2, 2005.
62. Wanebo HJ, Vezeridis MP. Treatment of gallbladder cancer. *Cancer Treat Res.* 1994;69:97–109.
63. American Cancer Society Web site. Detailed guide: bile duct cancer. Available at: http://www.cancer.org/docroot/CRI/CRI_2_3x.asp?dt=69. Accessed November 2, 2005.
64. Escott-Stump S. Biliary disorders: gallbladder disease. In: Escott-Stump S, ed. *Nutrition and Diagnosis-Related Care*. 5th ed. Philadelphia, Pa: Lippincott Williams & Williams; 2002:366–367.
65. Whang EE, Ashley SW, Zinner MJ. Small intestine. In: Brunicardi FR, Andersen DK, Billiar TR, Dunn DL, Hunter JG, Pollock RE, eds. *Scwhartz' Principles of Surgery.* 8th ed. New York, NY: McGraw-Hill Medical Publishers; 2005:1017–1054.
66. Ashley SW, Wells SA. Tumors of the small intestine. *Semin Oncol.* 1988;15:116–128.
67. Jeejeebhoy KN. Short bowel syndrome: a nutritional and medical approach. *CMAJ.* 2002;166:1297–1302.
68. American Cancer Society Web site. Detailed guide: colorectal cancer. Available at: http://www.cancer.org/docroot/CRI/CRI_2_3x.asp?dt=10. Accessed November 2, 2005.
69. American Dietetic Association, Dietitians of Canada. Ostomy. In: American Dietetic Association and Dietitians of Canada. *Manual of Clinical Dietetics.* 6th ed. Chicago, Ill: American Dietetic Association; 2000:422–424.

Chapter 11

Medical Nutrition Therapy in Pediatric Oncology

KAREN RINGWALD-SMITH, MS, RD, CARLA CARTWRIGHT, RD, CNSD, AND TEREZIE T. MOSBY, MS, RD, IBCLC

INTRODUCTION

Good nutrition is important for all children, especially for children diagnosed with cancer and undergoing antineoplastic therapy. In children, as in adults, the presence of cancer may cause systemic effects, including altered metabolism, anorexia, and electrolyte imbalances (1). Cancer and its treatment can also cause localized effects, such as typhlitis, an ileus or bowel obstruction, and malabsorption syndromes, such as pancreatic insufficiency that can result in weakness, weight loss, growth failure, and ultimately malnutrition (2). Malnutrition associated with cancer treatment predisposes children to increased morbidity, decreased immune function, poorer treatment outcomes, and diminished quality of life (3). For these reasons, early detection, prevention, and treatment of nutrition-related problems are very important. This chapter examines malnutrition in children with cancer, as well as nutrition screening and assessment methods and nutrition recommendations for the pediatric population.

MALNUTRITION AND NUTRITION IMPACT SYMPTOMS

Malnutrition at diagnosis is observed in 6% to 50% of children with cancer (4–7). The type of cancer diagnosed, its location, the extent of disease, or the methodology used to assess nutritional status may explain the varied incidence of malnutrition. Additionally, the child's age and stage in growth affect nutritional status at the time of diagnosis. Malnutrition in children with cancer also can occur during therapy and is observed in 8% to 32% of children with cancer at some point in their treatment (3).

As noted in Chapter 2, treatment modalities for pediatric cancers include chemotherapy, radiation therapy, surgery, and hematopoietic cell transplantation (HCT). There are numerous nutritional consequences associated with chemotherapeutic agents that can affect metabolism or cell reproduction and can result in gastrointestinal (GI) side effects. Treatment-related adverse effects depend on the drug type, dosage, duration of treatment, rate and mode of drug excretion, and individual susceptibility (8). For more on nutritional implications of chemotherapy, see Chapter 8.

In addition to treating malignant cells, radiation therapy can damage healthy tissue within the irradiated field. Early side effects of radiation therapy are generally related to the specific site being irradiated, and common side effects may include diarrhea, mucositis, nausea, and vomiting (8,9). Latent effects (eg, side effects occurring 3 months or longer after treatment has been completed) vary, depending on the location of the cancer and the age of the child, and can include cognitive impairment, altered bone development and growth, learning and hearing impairment, neuroendocrine problems, and secondary malignancies (10). In some instances, side effects of radiation therapy may not manifest for up to 10 years after treatment (10). For more information on radiation therapy, see Chapter 9.

Side effects of cancer-related surgery with nutritional implications may include postoperative ileus, nausea and vomiting, maldigestion, malabsorption, or alterations in substrate metabolism. Surgery can also have localized effects that may alter the child's ability to consume sufficient oral intake, including adequate energy, protein, and micronutrient requirements (9,11).

HCT may result in both oral and GI complications. For more information on these complications and for dietary guidelines on how to manage these complications, see Chapter 12.

PSYCHOLOGICAL CONSIDERATIONS

Psychological factors, such as depression and anxiety, can contribute to malnutrition and must be evaluated by the physician and appropriate behavioral medicine staff members. Illness, treatment, and their psychosocial effects on the family may affect a child's behavior and lead to depression-related anorexia (12). Anxious parents with a heightened concern about their child's intake can inadvertently contribute to malnutrition by making their children anxious about food. If a child is unable to eat, the registered dietitian (RD) can explain to the parents that this may be due to his or her medical condition and can assure them that the health care team is monitoring their child's nutritional status and will provide alternative means of nutrition support (eg, enteral or parenteral nutrition) if necessary.

NUTRITION SCREENING AND ASSESSMENT

Currently, there are no universally established, evidence-based guidelines for nutrition screening and assessment for pediatric oncology patients. The reason is that very few clinical nutrition trials are conducted on children with cancer, because of the complex ethical and clinical questions associated with this type of research and the lack of funding. In 2003, the Children's Oncology Group (COG) nutrition subcommittee surveyed its institutions to identify nutrition practices, assessment methods, and interventions used in managing children with cancer (13). This subcommittee found inconsistent nutrition care practices for this population among the institutions.

At this point, nutrition screening and assessment guidelines for pediatric oncology patients are institution specific. For example, St. Jude Children's Research Hospital in Memphis, Tennessee, emphasizes thorough nutrition screening for all children with cancer. Children identified as moderate to high risk require an in-depth nutrition assessment, including the child's past and current medical history, past and current nutrition history, treatment plan, and the risks associated with treatment. Children who are treated on an inpatient and outpatient basis are scheduled for regular follow-up and periodic reassessment.

The risk stratification protocol that clinicians at St. Jude Children's Research Hospital use to assess and reassess patients at risk for malnutrition is presented in Table 11.1. Boxes 11.1, 11.2, and 11.3 provide recommendations from the St. Jude Children's Research Hospital for identifying patients at nutritional risk (14–17).

The following assessment notes are based on a review of the literature and may be pertinent in situations where malnutrition may not be easily detected:

- A child is less likely to have signs of malnutrition when the diagnosis is a low- or standard-risk acute lymphocytic leukemia (ALL) than when it is stage IV neuroblastoma (18).
- Should the cancer include hepatosplenomegaly from tumor infiltrate, especially in a young child or infant, malnutrition may be overlooked because the hepatosplenomegaly may account for a substantial proportion of weight in the younger child (19).
- Solid tumor diagnoses identified as high nutritional risk may initially have a large tumor burden, hepatosplenomegaly, or ascites that push on the abdominal organs and interfere with a child's ability to consume adequate food (20).
- Malnutrition also may be more prevalent when a child is in a rapid growth stage, such as in infancy. An infant with GI symptoms has fewer body reserves and more nutritional requirements than an older child or an adolescent and may be more likely to have malnutrition. Because some tumors and their organ infiltrates may account for a fair amount of weight, close attention is needed with the nutrition screen to avoid missing malnutrition at the time of diagnosis (20).

Table 11.1 St. Jude Children's Research Hospital Risk Stratification Protocol for Pediatric Nutrition Screening and Assessment

Level	*Conditions*	*Assessment/Care Plan*	*Reassessment*
1	a. Nutrition support (enteral, parenteral) b. Bone marrow transplant—initial c. Weight loss (3%–5% in past month) d. NPO > 3 days	24 hours	Minimum 2 times per week
2	a. Non-chemotherapy-induced nausea/vomiting, diarrhea b. Mucositis/oral problems c. Modified diet	72 hours	Minimum 1 time a week
3	Newly diagnosed treatment on protocols known to result in nutrition problems based on chemotherapy used, diagnosis, location of disease (ie, head/neck/brain tumor) and age 3 years or less.	72 hours	As indicated

Abbreviation: NPO, nothing by os (nothing by mouth).

Source: Reprinted with the permission of the Department of Clinical Nutrition, St. Jude Children's Research Hospital, Memphis, Tennessee.

MACRONUTRIENT REQUIREMENTS

Energy and Protein

Children have greater energy requirements in proportion to their weight than do adults (21). This difference is due to children's distinctive body composition, proportionately smaller fat reserves (high water and low fat content), and constant energy demands for normal growth and development (21).

Nutrient requirements for infants, children, and adolescents with cancer are determined by a thorough assessment of a child's individual needs, disease state, and treatment course. The Dietary Reference Intakes (DRIs) (22) for age and gender can be used to estimate energy and protein requirements that are needed for optimal growth. See Tables 11.2–11.4 (21) for estimated energy requirements (EER) formulas for infants and for boys and girls. For overweight boys and girls between ages 3 and 19 years, clinicians should use total energy expenditure (TEE) equations in Tables 11.3 and 11.4. Tables 11.5 and 11.6 (21) give physical activity coefficients to use with the EER and TEE equations for boys and girls between 3 and 19 years of age.

Protein needs for infants up to age 6 months are calculated using the Adequate Intake (AI) established by the DRIs (22). For infants older than 6 months and for children and adolescents, protein needs are based on the individual's age (see Table 11.7) (21).

For children who weigh more than 120% ideal body weight (IBW), clinicians at St. Jude Children's Research Hospital use adjusted body weight ($A_{dj}BW$) in place of actual weight to calculate protein requirements (see Box 11.3 for more information on IBW). $A_{dj}BW$ is calculated as follows (23):

$$A_{dj}BW\ (kg) = [(\text{Actual Weight} - \text{IBW}) \times 0.25] + \text{IBW}$$

Assessment Tips in Determining Energy and Protein Needs

The following assessment tips are based on a review of the literature and evidence-based practice (12,24):

- Despite physical inactivity, energy needs may increase due to oncology treatment and/or the side effects of treatment.
- Children undergoing intensive therapy may have decreased energy needs because they are generally less active than usual. However, during times of stress and active infection, their energy needs may increase (24). Clinicians

Box 11.1

St. Jude Children's Research Hospital Nutrition Screening System

I. Risk Factors and Assigned Points

a. **Ideal body weight (IBW)***
1. > 90% (0 risk points)
2. 81%–90% (2 risk points)
3. ≤ 80% (3 risk points)

b. **Weight loss in 1 month**
1. < 5% (0 risk points)
2. 5%–10% in children or 1% in infants (2 risk points)
3. > 10% (3 risk points)

c. **Serum albumin (g/dL)** (indicator of visceral protein stores)
1. > 3.5 mg/dL (0 risk points)
2. 3.2-3.5 mg/dL (1 risk point)
3. < 3.2/mg dL (2 risk points)

d. **Impending therapy/treatment side effects** (2 risk points/each)
1. Surgery involving the gastrointestinal (GI) tract
2. Radiation therapy to the GI tract or central nervous system (CNS)
3. Bone marrow transplant
4. GI problems including but not limited to typhlitis, ileus, mucositis (≥ grade 3 based on National Cancer Institute [NCI] common toxicity criteria) (14)
5. Radiation enteritis and dumping syndrome

e. **Oral intake less than 50% of assessed needs, for ≥ 3 days.** (2 risk points)

f. **Change in growth percentile curve:** Any decrease in the curve by 2 or more growth percentile channels (stature-for-age percentiles, weight-for age percentiles, weight-for-stature percentiles) (15). (2 risk points)

g. **High nutritional risk cancer diagnosis** (1 risk point)
1. Wilms' Tumor (Stages III and IV, unfavorable histology, and relapsed)
2. Neuroblastoma (Stages III and IV)
3. Metastatic solid tumors
4. Non-Hodgkin's lymphoma (Stages III and IV, and relapsed)
5. Acute myelogenous leukemia and chronic myelogenous leukemia (newly diagnosed, relapsed)
6. Acute lymphocytic leukemia with poor prognosis (high-risk categories and relapsed)
7. Medulloblastoma and other brain tumors

h. **Lower nutritional risk cancer diagnosis** (0 risk points)
1. Acute lymphocytic leukemia with good prognosis
2. Nonmetastatic solid tumors
3. Advanced diseases in remission during maintenance treatment

II. Categories of Risk and Point Designations

a. **0-1** risk factor points . . . 1st degree—**low risk**
b. **2-3** risk factor points . . . 2nd degree—**moderate risk**
c. **3+** risk factors points . . . 3rd degree—**high risk**

*See Box 11.3 for methods to determine IBW.

Source: Adapted with the permission of the Department of Clinical Nutrition, St. Jude Children's Research Hospital, Memphis, Tennessee. Data are from references 14 and 15.

Box 11.2

St. Jude Children's Research Hospital Nutrition Assessment Parameters

All patients identified at moderate or high risk should receive an in-depth nutrition assessment, which may include gathering information on, but not be limited to:

- Anthropometric measurements
- Biochemical parameters indicative of nutritional status based on available laboratory data, such as electrolytes, albumin, prealbumin, liver enzymes
- In-depth diet, appetite, and nutrition history, noting physical, cognitive, emotional and psychological alterations related to eating
- Assessment of nutrient deficiencies and nutrient needs
- Food/drug interactions
- Food intolerances or allergies
- Conditions that could affect gastrointestinal (GI) tract function, such as changes in digestion and absorption
- Food preferences based on likes, culture, and religion
- Any information provided by other disciplines (eg, social work, speech therapy, pastoral care, physical therapy) that is pertinent to the nutrition care plan
- Language and educational barriers
- Recommended rationale and goals of medical nutrition therapy
- Monitoring of patient's ability and willingness to comply with nutrition plan

Source: Adapted with the permission of the Department of Clinical Nutrition, St. Jude Children's Research Hospital, Memphis, Tennessee.

should use physical activity coefficients when assessing energy and protein needs.
- To ensure that the patient receives sufficient nutrition for growth and development during treatment and recovery from treatment, clinicians should monitor growth on Centers for Disease Control and Prevention (CDC) clinical growth charts.
- Because of medical stress, protein requirements for children with cancer may be greater than for healthy children. Serum prealbumin and albumin levels can be indicators of protein status, but they can also be affected by liver and renal function. These levels should be monitored, and protein intake should be adjusted as needed to promote anabolism (12).

Energy and Protein Needs in Failure to Thrive

Failure to thrive (FTT) is "a description applied to children whose current weight or rate of weight gain is significantly below that of other children of similar age and sex" (25). Children are considered to have FTT if they meet one of any of the following criteria (26–28):

- Weight-for-stature below 5th percentile on CDC clinical growth charts (15).
- Weight or height deficit of more than 2 percentiles from usual percentile channel on CDC clinical growth charts (15).
- Weight less than 80% of IBW for height.
- Body mass index less than 5th percentile on CDC clinical growth charts.

For children with FTT, the time to address catch-up growth (growth that occurs at a rate greater than expected for age and sex to catch up to the child's normal growth curve) is dependent on the stage and intensity level of therapy (eg, high-dose vs low-dose chemotherapy, or recovery vs intensive therapy), and age in relation to anticipated growth. Children who are

Box 11.3

St. Jude Children's Research Hospital Guidelines for Assessment of Body Weight

Infants, Birth to 36 Months

To find a child's ideal body weight (IBW), measure his or her length and then look up this measurement on the appropriate Centers for Disease Control and Prevention (CDC) growth chart for weight-for-length (there are separate charts for boys and girls) (15). The weight given on the 50th percentile curve for that length is the IBW.

Children and Adolescents, 3 to 20 Years

To find a patient's IBW, use the CDC body mass index (BMI)-for age growth chart (there are separate charts for boys and girls) (15). Locate the BMI at the 50th percentile for the child's age and multiply that BMI by the square of the child's height in centimeters. Divide that number by 10,000 to get the IBW. For example, a 7-year-old boy is 124.4 cm in height and weighs 21.8 kg. The BMI at the 50th percentile for boys his age is 15.5. His IBW = (15.5 × 124.4 × 124.4)/10,000 = 24 kg. This boy's weight is therefore 2.2 kg below his IBW.

Children With Amputations

Pediatric cancer treatments for osteosarcoma and other bone-related cancers may include the surgical removal of long bones in children and adolescents. For children with amputations, calculate IBW and then adjust this weight for the body part that has been amputated. The following table lists amputation sites and the estimated percentage of total body weight contributed by each body part (16).

Body Part	*Percentage of Total Body Weight*
Entire arm	5.0
Upper arm	2.7
Forearm	2.3
Hand	0.7
Entire leg	16
Upper leg	10.1
Lower leg	5.9
Foot	1.5

In assigning risk factor points (see Box 11.1), use the following formula to calculate IBW adjusted for amputation (IBW_{adj}) (17):

$$IBW_{adj}\ (kg) = \frac{\text{Current weight (kg)} \times 100}{100 - \%\ \text{Amputation}}$$

For patients with amputations who weigh more than 120% IBW_{adj}, an adjusted body weight ($A_{dj}BW$) is used in place of IBW_{adj} when assigning risk factor points. Use the following formula to calculate adjusted body weight ($A_{dj}BW$) for individuals with amputations who weigh more than 120% IBW_{adj}:

$$A_{dj}BW\ (kg) = [(\text{Actual weight (kg)} - IBW_{adj}) \times 0.25] + IBW_{adj}$$

Source: The content of this box is adapted with the permission of the Department of Clinical Nutrition, St. Jude Children's Research Hospital, Memphis, Tennessee. Data are from references 15–17.

Table 11.2 Formulas for Calculating Estimated Energy Requirements (EER) (kcal/d) for Infants and Toddlers

Age, months	*Equation*
0–3	(89 × Wt – 100) + 175
4–6	(89 × Wt – 100) + 56
7–12	(89 × Wt – 100) + 22
13–35	(89 × Wt – 100) + 20

Abbreviation: Wt, weight (kg).

Source: Reprinted with permission from Pediatric Nutrition Practice Group and Dietetics in Developmental and Psychiatric Disorders. *Children With Special Health Care Needs: Nutrition Care Handbook*. Chicago, Ill: American Dietetic Association; 2005.

recovering from illness need aggressive intervention because catch-up growth is desirable. Children undergoing intensive therapy present more of a challenge because a child's capacity for catch-up growth depends on how many calories he or she is able to consistently consume. The timing, severity, nature, and duration of the nutritional deficit may directly affect potential for catch-up growth (27). Once a nutrition care plan has been implemented, the child's progress must be closely monitored. If the child exhibits suboptimal growth and weight gain, the RD should reassess the nutritional needs, implement a new care plan to enhance energy and nutrient intake, consult with other disciplines (endocrinology, speech/language pathology, behavioral medicine), and continue to monitor closely.

The American Academy of Pediatrics (AAP) (28) recommends calculating the energy needs of infants with FTT as kcal/kg/day using the RDAs (29), not the DRIs (22). The AAP provides the following formula as a general guideline for calculating daily catch-up energy needs for infants and children with FTT:

$$\text{Energy Intake (kcal/kg)} = \frac{\text{RDA (kal/kg} \times \text{Ideal weight for height (kg)}}{\text{Actual weight (kg)}}$$

Where: RDA = Recommended Dietary Allowance for energy for age (29); Ideal weight for height = median weight (kg) for the patient's height (cm), as indicated on CDC weight-for-height growth chart (15).

The formula for calculating daily protein requirements of the child with FTT is as follows (27):

$$\text{Protein requirements (g/kg)} = \frac{\text{RDA (g/kg)} \times \text{Ideal weight for height (kg)}}{\text{Actual weight (kg)}}$$

Where: RDA = Recommended Dietary Allowance for protein for age (29); Ideal weight for height = median weight (kg) for the patient's height (cm), as indicated on CDC weight-for-height growth chart (15).

Fat

Fat is an especially critical nutrient for children. When fat is available in the body as an energy source, the body will use it for energy, thus sparing the protein (30). Fat also facilitates the absorption of fat-soluble vitamins (A, D, E, and K) and provides the essential fatty acids that cannot be synthesized endogenously by humans (30).

For children younger than 6 months, the DRI for fat is 30 g/day; for children 7 to 12 months of age, the DRI is 31 g/day (22,31). For children 1 to 3 years of age, the Acceptable Macronutrient Distribution Range (AMDR) of energy supplied from fat should be 30% to 40%; for children between the ages of 3 and 18 years, the AMDR is 25% to 35% (22).

FLUIDS

In 2004, the Food and Nutrition Board released DRIs for water (32). The report did not outline specific water requirements but established AIs, which are based on median intakes of generally healthy individuals who are adequately hydrated and do not take into account the individual's weight. At St. Jude Children's Research Hospital, clinicians calculate fluid requirements according to the individual's weight (Table 11.8) (33). These calculations take into account that the requirement for maintenance fluids varies with the weight of the child. In our clinical practice, we have found that infants need more fluid per kilogram of body weight than do older children.

MICRONUTRIENT REQUIREMENTS

Vitamins and minerals are necessary for normal growth and development. Insufficient energy and macronutrient intake can put children at risk for

Table 11.3 Formulas for Calculating Estimated Energy Requirements and Total Energy Expenditures for Boys

Age, y	*Equation*
3–8	EER = 88.5 – 61.9 × Age (y) + PA × (26.7 × Wt + 903 × Ht) + 20
9–19	EER = 88.5 – 61.9 × Age (y) + PA × (26.7 × Wt + 903 × Ht) + 25
3–19, overweight	TEE = – 114 – 50.9 × Age (y) + PA × (19.5 × Wt + 1161.4 × Ht)

Abbreviations: EER, estimated energy requirement (kcal/d); Ht, height (meters); PA, physical activity coefficient; TEE, total energy expenditure (kcal/d); Wt, weight (kg).

Source: Reprinted with permission from Pediatric Nutrition Practice Group and Dietetics in Developmental and Psychiatric Disorders. *Children With Special Health Care Needs: Nutrition Care Handbook.* Chicago, Ill: American Dietetic Association; 2005.

Table 11.4 Formulas for Calculating Estimated Energy Requirements and Total Energy Expenditures for Girls

Age, y	*Equation*
3–8	EER = 135.3 – 30.8 × Age (y) + PA × (10.0 × Wt + 934 × Ht) + 20
9–19	EER = 135.3 – 30.8 × Age (y) + PA × (10.0 × Wt + 934 × Ht) + 25
3–19, overweight	TEE = 389 – 41.2 × Age (y) + PA × (15.0 × Wt + 701 × Ht)

Abbreviations: EER, estimated energy requirement (kcal/d); Ht, height (meters); PA, physical activity coefficient; TEE, total energy expenditure (kcal/d); Wt, weight (kg).

Source: Reprinted with permission from Pediatric Nutrition Practice Group and Dietetics in Developmental and Psychiatric Disorders. *Children With Special Health Care Needs: Nutrition Care Handbook.* Chicago, Ill: American Dietetic Association; 2005.

impaired growth and deficiency diseases. According to the AAP (34), children at risk for inadequate nutrition intake may benefit from vitamin and mineral supplementation. In general, it is recommended that the DRIs/RDAs be used as a guide for providing age-appropriate micronutrient needs.

Calcium and vitamin D may be two micronutrients of concern for pediatric oncology patients because a child's bone health may be compromised during the course of cancer treatment (35). The AI for calcium needs is shown in Table 11.9 (36). The AI for vitamin D is 200 IU per day for infants 0 to 12 months and children 1 to 18 years of age (36). The AAP recommends a daily supplement of 200 IU of vitamin D for breast-fed infants (37). When children are weaned from breastmilk, or if they consume at least 500 mL vitamin D-fortified formula per day, supplementation is usually unnecessary.

If a child undergoes multiple transfusions during treatment, iron supplementation is not recommended because it could increase the risk of iron overload.

NUTRITION INTERVENTIONS: FROM ORAL INTAKE TO NUTRITION SUPPORT

Methods for preventing or treating nutritional deficiency and depletion in children with cancer vary; they range from nutrition counseling that encourages high-quality oral intake to aggressive nutrition support via enteral or parenteral access. A multidisciplinary team approach is the best way to integrate nutrition planning into oncology treatment.

Table 11.5 Physical Activity (PA) Coefficients for Boys Ages 3 to 19 Years

	Coefficient	
Activity Level	*Normal Weight*	*Overweight*
Sedentary	1.0	1.00
Low active	1.13	1.12
Active	1.26	1.24
Very active	1.42	1.45

Source: Reprinted with permission from Pediatric Nutrition Practice Group and Dietetics in Developmental and Psychiatric Disorders. *Children With Special Health Care Needs: Nutrition Care Handbook.* Chicago, Ill: American Dietetic Association; 2005.

Table 11.6 Physical Activity (PA) Coefficients for Girls Ages 3 to 19 Years

	Coefficient	
Activity Level	*Normal Weight*	*Overweight*
Sedentary	1.0	1.00
Low active	1.16	1.18
Active	1.31	1.35
Very active	1.56	1.60

Source: Reprinted with permission from Pediatric Nutrition Practice Group and Dietetics in Developmental and Psychiatric Disorders. *Children With Special Health Care Needs: Nutrition Care Handbook.* Chicago, Ill: American Dietetic Association; 2005.

Table 11.7 Daily Protein Needs

Age	*Protein, g/kg**
0–6 mo	1.52
7–12 mo	1.2
1–3 y	1.05
4–8 y	0.95
9–13 y	0.95
14–18 y	0.85

*For infants ages up to age 6 months, Adequate Intake value is shown. For children of other ages, values are Recommended Dietary Allowances.

Source: Data are from reference 22.

Table 11.8 Daily Fluid Requirements

Body Weight, kg	*Fluid*
1–10	100 mL/kg
10–20	1000 mL + 50 mL/kg for each kg > 10
> 20	1500 mL + 20 mL/kg for each kg > 20

Source: Data are from reference 33.

Table 11.9 Daily Calcium Requirements

Age	*Calcium, mg*
0–6 mo	210
7–12 mo	270
1–3 y	500
4–8 y	800
9–18 y	1300

Source: Data are from reference 36.

Effective nutrition strategies will depend on the support and involvement of the family and/or caregivers. A comprehensive care plan that includes nutrition support and addresses the psychological and physical needs of the child is likely to be successful (12,34).

Institution-specific criteria regarding the route of support and appropriate time for intervention are recommended. An algorithm for nutrition support is shown in Figure 11.1 (38).

Considerations With Oral Intake

RDs should make every attempt to encourage oral food intake for children diagnosed with cancer. Instruction can be given to caregivers for suggestions on how to alter food consistencies or ways to make food more energy- and nutrient-dense. In addition, there are many commercially available pediatric nutrition supplements that can be used to supplement oral intake. See Boxes 11.4–11.8.

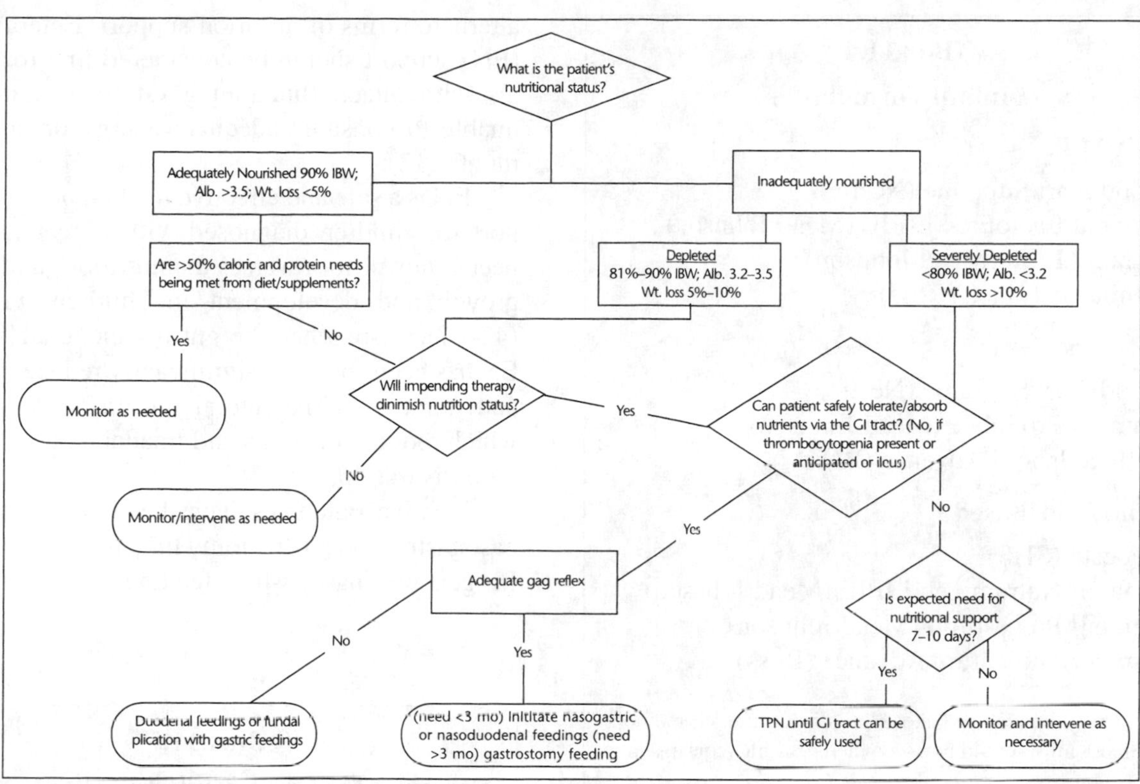

Figure 11.1 St. Jude Children's Research Hospital algorithm for nutrition support. Abbreviations: Alb, albumin; GI, gastrointestinal; IBW, ideal body weight; PN parenteral nutrition; Wt, weight. Reprinted from: Algorithm for nutritional support: experience of the Metabolic and Infusion Support Service of St. Jude Children's Research Hospital, Bowman LC, Williams R, Sanders M, Ringwald-Smith K, Baker D, Gajjar A, Copyright 1998, *International Journal of Cancer.* Reprinted by permission of Wiley-Liss, Inc., a subsidiary of John Wiley & Sons, Inc.

Food Safety

Children with cancer and their caregivers should be encouraged to follow food safety guidelines throughout the entire treatment course. In immunocompromised individuals, food-borne illnesses can be especially serious (11). Children and their families should be educated about food-borne illnesses, the foods that pose the greatest risk, and guidelines for buying, storing, and preparing foods safely. The COG survey reported a wide variation in the use of the neutropenic diet (13). Of those institutions responding, 33% incorporate education on this diet for both the oncology and HCT populations. For sample dietary guidelines, see Box 11.9 (8). Additional information about neutropenic or low-bacteria diet is available from the St. Jude's Children Research Hospital Clinical Nutrition Department (http://www.stjude.org) (39) or in Chapter 12.

Cancer-Related Cachexia and Anorexia and Appetite Stimulants

Cancer-related cachexia and anorexia are common in children who receive cancer treatment (40,41). Cachexia is a syndrome that includes anorexia, tissue wasting, and physical weakness, and it may affect quality of life (see Chapter 3). Factors that may contribute to cancer-related cachexia are the malignant process, medications, food aversions, malabsorption, emesis, mucositis, diarrhea, and energy expenditure (40). See Appendix A for suggestions on ways to im-

Box 11.4

Infant Formulas*

Cow's Milk

- Good Start Supreme (Nestle)
- Enfamil LactoFree LIPIL (Mead Johnson)
- Enfamil Lipil (Mead Johnson)
- Similac Advance (Ross)

Soy

- Good Start Supreme (Nestle)
- Enfamil ProSobee (Mead Johnson)
- Similac Isomil Advance (Ross)

Amino Acid-Based

- Neocate (SHS)
- Enfamil Nutramigen LIPIL (Mead Johnson)
- Enfamil Pregestimil (Mead Johnson)
- Similac Alimentum Advance (Ross)

*Infants may experience lactose intolerance after chemotherapy. Breast-milk should be used when possible (contains lactose).
Manufacturers: Nestle USA, Glendale, CA 91203; Mead Johnson, Evansville, IN 47721; Ross Products Division, Abbott Laboratories, Abbott Park, IL 60064; SHS North America, Gaithersburg, MD 20884.

prove oral intake in patients with anorexia and cancer-related cachexia.

There is limited research on the use of appetite stimulants in children diagnosed with cancer, and their use should only be considered after all other attempts to increase oral intake have been unsuccessful (42). Of note, researchers undertaking a review of pediatric cancer patients who had received the appetite stimulant megestrerol acetate (MA) found that MA significantly improved nutritional status, but its use resulted in severe adrenal suppression in almost all patients tested (42). See Chapter 15 for more information on appetite stimulants.

Specialized Nutrition Support

Enteral Nutrition

Cancer and the side effects and toxicities of cancer treatment can contribute to inadequate oral intake (12,33). If this is the case, the RD should consider alternate forms of nutrition support. Enteral nutrition (EN) support should be considered first for individuals with intact, functioning GI tracts but who are unable to consume adequate energy or nutrients by mouth (12).

EN is a safe and effective method of nutrition support for children diagnosed with cancer (12). It has been shown to reverse malnutrition and promote growth and development in children with cancer (43–47). Also, when the gut is functional, the use of EN has been shown to significantly reduce the amount and duration of parenteral nutrition (PN) required, which reduces the risks and financial costs associated with PN (43,46,48).

Positive outcomes have been reported for both nasogastric and gastrostomy tube feedings (46,48,49). In general, nasogastric feeding tubes are recom-

Box 11.5

Formulas for Use in Children Ages 1–10 years

Standard

- Boost Breeze (Novartis)
- Compleat Pediatric (Novartis)
- Enfamil Kindercal (Mead Johnson)
- Nutren Junior (Nestle)
- PediaSure (Ross)
- RESOURCE Just For Kids (Novartis)

Soy

- Bright Beginnings (PBM)

Calorie-Dense

- Nutren 1.5 (Nestle)
- Nutren 2.0 (Nestle)
- RESOURCE Just For Kids 1.5 (Novartis)

Modified Protein or Elemental

- Neocate Junior (SHS)
- Pediatric Peptinex DT (Novartis)
- Peptamen Junior (Nestle)
- Vivonex Pediatric (Novartis)

Manufacturers: Mead Johnson, Evansville, IN 47721; Novartis Medical Nutrition, Minneapolis, MN 55416; Nestle USA, Glendale, CA 91203; Ross Products Division, Abbott Laboratories, Abbott Park, IL 60064; PBM Products, Gordonsville, VA 22942; SHS America, Gaithersburg, MD 20884.

Box 11.6

Formulas for Use in Individuals Older Than 10 Years

Standard

- Compleat (Novartis)
- Isocal (Novartis)
- Nutren (Nestle)
- Osmolite (Ross)

High Nitrogen

- Isocal HN (Novartis)
- IsoSource HN (Novartis)
- Replete (Nestle)

Calorie-Dense

- Deliver 2.0 (Novartis)
- IsoSource 1.5 Cal (Novartis)
- Nutren 1.5 (Nestle)
- Nutren 2.0 (Nestle)
- TwoCal HN (Ross)

Modified Protein or Elemental

- Criticare HN (Novartis)
- Peptamen (Nestle)
- Peptamen 1.5 (Nestle)
- Peptamen VHP (Nestle)
- Peptinex DT (Novartis)
- TOLEREX (Novartis)
- Vital HN (Ross)
- VIVONEX PLUS (Novartis)
- VIVONEX T.E.N. (Novartis)

Manufacturers: Novartis Medical Nutrition, Minneapolis, MN 55416; Nestle USA, Glendale, CA 91203; Ross Products Division, Abbott Laboratories, Abbott Park, IL 60064.

mended for short-term use (less than 3 months) (34). Gastrostomy feeding tubes are recommended for children who require enteral support for more than 3 months (34).

The best time to initiate enteral feedings will depend on the child's current medical condition, diagnosis, and response to treatment. Consider the following factors to select the best method for tube placement and to help prevent complications (34,45):

- Mucosal integrity: presence of ulcers and mucositis may inhibit tube placement.
- Tumor location: placement of feeding tube may be difficult in children with masses involving the GI tract or abdomen.
- Platelet count: presence of thrombocytopenia places children at risk for bleeding from the procedure. The platelet count should be greater than 50,000/mm^3 before tube is placed (34,45).
- Immune function: presence of neutropenia places children at risk for infection. In general, the phagocyte count should be at least 500/mm^3 before tube is placed (34,45).
- Impending therapy and child's tolerance to initiation of enteral feeding. High-dose chemotherapy, radiation therapy, and surgery may affect the GI tract or cause nausea and vomiting and therefore may result in poor tolerance of enteral feedings. Review the child's planned treatment before commencing enteral feedings.

Box 11.7

Modular Components

Protein

- Casec (Novartis)
- Nonfat dry milk powder
- ProMod (Ross)
- RESOURCE Beneprotein (Novartis)

Carbohydrate

- Moducal (Novartis)
- Polycose (powder or liquid) (Ross)
- RESOURCE Benecalorie (Novartis)
- Super Soluble Duocal (fat and carbohydrate) (SHS)

Fat

- Microlipid (Novartis)
- MCT oil (Novartis)
- Vegetable oil (LCT)

Fiber

- Pectin
- RESOURCE Benefiber (Novartis)

Manufacturers: Novartis Medical Nutrition, Minneapolis, MN 55416; Ross Products Division, Abbott Laboratories, Abbott Park, IL 60064; 3. SHS America, Gaithersburg, MD 20884.

Box 11.8
Oral or Enteral Electrolyte Solutions*

- Pedialyte
- Rehydralyte

*Rehydration solutions designed to provide electrolytes, calories, and water to prevent mild to moderate dehydration. Both products are manufactured by Ross Products Division, Abbott Laboratories, Abbott Park, IL 60064.

When selecting the appropriate EN support formula for a child, several factors must be considered, including the age, nutritional status, diagnosis, and organ function of the individual. In general, most children with cancer tolerate standard or polymeric formulas, but a full assessment of the individual's medical history is needed to make the appropriate formula choice.

Parenteral Nutrition

In children with cancer, the GI tract may become unusable for nutrition support because of surgery, persistent vomiting, intractable diarrhea, graft-versus-host disease of the GI tract, ileus, or radiation enteritis requiring NPO status. PN is indicated when the GI tract cannot be used for a prolonged period (11), which is defined in the American Dietetic Association *Pediatric Manual of Clinical Dietetics,* 2nd edition (50), as:

- Preterm infants: in the first 3 days of life
- Term infants: in the first 5 days of life
- Children with GI dysfunction due to disease or injury: ≥ 3 days
- Children with suboptimal nutritional status: ≤ 3 days

Although PN is widely used for nutrition support in children with cancer, its benefits are questionable. Short-term (for less than 7days) PN support is not generally recommended in any patient population for several reasons. In a study of PN in children with cancer, an improvement of measurable nutrition parameters (eg, weight, albumin, prealbumin) were noted only

Box 11.9
Sample Food Safety Guidelines for Immunosuppressed Patients

- Wash your hands with soap and water before eating or handling food.
- Clean all preparation items before and after use, to prevent cross-contamination.
- Avoid foods from deli counters and street vendors.
- Cook all meats until well done.
- Avoid raw eggs or food prepared with raw eggs.
- Avoid unpasteurized milk and milk products.
- Avoid powdered milk-based infant formulas and supplements that are not sterile, because of the possibility of bacterial growth from the product.
- Avoid raw or unpasteurized honey.
- Avoid fruit and vegetables that cannot be peeled. Canned fruit and vegetables are allowed.
- Avoid miso products, tempeh, moldy and outdated food products.
- Drink only bottled water processed by reverse osmosis, distillation, or 1-µm particulate absolute filtration, tap water from a safe source, and shelf-stable drink.
- Keep foods at safe temperatures, to minimize growth of bacteria. Cold food should be kept at < 40ºF; hot food at > 140ºF.
- Keep refrigerated leftovers for no more than 1 day.
- Do not eat food that has been kept out of the refrigerator for more than 2 hours.
- Heat hot foods to at least 165ºF; remember to hold hot foods at > 140ºF.
- Do not eat foods from dented or bulging food cans, torn boxes, or leaky plastic wrappers.
- Avoid all fresh fruit and vegetables until approximately 100 days after transplant.
- Avoid aged cheeses like brie, camembert, and blue cheese.
- Avoid fresh herbs and spices.
- Avoid unpasteurized juices.
- Allow *only* canned roasted or dry roasted nuts.

Source: Data are from reference 4.

after 28 days of PN use (51). PN has also been shown to slow the transition to oral intake in pediatric cancer patients. In a study of the effects of PN on oral intake in children and young adults after hematopoietic stem cell transplant, the transition to oral intake took 6 days longer in those patients receiving PN than those receiving 5% dextrose hydration (51). Prolonged parenteral support with minimal or no enteral intake has been associated with adverse effects on the intestinal mucosa, including increased incidence of bacterial translocation (52). In addition, PN has been associated with an increased rate of infection in children with cancer (53).

Hematopoietic stem cell transplantation is one clinical situation in which PN has been demonstrated to be of benefit. One study indicates that overall survival rate may be improved in children receiving PN both before and during the transplantation period (54).

Risks associated with PN include infections, hepatotoxicity, suppression of oral intake, and metabolic abnormalities (51). In addition, the use of PN in conjunction with many of the medications used to treat children with cancer can cause biliary dysfunction or steatosis (55). Therefore, having a nutrition support team and a policy (eg, specific monitoring guidelines) regarding the use of PN is invaluable. Every institution should develop an algorithm for nutrition support similar to the one shown in Figure 11.1. At St. Jude Children Research Hospital, implementation of this algorithm has increased the use of EN support at least threefold (26).

REFERENCES

1. Falcone RA, Warner BW. Pediatric parenteral nutrition. In: Rombeau JL, Rolandelli RH, eds. *Clinical Nutrition: Parenteral Nutrition.* 3rd ed. Philadelphia, Pa: WB Saunders; 2001:476–496.
2. *Practice Guidelines and Diet Manual for the Care of the Patient With Cancer.* Houston, Tex: University of Texas MD Anderson Cancer Center; 2001.
3. Han-Markey T. Nutritional considerations in pediatric oncology. *Semin Oncol Nurs.* 2000;16:146–151.
4. Coates TD, Rickard KA, Grosfeld JL, Weetman RM. Nutritional support of children with neoplastic diseases. *Surg Clin North Am.* 1986;66:1197–1212.
5. Donaldson SS, Wesley MN, DeWys WD, Suskind RM, Jaffe N, vanEys J. A study of the nutritional status of pediatric cancer patients. *Am J Dis Child.* 1981;135:1107–1112.
6. Mauer AM, Burgess JB, Donaldson SS, Rickard KA, Stallings VA, van Eys J, Winick M. Special nutritional needs of children with malignancies: a review. *JPEN J Parenter Enteral Nutr.* 1990;14:315–324.
7. van Eys J. Malnutrition in children with cancer: incidence and consequence. *Cancer.* 1979;43:2030–2035.
8. Sheard NF, Clark NG. Nutrition management of pediatric oncology patients. In: Baker SB, Baker RD, Davis A, eds. *Pediatric Enteral Nutrition.* New York: Chapman & Hall; 1994:387–398.
9. Barale KV, Charuhas PM. Oncology and marrow transplantation. In: Samour PQ, Helm KK, Lang CE, eds. *Handbook of Pediatric Nutrition.* 2nd ed. Gaithersburg, Md: American Society for Parenteral and Enteral Nutrition; 1999:465–491.
10. Dreyer ZE, Blatt J, Bleyer A. Late effects of childhood cancer and its treatment. In: Pizzo PA, Poplack DG, eds. *Principles and Practice of Pediatric Oncology.* Philadelphia, Pa: Lippincott Williams & Wilkins; 2001:1431–1461.
11. Nutrition management of oncology and marrow/hematopoietic stem cell transplantation. In: Nevin Folino NL, ed. *Pediatric Manual of Clinical Dietetics.* 2nd ed. Chicago, Ill: American Dietetic Association; 2003:175–184.
12. Bechard LJ, Adiv OE, Jaksic T, Duggan C. Nutritional supportive care. In: Pizzo PA, Poplack DG, eds. *Principles and Practice of Pediatric Oncology.* Philadelphia, Pa: Lippincott Williams & Wilkins; 2001.
13. Ladas EJ, Sacks N, Meacham L, Henry D, Enriquez L, Lowry G, Hawkes R, Dadd G, Rogers P. A multidisciplinary review of nutrition considerations in the pediatric oncology population: a perspective from children's oncology group. *Nutr Clin Pract.* 2005;20: 377–393.
14. Cancer Therapy Evaluation Program. Common Toxicity Criteria Document for Adverse Events, Version 3.0. DCTD, NCI, NIH, DHHS. Available at: http://ctep.cancer.gov. Accessed October 26, 2005.
15. Centers for Disease Control and Prevention. Growth Charts. Developed by the National Center for Health Statistics in collaboration with the National Center for Chronic Disease Prevention and Health Promotion (2000). Available at: http://www.cdc.gov/growthcharts. Accessed October 20, 2005.
16. Osterkamp LK. Current perspective on assessment of human body proportions of relevance to amputees. *J Am Diet Assoc.* 1995;95:215–218.
17. Anthropometry. In: Lee RD, Nieman DC, eds. *Nutritional Assessment.* 2nd ed. St. Louis, Mo: Mosby-Year Book; 1996:223–288.

18. Sala A, Pencharz P, Barr RD. Children, cancer, and nutrition—a dynamic triangle in review. *Cancer.* 2004;100:677–687.
19. Lanzkowsky P, ed. *Manual of Pediatric Hematology and Oncology.* 4th ed. Burlington, Mass: Elsevier Academic Press; 2005.
20. Hanigan MJ, Walter GA. Nutritional support of the child with cancer. *J Pediatr Oncol Nurs.* 1992;9: 110–118.
21. Lucas B. Nutrition in childhood. In: Mahan LK, Escott-Stump S, eds. *Krause's Food, Nutrition, & Diet Therapy.* 10th ed. Philadelphia, Pa: WB Saunders; 2000:239–256.
22. Institute of Medicine. *Dietary Reference Intakes for Energy, Carbohydrate, Fiber, Fat, Fatty Acids, Cholesterol, Protein, and Amino Acids (Macronutrients) (2005).* Washington, DC: National Academy Press; 2005.
23. Wiggins KL, ed. *Suggested Guidelines for Nutrition Care of Renal Patients.* Chicago, Ill: American Dietetic Association; 1986.
24. American Academy of Pediatrics. Energy. In: Kleinman RE, ed. *Pediatric Nutrition Handbook.* 5th ed. Elk Grove, Ill: American Academy of Pediatrics; 2004:241–246.
25. Medline Plus Medical Encyclopedia. Failure to thrive. Available at: http://www.nlm.nih.gov/medlineplus/ency/article/Definition. Accessed October 20, 2005.
26. Nutrition management of failure to thrive. In: Nevin-Folino NL, ed. *Pediatric Manual of Clinical Dietetics.* 2nd ed. Chicago, Ill: American Dietetic Association; 2003:243–257.
27. Corrales KM, Utter SL. Growth failure. In: Samour PQ, King K, eds. *Handbook of Pediatric Nutrition.* 3rd ed. Sudbury, Mass: Jones and Bartlett Publishers; 2005:391–406.
28. American Academy of Pediatrics. Failure to thrive (pediatric undernutrition). In: Kleinman RE, ed. *Pediatric Nutrition Handbook.* 5th ed. Elk Grove, Ill: American Academy of Pediatrics; 2004:443–457.
29. Institute of Medicine. *Recommended Dietary Allowances.* 10th ed. Washington, DC: National Academy Press; 1989.
30. Ettinger S. Macronutrients: carbohydrates, proteins, and lipids. In: Mahan KL, Escott-Stump S, eds. *Krause's Food, Nutrition, & Diet Therapy.* 11th ed. Philadelphia, Pa: WB Saunders; 2004:37–74.
31. Trahms CM. Nutrition during infancy. In: Mahan KL, Escott-Stump S, eds. *Food, Nutrition, and Diet Therapy.*11th ed. Philadelphia, Pa: WB Saunders; 2004: 214–233.
32. Institute of Medicine. *Dietary Reference Intakes: Water, Potassium, Sodium, Chloride, and Sulfate.* Washington, DC: National Academy Press; 2004.
33. Robertson J, Shilkofski N, eds. *Harriet Lane Handbook: A Manual for Pediatric House Officers.* 17th ed. St. Louis, Mo: Mosby; 2005.
34. Nutritional management of children with cancer. In: Kleinman RE, ed. *Pediatric Nutrition Handbook.* 5th ed. Elk Grove, Ill: American Academy of Pediatrics; 2004:709–720.
35. Atkinson SA, Halton JM, Bradley C, Wu B, Barr RD. Bone and mineral abnormalities in childhood acute lymphoblastic leukemia: influence of disease, drugs and nutrition. *Int J Cancer Suppl.* 1998;11:35–39.
36. Institute of Medicine. *Dietary Reference Intakes for Calcium, Phosphorus, Magnesium, Vitamin D, and Fluoride.* Washington, DC: National Academy Press; 1997.
37. Gartner LM, Greer FR; Section on Breastfeeding and Committee on Nutrition. American Academy of Pediatrics. Prevention of rickets and vitamin D deficiency: new guidelines for vitamin D intake. *Pediatrics.* 2003;111:908–910.
38. Bowman LC, Williams R, Sanders M, Ringwald-Smith K, Baker D, Gajjar A. Algorithm for nutritional support: experience of the Metabolic and Infusion Support Service of St. Jude Children's Research Hospital. *Int J Cancer Suppl.* 1998;11:76–80.
39. St. Jude Children's Research Hospital Clinical Nutrition Department Web site. Available at: http://www.stjude.org/clinical-nutrition. Accessed April 26, 2005.
40. Potter J, Hami F, Bryan T, Quigley C. Symptoms in 400 patients referred to palliative care services: prevalence and patterns. *Palliat Med.* 2003;17:310–314.
41. Andrassy RJ, Chwals WJ. Nutrition support of the pediatric cancer patient. *Nutrition.* 1998;14:124–129.
42. Orme LM, Bond JD, Humphrey MS, Zacharin MR, Downie PA, Jamsen KM, Mitchell SL, Robinson JM, Grapsas NA, Ashley DM. Megestrol acetate in pediatric oncology patients may lead to severe, symptomatic adrenal suppression. *Cancer.* 2003;98:397–405.
43. Mathew P, Bowman L, Williams R, Jones D, Rao B, Schropp K, Warren B, Klyce MK, Whitington G, Hudson M. Complications and effectiveness of gastrostomy feedings in pediatric cancer patients. *J Pediatr Hematol Oncol.* 1996;18:81–85.
44. Ringwald-Smith K, Krance R, Stricklin L. Enteral nutrition support in a child after bone marrow transplantation. *Nutr Clin Pract.* 1995;10:140–143.
45. Barron MA, Duncan DS, Green GJ, Modrusan D, Connolly B, Chait P, Saunders EF, Greenberg M. Effi-

cacy and safety of radiologically placed gastrostomy tubes in paediatric hematology/oncology patients. *Med Pediatr Oncol.* 2000;34:177–182.

46. Aquino VM, Smyrl CB, Hagg R, McHard KM, Prestridge L, Sandler ES. Enteral nutritional support by gastrostomy tube in children with cancer. *J Pediatr.* 1995;127:58–62.
47. Bakish J, Hargrave D, Tariq N, Laperriere N, Rutka JT, Bouffet E. Evaluation of dietetic intervention in children with medulloblastoma or supratentorial primitive neuroectodermal tumors. *Cancer.* 2003;98: 1014–1020.
48. Pietsch JB, Ford C, Whitlock JA. Nasogastric tube feedings in children with high-risk cancer: a pilot study. *J Pediatr Hematol Oncol.* 1999;21:111–114.
49. den Broeder E, Lippens RJ, van't Hof MA, Tolboom JJ, Sengers RC, van den Berg AM, van Houdt NB, Hofman Z, van Staveren WA. Nasogastric tube feeding in children with cancer: the effect of two different formulas on weight, body composition, and serum protein concentrations. *JPEN J Parenter Enteral Nutr.* 2000;24:351–360.
50. Klawitter B. Pediatric enteral nutrition support. In: Nevin-Folino NL, ed. *Pediatric Manual of Clinical Dietetics.* 2nd ed. Chicago, Ill: American Dietetic Association; 2003: 471–493.
51. Charuhas PM, Fosberg KL, Bruemmer B, Aker SN, Leisenring W, Seide K, Sullivan KM. A double-blind randomized trial comparing outpatient parenteral nutrition with intravenous hydration: effect on resumption of oral intake after marrow transplantation. *JPEN J Parenter Enteral Nutr.* 1997;21:157–161.
52. Wang TW, Sax HC. Total parenteral nutrition: effects on the small intestine. In: *Clinical Nutrition Parenteral Nutrition.* 3rd ed. Philadelphia, Pa: WB Saunders; 2001:353–365.
53. Christensen ML, Hancock ML, Gattuso J, Hurwitz CA, Smith C, McCormick J, Mirro J Jr. Parenteral nutrition associated with increased infection rate in children with cancer. *Cancer.* 1993;72:2732–2738.
54. Uderzo C, Rovelli A, Bonomi M, Fomia L, Pirovano L, Masera G. Total parenteral nutrition and nutritional assessment and leukaemic children undergoing bone marrow transplantation. *Eur J Cancer.* 1991;27: 758–762.
55. Copeman MC. Use of total parenteral nutrition in children with cancer: a review and some recommendations. *Pediatr Hematol Oncol.* 1994;11:463–470.

Chapter 12

Medical Nutrition Therapy in Hematopoietic Cell Transplantation

PAULA M. CHARUHAS, MS, RD, FADA, CNSD

INTRODUCTION

Hematopoietic cell transplantation (HCT) has become an established therapeutic modality for certain hematologic malignancies, some solid tumors, and several nonmalignant disorders. The goals of HCT are to replace the malignant or defective marrow and to restore normal hematopoiesis and immunologic function. Treatment consists of a preparative regimen that includes cytotoxic chemotherapy to eradicate the malignant or defective stem cells and may also include total body irradiation (1). This chapter reviews the diseases and conditions treated by HCT, nutrient considerations for patients undergoing HCT therapy, and complications associated with HCT.

DISEASES AND CONDITIONS TREATED BY HCT

HCT is a treatment modality for a variety of malignant and nonmalignant disorders, including the following (1):

- Hematologic malignancies—acute leukemias, chronic leukemias, lymphomas, multiple myeloma, myelodysplastic syndromes (ie, refractory anemias)
- Malignant solid tumors—advanced-stage neuroblastoma, refractory Ewing's sarcoma, ovarian cancer, prostate cancer, testicular cancer, renal cell carcinoma
- Immunologic disorders—severe combined immunodeficiency disease, Wiskott-Aldrich syndrome, other cellular immunodeficiencies
- Nonneoplastic disorders of hematopoiesis—severe aplastic anemia, β-thalassemia major, Fanconi's anemia, paroxysmal nocturnal hemoglobinuria
- Nonmalignant congenital disorders—storage diseases (eg, Gaucher's disease), lysosomal diseases (eg, Lesch-Nyhan syndrome), mucopolysaccharidoses (eg, Hurler's syndrome, Hunter's disease), mucolipidoses (eg, metachromatic leukodystrophy, Niemann-Pick disease), infantile osteopetrosis
- Autoimmune disorders—multiple sclerosis, systemic lupus erythematous, systemic sclerosis

PREPARATIVE TRANSPLANT CONDITIONING REGIMENS

There are two types of HCT preparative conditioning regimens: myeloablative and nonmyeloablative. Myeloablative transplant conditioning regimens use both high-dose chemotherapy and radiation to ablate bone marrow. Nonmyeloablative conditioning regimens deliver low-dose chemotherapy and radiation. Older patients, patients with relapsed malignancy after myeloablative HCT, and patients with pretransplant comorbidities (eg, hepatic compromise) are often candidates for nonmyeloablative conditioning regimens

(2). An intravenous infusion of autologous (self), syngeneic (genetically identical twin), or allogeneic (from a histocompatible-related or -unrelated donor) stem cells follows the conditioning regimen. The source of the stem cells may be bone marrow, peripheral blood, or umbilical cord blood (1).

After the conditioning regimen and stem cell infusion, the patient is often neutropenic and immunosuppressed for a period of 2 to 3 weeks, until marrow engraftment. Multiple oral and gastrointestinal (GI) effects, infections, major organ toxicities, and graft-versus-host disease (GVHD) are common posttransplant and may affect oral intake and nutritional status. In view of these implications, parenteral nutrition (PN) is usually instituted in the conditioning phase and is an important component of the overall treatment plan.

NUTRITION ASSESSMENT

Nutrition assessment should begin pretransplant and should continue throughout the transplant course, because the complications associated with HCT may have profound implications on the patient's nutritional status. The nutrition assessment includes a comprehensive evaluation of the patient's nutrition history, anthropometric parameters, blood chemistries, and other factors.

Nutrition History

As a component of the patient's nutrition history, current oral and GI symptoms should be assessed and include the following (3):

- Chewing and swallowing ability
- Mucositis and esophagitis
- Taste alterations
- Xerostomia
- Heartburn
- Nausea
- Vomiting
- Early satiety
- Anorexia
- Changes in bowel habits

The patient's current dietary modifications and special diets should be examined in addition to the current use of nutritional supplements, which includes vitamin and mineral supplements and herbal preparations. Food allergies or intolerances should be evaluated and prior need and use of enteral nutrition or PN support should also be assessed. For pediatric patients, stage of eating development and use of infant formulas should be reviewed.

Anthropometry

Baseline anthropometry during HCT provides landmark data for serial measurements. A measured standing height (measured length in children younger than 2 years) should be obtained in all patients (3). Weight changes from pre-illness weight and percent of usual weight should be determined, and ideal body weight (IBW) and percent of IBW should be calculated. For obese patients (patients who are ≥125% IBW), an adjusted weight should be determined using the following formula (4):

$$\text{Adjusted weight} = [(\text{Actual weight} - \text{IBW})\ (0.25)] + \text{IBW}$$

Arm anthropometry may also be obtained for some patient populations, to evaluate somatic muscle protein and adipose reserves. Skinfold measurements obtained pretransplant provide baseline data for serial measurements. Body surface area, which is often used in determining medication dosages, is also calculated. The formula for calculating body surface area is provided below:

$$\text{Body surface area (m}^2\text{)} = \frac{\sqrt{\text{Actual weight (kg)} \times \text{Height (cm)}}}{60}$$

For pediatric patients, growth history, which may be affected by disease and prior therapy, should be assessed. Children younger than 2 years should have their occipital head circumference measured (3).

Blood Chemistries

An evaluation of the patient's blood chemistries should include the following serum measurements:

- Renal parameters (creatinine, blood urea nitrogen)

- Electrolytes (sodium, potassium, magnesium, calcium, phosphate)
- Liver function enzymes (bilirubin, serum glutamic oxaloacetic transaminase, alkaline phosphatase)
- Visceral protein parameters (albumin and/or prealbumin)
- Blood lipids (cholesterol, triglycerides)

Other Considerations

Additional considerations in the nutrition assessment include the patient's medical history, presence of comorbidities (eg, diabetes mellitus, GI surgery), prior therapy, and current medications for drug-nutrient interactions. The patient's physical strength and activity level, as well as the level of pain and pain control that may interfere with oral intake, should also be assessed.

NUTRIENT REQUIREMENTS

Energy

Energy requirements are increased early post-HCT to account for the metabolic stress induced by the preparative regimen, fever, infections, and other metabolic complications (3).

Pediatric Patients

For children younger than 16 years and weighing less than 75 kg, recommended energy guidelines are as follows (3,5):

- Stress needs: Basal metabolic rate (BMR) multiplied by 1.6 to 1.8
- Baseline needs: BMR multiplied by 1.4 to 1.6

Adult and Adolescent Patients

For adults and pediatric patients who are older than16 years or weigh more than 75 kg, recommended energy guidelines are as follows (3,6):

- Stress needs: basal energy expenditure (BEE) multiplied by 1.5 to 1.6
- Baseline needs: BEE multiplied by 1.3 to 1.4

Energy needs are adjusted downward to baseline levels for patients with evidence of hematologic engraftment (blood neutrophil count > 500/cm^3), without metabolic complications (3).

Protein

Protein requirements are increased to twice baseline needs, to promote tissue repair after cytoreduction and to spare breakdown of lean body mass (3). Protein needs may be further increased with catabolic corticosteroid therapy, whereas needs may decrease with renal or hepatic dysfunction.

Daily protein requirements are generally based on actual weight; however, an adjusted body weight may be used in patients ≥ 125% ideal weight. Recommended guidelines for protein intake by age are as follows (3):

- 1 to 6 years: 2.5–3 g/kg/day
- 7 to 10 years: 2.4 g/kg/day
- 11 to 14 years: 2 g/kg/day
- 15 to 18 years: 1.8 g/kg/day
- Adults: 1.5 g/kg/day

Fluids

Fluid needs are highly individualized and based on clinical status. Fever, excessive GI losses, hypermetabolism, high-output renal failure, and nephrotoxic medications increase patients' fluid needs (3). Fluid restrictions may be necessary during compromised organ function and iatrogenic fluid overload. Calculations for daily maintenance fluid needs based on body weight are provided below (7):

- < 10 kg: 100 mL/kg
- 11–20 kg: 1,000 mL + 50 mL/kg for each kg > 10 kg
- 21–40 kg: 1,500 mL + 20 mL/kg for each kg > 20 kg
- > 40 kg: 1,500 mL/m^2 body surface area

Vitamins

Oral

To ensure that micronutrient needs are met, an oral multivitamin-mineral supplement with 100% of the Dietary Reference Intake (without iron to prevent iron overload, which often develops after multiple red blood cell transfusions during therapy) is recommended after discontinuation of PN for 1 year posttransplant and longer in patients who remain on long-term immunosuppressive medications (3).

Parenteral

Parenteral vitamin recommendations are based on guidelines provided by the Food and Drug Administration (8). Additional vitamin C (250 mg/day for patients weighing less than 31 kg; 500 mg/day for patients weighing 31 kg or more) should be provided to promote tissue recovery via collagen biosynthesis after cytoreductive therapy (3). However, to decrease oxidative damage from release of free iron, additional vitamin C (a pro-oxidant in the presence of free iron) is contraindicated in patients with serum ferritin levels greater than 1,000 μg/L (3,9). If vitamin K is not included in the IV vitamin formulation, 10 mg/wk should be provided (3).

Trace Mineral Supplementation in PN

Daily parenteral trace mineral recommendations are based on guidelines provided by the Nutrition Advisory Group of the American Medical Association (10). Patients with diarrhea may experience zinc losses. During episodes of diarrhea, additional zinc should be added to the PN at a suggested dose of 1 mg/100 mL. Zinc replacement should be initiated when stool volume exceeds 250 mL for patients weighing less than 20 kg; when volume exceeds 500 mL for patients weighing between 20 and 40 kg; and when volume exceeds 1,000 mL for patients weighing more than 40 kg. Biliary excreted trace elements, copper and manganese, should be removed from PN for patients with persistent hyperbilirubinemia (serum bilirubin > 10 mg/dL) (3).

Electrolytes

Electrolyte requirements vary widely and are influenced by GI losses, altered renal function, aggressive nutrient repletion, and medications. Serum electrolyte levels should be closely monitored, and the following should be noted:

- Hypomagnesemia is associated with cyclosporine, tacrolimus, amphotericin, and foscarnet therapy.
- Hypokalemia is observed with administration of amphotericin, corticosteroids, potassium-wasting diuretics, and excessive GI losses.
- Hypophosphatemia may occur with corticosteroids, foscarnet, and sirolimus therapy.

NUTRITION SUPPORT

Oral Feedings

Oral feedings are indicated for patients with a functional GI tract. Most transplant centers use some type of low-bacteria diet to decrease the risk of food-related infections (11). An example of a diet for immunosuppressed HCT patients is presented in Box 12.1.

As explained in these guidelines, dietary counseling about high-risk foods and safe food handling is also recommended (12). The protective benefits of a neutropenic diet, however, are unknown and warrant further research (13).

Enteral Nutrition

Enteral nutrition is indicated for patients with a functional GI tract who are either malnourished or who have a prolonged poor oral intake (2). Enteral feedings have been used with limited success early posttransplant, because of GI dysfunction associated with regimen-related toxicities, thrombocytopenia, and neutropenia. Complications such as dislodgment of nasoenteral tubes (14,15), delayed gastric emptying (16), and inadequate energy support with subsequent weight loss (14) have been reported. The combined use of enteral feedings with PN is an acceptable and cost-effective alternative (17). Enteral nutrition should be considered in patients with the following (18):

- Mild intestinal GVHD (defined by the institution based on stool output)
- Low-risk HCT (autologous or matched sibling) with long-term eating problems
- Adequate platelet recovery (as defined by the institution)
- Need for long-term nutrition support
- Adequate family support

Patients undergoing nonmyeloablative conditioning regimens may also be candidates for enteral feedings (2). Issues surrounding optimum time for initiation of feedings, enteral access routes, administration

Box 12.1

Dietary Guidelines for Immunosuppressed Patients

These guidelines are intended to minimize the introduction of pathogenic organisms into the gastrointestinal tract by food while maximizing healthy food options for immunosuppressed patients. The guidelines should be coupled with food safety education to assure proper food preparation and storage in the home and hospital kitchen. High-risk foods identified as potential sources of organisms known to cause infection in immunosuppressed patients are restricted.

In general, autologous transplant patients follow the diet during the first 3 months after HCT. Allogeneic transplant patients should follow the diet until off all immunosuppressive therapy (ie, cyclosporine, tacrolimus, prednisone).

Food Restrictions

- Raw and undercooked: meat (including game), fish, shellfish, poultry, eggs, hot dogs, tofu, sausage, bacon
- Raw tofu, unless pasteurized or aseptically packaged
- Luncheon meats (including salami, bologna, hot dogs, ham, other) unless heated until steaming
- Refrigerated smoked seafood typically labeled as lox; kippered, nova-style, smoked or fish jerky (unless contained in a cooked dish)
- Pickled fish
- Nonpasteurized milk and raw milk products, nonpasteurized cheese, and nonpasteurized yogurt
- Soft and blue-veined cheese, including brie, camembert, feta, farmer's, blue, gorgonzola, Roquefort, Stilton
- Mexican-style soft cheese including quesco blanco and quesco fresco
- Cheese containing chili peppers or other uncooked vegetables
- Fresh salad dressings (stored in the grocer's refrigerated case) containing raw eggs or contraindicated cheeses
- Unwashed raw vegetables and fruits and those with visible mold
- Commercial unpasteurized fruit and vegetable juices
- Raw honey
- All miso products (eg, miso soup), tempeh, maté tea
- Raw, uncooked brewer's yeast
- All moldy and out-dated food products
- Well water, unless boiled for 1 minute

Source: Reprinted with permission from the Nutrition Program, Seattle Cancer Care Alliance, Seattle, WA.

methods, and appropriate formulas need to be further explored.

Parenteral Nutrition

PN is generally the standard nutrition support therapy in the immediate posttransplant period for patients undergoing conventional HCT with myeloablative conditioning regimens who experience multiple adverse oral and GI manifestations (12). Administration of carbohydrate typically comprises 50% to 60% of total energy; however, it should be individualized (3). A lower dextrose PN concentration, coupled with intravenous lipid infusions to balance substrates, is indicated during glucose intolerance (ie, serum glucose > 180 mg/dL).

Protein, in the form of crystalline amino acids, usually comprises 15% to 20% of total energy (3). Specialized pediatric amino acid formulas, which contain an amino acid profile similar to that of breast-fed infants, may be used for young transplant patients. Glutamine-enriched PN solutions used during HCT have been reported to improve nitrogen balance and immune recovery, to reduce infectious complications, and to decrease length of hospital stay (19,20). A recent study, however, observed that parenteral glutamine supplementation during autologous HCT was associated with more relapses and deaths (21). Larger, controlled clinical trials are needed to define the efficacy of glutamine supplementation during HCT before specific recommendations can be made (22).

Intravenous lipids typically comprise 20% to 30% of total energy and supply a concentrated source of calories and essential fatty acids (3). For pediatric patients, the maximum lipid dosage is 3 g/kg/day (23).

MONITORING NUTRITION SUPPORT

Daily monitoring of the patient's medical condition, nutritional status, blood chemistries, and treatment-related symptoms is necessary because changes may require modifications in nutrient and fluid support. During the early posttransplant period (from conditioning through the neutropenic phase), the patient's weight, total intake, and output volumes should be monitored on a daily basis. Oral and intravenous calorie, protein, and fluid intake levels also should be evaluated daily so that appropriate nutrition support can be provided. Monitoring the patient's oral and GI tolerance is necessary when oral feedings or enteral nutrition support is instituted.

NUTRITIONAL CONSIDERATIONS DURING HCT

Oral and GI Complications

Oral and GI complications associated with HCT are numerous, varying from oral and esophageal mucositis to impaired taste to anorexia. Dietary guidelines for managing common oral and GI complications are shown in Box 12.2 (24).

Sinusoidal Obstructive Syndrome

The condition of sinusoidal obstructive syndrome (SOS; also known as hepatic veno-occlusive disease) is a common problem in the first month posttransplant. The incidence of SOS varies from 1% to 2% to as high as 50% in some patient populations (25).

SOS is characterized by a fibrous obstruction of the hepatic venules and is associated with chemoradiotherapy (26). Clinical characteristics of SOS include sudden weight gain with concomitant ascites, abdominal pain, hepatomegaly, hyperbilirubinemia (serum bilirubin > 2 mg/dL) and jaundice, and, in severe cases, encephalopathy (27). Nutrition management of SOS consists of the following (3):

- Concentrating PN fluids and reducing sodium additives to minimize fluid retention
- Removing copper and manganese from PN for patients with persistent hyperbilirubinemia (serum bilirubin > 10 mg/dL)
- Monitoring serum triglyceride level if serum bilirubin increases to more than 10 mg/dL

Renal Complications

Impaired renal function may be related to hemolytic syndromes, SOS, intravascular volume depletion, medications, and sepsis. Nutrition management during impaired renal function includes the following (3):

- Maximizing nutrition support within fluid allowance
- Correcting electrolyte imbalances
- During dialysis, providing 50% of standard IV multivitamin dose with complete complex of water-soluble vitamins; if patient is on long-term dialysis, re-evaluate the need for increased supplementation of fat soluble vitamins

Graft-Versus-Host Disease

GVHD is a T-cell-mediated immunologic reaction of engrafted lymphoid cells against the host tissues (28). The major target organs affected are the skin, liver, and GI tract. Measures used to prevent or treat GVHD often include multidrug immunosuppressive therapies, many of which have nutritional implications (Table 12.1) (3).

Clinical manifestations of GI GVHD include nausea, vomiting, anorexia, diarrhea, and/or abdominal pain. Voluminous, secretory diarrhea, and intestinal bleeding occur in advanced disease (28). Malabsorption and intestinal protein losses are also characteristic of the mucosal degeneration associated with intestinal GVHD. In addition to immunosuppressive drug

Box 12.2

Management of Common Nutrition Problems Associated With Hematopoietic Cell Transplantation

Oral and esophageal mucositis

- Try soft/puree-textured or blenderized liquid diet.
- Try smooth, bland, moist foods (custard, cream soups, mashed potatoes).
- Offer soft, non-irritating, cold foods (popsicles, ice cream, frozen yogurt, slushes).
- Encourage frequent mouth rinsing to remove food and bacteria and promote healing, using a solution of 1 quart water and ½ to ¾ level teaspoon salt. If the salt solution causes stinging or burning, this may be relieved by adding 1 to 2 teaspoons of baking soda.

Xerostomia (oral dryness)

- Offer moist foods (stews, casseroles, canned fruit) and liquids.
- Add extra sauces, gravies, margarine, butter, and broth to foods.
- Encourage liquids with meals.
- Add vinegar and pickles to foods to help lessen xerostomia.
- Offer lemon-flavored, sugarless candy to help stimulate saliva.
- Encourage good oral hygiene (rinsing mouth often with salt-water solution, brushing teeth with a soft-bristle toothbrush or sponge brush, flossing as long as it is comfortable).
- Try commercial saliva substitutes.

Thick, viscous saliva and mucous

- Encourage adequate fluid intake.
- Offer clear liquids (tea, popsicles, slushes, warm broth).
- Encourage good oral hygiene (as described above).

Dysgeusia (impaired taste)

- Flavor poultry, fish, eggs, or dairy products.
- Enhance food taste with herbs, spices, flavor extracts, and marinades.
- Offer cold, non-odorous foods.
- Offer fruit-flavored beverages.
- Try highly aromatic foods; add extra herbs and spices to foods while cooking or at the table.
- Try tart foods like oranges or lemonade, which may have more taste.
- Encourage good oral hygiene (as described above).
- Offer fluids with meals to help remove a bad taste in the mouth.

Anorexia

- Offer small, frequent meals of nutrient-dense foods.
- Use carbohydrate supplements and protein powders.
- Create a pleasant mealtime atmosphere with enhancing food aromas, colorful place settings, and varied color and textures of foods.
- Involve the patient in grocery shopping, meal planning, and simple meal preparation.
- Encourage relaxation techniques and light exercise before meals, which may help to improve food intake.

Nausea and vomiting

- Try high carbohydrate foods and fluids (crackers, toast, gelatin) and nonacidic juices.
- Try small, frequent feedings.
- Offer cold, clear liquids and solids.
- Avoid overly sweet or high-fat foods.

(*continued*)

(continued)

- Avoid feeding in a stuffy, too-warm room or one filled with cooking odors or other odors that might be disagreeable.
- Encourage drinking or sipping liquids frequently throughout the day; using a straw through a lid on the cup may help.
- Encourage rest periods after meals.
- Avoid offering favorite foods when nauseated; it may cause a permanent dislike of the food.
- Observe if there is a pattern or regularity to when nausea occurs and what causes it (specific foods, events, surroundings); suggest appropriate changes in diet or schedule.
- Avoid reclining after meals.

Diarrhea

- Try a low-fat, low-fiber diet.
- Avoid caffeine.
- Offer cold or room-temperature foods and beverages, which may be better tolerated than hot foods.
- Try a low-lactose diet.
- Encourage adequate fluids to prevent dehydration.
- Avoid excessive fruit juice.

Constipation

- Encourage fluids.
- Offer a hot beverage in the morning or evening, which may stimulate a bowel movement.
- Offer high-fiber foods.

Source: Adapted with permission from Charuhas PM. Introduction to marrow transplantation. *Oncology Nutrition Dietetic Practice Group Newsletter.* 1994;2:2–9.

therapy, a specialized five-phase dietary regimen should be instituted (Table 12.2) (29).

Infection

Infection may be a major source of morbidity and mortality during HCT (30). Treatment includes antibiotics and antifungal agents, which may induce oral and GI symptoms, thereby affecting oral intake and nutritional status. Intravenous lipids have been implicated as being immunosuppressive; however, lipids provided during HCT have not been reported to increase the incidence of bacterial or fungal infections (31).

LONG-TERM COMPLICATIONS AND MANAGEMENT

Chronic Graft-Versus-Host Disease

Chronic GVHD develops after day 70 posttransplant, with increased frequency in transplants from nonidentical related and unrelated donors (32). Nutrition problems reported at 1 year posttransplant in patients with chronic GVHD include weight gain, weight loss, oral sensitivity, xerostomia, stomatitis, anorexia, reflux symptoms, and diarrhea (33). Regular monitoring of oral and GI symptoms, as well as weight, is necessary after discharge home from transplant centers (33).

Osteoporosis

Osteoporosis is a recognized complication of long-term corticosteroid therapy, often used for treatment of GVHD (34,35). Prevention and management of osteoporosis includes supplemental calcium and vitamin D. Supplemental calcium and vitamin D guidelines by age are as follows (3,35):

- 1 to 5 years: 800–1,200 mg/day of calcium; 400 IU/day of vitamin D
- 6 to 8 years: 1,200 mg/day of calcium; 400 IU/day of vitamin D

Table 12.1 Nutritional Implications of Therapies Used for Prophylaxis and Treatment of GVHD

Therapy	*Nutritional Implications*
Anti-thymocyte globulin	Nausea and vomiting, diarrhea, stomatitis
Azathioprine	Nausea and vomiting, anorexia, diarrhea, mucosal ulceration, esophagitis, steatorrhea
Beclomethasone dipropionate	Xerostomia, dysgeusia, nausea
Budesonide	None known
Corticosteroids	Sodium and fluid retention resulting in weight gain or hypertension, hyperphagia, weight gain, hypokalemia, skeletal muscle catabolism and atrophy, gastric irritation and peptic ulceration, osteoporosis, growth retardation in children, decreased insulin sensitivity and impaired glucose tolerance resulting in hyperglycemia or steroid-induced diabetes, hypertriglyceridemia
Cyclosporine	Nausea and vomiting, renal insufficiency, magnesium wasting, potassium wasting
Extra corporeal photopheresis	Intravenous fluid may be necessary to maintain adequate hydration status; if citrate anticoagulant is used, calcium status should be monitored because the medication may bind calcium and induce hypocalcemia
Methotrexate	Nausea and vomiting (mild to moderate); anorexia; mucositis and esophagitis; diarrhea; renal and hepatic changes; decreased absorption of vitamin B-12, fat, and D-xylose; hepatic fibrosis; change in taste acuity
Methoxsalen (in conjunction with psoralen + ultraviolet A light)	Nausea, hepatotoxicity
Monoclonal antibodies	Nausea and vomiting
Mycophenolate mofetil	Nausea and vomiting, diarrhea
Sirolimus	Hypertriglyceridemia
Tacrolimus	Nephrotoxicity, hyperglycemia, hyperkalemia, hypomagnesemia
Thalidomide	Constipation, nausea, xerostomia
Ursodeoxycholic acid	Nausea and vomiting, diarrhea, dyspepsia

Source: Data are from reference 3.

Table 12.2 Gastrointestinal GVHD Diet Progression

Phase	*Clinical Symptoms*	*Diet*	*Nutrition Support*
1. Bowel rest	GI cramping, large volume of watery diarrhea or active GI bleeding, depressed serum albumin, severely reduced transit time, small-bowel obstruction or diminished bowel sounds, nausea and vomiting	Oral: NPO.	TPN with multivitamins, add trace elements, supplemental zinc, and possibly copper.
2. Introduction of oral feeding	Minimal GI cramping, diarrhea < 500 mL/day, guaiac-negative stools, improved transit time (minimum 1.5 hours), infrequent nausea and vomiting	Oral: isotonic, low-residue, low-lactose beverages, initially 60 mL every 2 to 3 hours, for several days.	TPN: trophic enteral feeds of semi-elemental formula if patient is unable to eat.
3. Introduction of solids	Minimal or no GI cramping, formed stool	Oral: allow introduction of solid food, once every 3 to 4 hours: minimal lactose, low-fiber, low-fat (20 to 40 g/day) diet; avoid high-acid foods, no gastric irritants.	Begin to cycle and decrease TPN; advance feeds slowly (small boluses or continuous infusion) if patient is unable to eat.
4. Expansion of diet	Minimal or no GI cramping; formed stool	Oral: minimal lactose, low fiber, low total acidity, no gastric irritants; if stools indicate fat malabsorption, use low-fat diet.	Nighttime supplemental TPN if oral intake is less than needs or if patient is unable to maintain weight from malabsorption. Enteral feed schedule and formula is dependent on any residual GI symptoms.
5. Resumption of regular diet	No GI cramping; normal stool, normal transit time, normal albumin	Oral: progress to regular diet by introducing one restricted food per day: acid foods with meals, fiber-containing foods, lactose-containing foods; order of addition will vary, depending on individual tolerances and preferences. Patients no longer exhibiting steatorrhea should have the fat restriction liberalized slowly.	Discontinue TPN; supplemental enteral feeds if patient is unable to eat adequate nutrients.

Abbreviations: GI, gastrointestinal; NPO, nothing per os (nothing by mouth); TPN, total parenteral nutrition.

Source: Adapted with permission from Gauvreau JM, Lenssen P, Cheney CL, Aker SN, Hutchinson ML, Barale KV. Nutritional management of patients with intestinal graft-versus-host disease. *J Am Diet Assoc.* 1981;79:673-677.

- > 9 years: 1,500 mg/day of calcium; 600–800 IU/day of vitamin D

For best absorption, single doses of calcium should be ≤ 500 mg (36). Weight-bearing exercise, bisphosphonate therapy, and hormone replacement therapy are also recommended (35).

Growth and Development Issues

Compromised growth and development (eg, decreased growth velocity, growth hormone deficiency, and delayed onset of puberty) are frequent in the pediatric population after HCT (37). An annual evaluation with assessment of growth and development is appropriate for children after discharge from the transplant center.

REFERENCES

1. Horowitz MM. Uses and growth of hematopoietic cell transplantation. In: Blume KG, Forman SJ, Appelbaum FR, eds. *Thomas' Hematopoietic Cell Transplantation.* 3rd ed. Malden, Mass: Blackwell Publishing; 2004:9–15.
2. Charuhas PM, Lipkin A, Lenssen P, McMillen K. Hematopoietic stem cell transplantation. In: Merritt R, ed. *The American Society for Parenteral and Enteral Nutrition Support Practice Manual.* 2nd ed. Silver Spring, Md: American Society for Parenteral and Enteral Nutrition. In press.
3. Seattle Cancer Care Alliance. *Hematopoietic Stem Cell Transplantation Nutrition Care Criteria.* 2nd ed. Seattle, Wash: Seattle Cancer Care Alliance; 2002.
4. Adjustment in body weight (Appendix B). In: Wiggins KL. *Guidelines for Nutrition Care of Renal Patients.* 3rd ed. Chicago, Ill: American Dietetic Association; 2002:113–116.
5. Altman PL, Dittmer DS. *Metabolism.* Bethesda, Md: Federation of American Societies for Experimental Biology; 1968.
6. Harris JA, Benedict FG. *Biometric Studies of Basal Metabolism in Man.* Washington, DC: Carnegie Institution; 1919.
7. Holliday MA, Seger WE. The maintenance need for water in parenteral fluid therapy. *Pediatrics.* 1957; 19:823–832.
8. Parenteral multivitamins products; drugs for human use; drug efficacy study implementation: amendment. *Federal Register*. 2000;65:21200–21201.
9. Gordon LI, Brown SG, Tallman MS, Rademaker AW, Weitzman SA, Lazarus HM, Kelley CH, Mangan C, Rubin H, Fox RM, Creger RJ, Winter JN. Sequential changes in serum iron and ferritin in patients undergoing high-dose chemotherapy and radiation with autologous bone marrow transplantation: possible implications for treatment related toxicity. *Free Radic Biol Med.* 1995;18:383–389.
10. Guidelines for essential trace element preparations for parenteral use. A statement by the Nutrition Advisory Group. American Medical Association. *JPEN.* 1979;3: 263–267.
11. French MR, Levy-Milne R, Zibrik D. A survey of the use of low microbial diets in pediatric bone marrow transplant programs. *J Am Diet Assoc.* 2001;101: 1194–1198.
12. ASPEN Board of Directors and the Clinical Guidelines Task Force. Guidelines for the use of parenteral and enteral nutrition in adult and pediatric patients. *JPEN J Parenter Enteral Nutr.* 2002;26(Suppl 1): SA1-SA138.
13. Moody K, Charlson ME, Finlay J. The neutropenic diet: what's the evidence? *J Pediatr Hematol Oncol.* 2002;24:717–721.
14. Sefcick A, Anderton D, Byrne JL, Teahon K, Russell NH. Naso-jejunal feeding in allogeneic bone marrow transplant recipients: results of a pilot study. *Bone Marrow Transplant.* 2001;28:1135–1139.
15. Lenssen P, Bruemmer B, Aker S, McDonald GB. Nutrient support in hematopoietic cell transplantation. *JPEN J Parenter Enteral Nutr.* 2001;25:219–228.
16. Eagle DA, Gian V, Lauwers GY, Manivel JC, Moreb JS, Mastin S, Wingard JR. Gastroparesis following bone marrow transplantation. *Bone Marrow Transplant.* 2001;28:59–62.
17. Szeluga DJ, Stuart RK, Brookmeyer R, Utermohlen V, Santos GW. Nutritional support of bone marrow transplant recipients: a prospective randomized clinical trial comparing total parenteral nutrition to an enteral feeding program. *Cancer Res.* 1987;47:3309–3316.
18. Ringwald-Smith K, Krance R, Strickin L. Enteral nutrition support in a child after bone marrow transplantation. *Nutr Clin Pract.* 1995;10:140–143.
19. Ziegler TR, Young LS, Benfall K, Scheltinga M, Hortos K, Bye R, Morrow FD, Jacobs DO, Smith RJ, Antin JH, Wilmore DW. Clinical and metabolic efficacy of glutamine- supplemented parenteral nutrition following bone marrow transplantation: a randomized, double-blind, controlled study. *Ann Intern Med.* 1992; 116:821–828.

20. Piccirillo N, De Matteis S, Laurenti L, Chiusolo P, Sora' F, Pittiruti M, Rutella S, Cicconi S, Fiorini A, D'Onofrio G, Leone G, Sica S. Glutamine-enriched parenteral nutrition after autologous peripheral blood stem cell transplantation: effects on immune reconstitution and mucositis. *Haematologica.* 2003;88: 192–200.
21. Pytlik R, Benes P, Patorkova M, Chocenska E, Gregora E, Prochazka B, Kozak T. Standardized parenteral alanyl-glutamine dipeptide supplementation is not beneficial in autologous transplant patients: a randomized, double-blind, placebo controlled study. *Bone Marrow Transplant.* 2004;33:953–961.
22. Ziegler TR. Glutamine supplementation in bone marrow transplantation. *Br J Nutr.* 2002;87(Suppl 1):S9-S15.
23. Commentary on parenteral nutrition. Committee on Nutrition. *Pediatrics.* 1983;71:547–552.
24. Charuhas PM. Introduction to marrow transplantation. *Oncology Nutrition Dietetic Practice Group Newsletter.* 1994;2:2–9.
25. Shulman HM, Hinterberger W. Hepatic veno-occlusive disease—liver toxicity syndrome after bone marrow transplantation. *Bone Marrow Transplant.* 1992; 10:197–214.
26. Baglin TP. Veno-occlusive disease of the liver complicating bone marrow transplantation. *Bone Marrow Transplant.* 1994;13:1–4.
27. Vogelsang GB, Dalal J. Hepatic venoocclusive disease in blood and bone marrow transplantation in children: incidence, risk factors, and outcome. *J Pediatr Hematol Oncol.* 2002;24:706–709.
28. Vogelsang GB, Lee L, Bensen-Kennedy DM. Pathogenesis and treatment of graft-versus-host disease after bone marrow transplant. *Ann Rev Med.* 2003;54: 29–52.
29. Gauvreau JM, Lenssen P, Cheney CL, Aker SN, Hutchinson ML, Barale KV. Nutritional management of patients with intestinal graft-versus-host disease. *J Am Diet Assoc.* 1981;79:673–677.
30. Nichols WG. Combating infections in hematopoietic stem cell transplant recipients. *Expert Rev Anti Infect Ther.* 2003;1:57–73.
31. Lenssen P, Bruemmer B, Bowden RA, Gooley T, Aker SN, Mattson D. Intravenous lipid dose and incidence of bacteremia and fungemia in patients undergoing bone marrow transplantation. *Am J Clin Nutr.* 1998; 67:927–933.
32. Stewart BL, Storer B, Storek J, Deeg HJ, Storb R, Hansen JA, Appelbaum FR, Carpenter PA, Sanders JE, Kiem HP, Nash RA, Petersdorf EW, Moravec C, Morton AJ, Anasetti C, Flowers ME, Martin PJ. Duration of immunosuppressive treatment for chronic graft-versus-host disease. *Blood.* 2004;104:3501–3506.
33. Lenssen P, Sherry ME, Cheney CL, Nims JW, Sullivan KM, Stern JM, Moe G, Aker SN. Prevalence of nutrition-related problems among long-term survivors of allogeneic marrow transplantation. *J Am Diet Assoc.* 1990;90:835–842.
34. Stern JM, Chesnut CH III, Bruemmer B, Sullivan KM, Lenssen P, Aker SN, Sanders J. Bone density loss during treatment of chronic GVHD. *Bone Marrow Transplant.* 1996;17:395–400.
35. Recommendations for the prevention and treatment of glucocorticoid-induced osteoporosis: 2001 update. American College of Rheumatology Ad Hoc Committee on Glucocorticoid-Induced Osteoporosis. *Arthritis Rheum.* 2001;44:1496–1503.
36. Allen L. Calcium. In: Sadler MJ, Strain JJ, Caballero B, eds. *Encyclopedia of Human Nutrition.* San Diego, Calif: Academic Press; 1999:214–218.
37. Sanders JE. Growth and development after hematopoietic cell transplantation. In: Blume KG, Forman SJ, Appelbaum FR, eds. *Thomas' Hematopoietic Cell Transplantation.* 3rd ed. Malden, Mass: Blackwell Publishing; 2004:929–943.

Chapter 13

Enteral Nutrition in Adult Oncology

CARRIE A. ROBINSON, RD, CNSD

INTRODUCTION

Approximately 50% to 80% of patients with invasive cancers may develop malnutrition or cachexia during the course of their illness (1,2). Malnutrition during cancer treatment has been associated with increased morbidity and mortality, as well as decreased response to therapy (3,4). Malnourished individuals receiving antineoplastic therapy should be evaluated for specialized nutrition support (5). Specialized nutrition support, which includes the provision of nutrients and fluids with therapeutic intent, may help to prevent or diminish the progression of malnutrition in a patient who is unable to consume sufficient nutrients to maintain weight, strength, and well-being (2). If the patient's gastrointestinal (GI) tract is functional and can be accessed safely, enteral nutrition (EN) is the preferred method of specialized nutrition support (6,7).

BENEFITS OF ENTERAL FEEDING

For oncology patients who are candidates for EN, it does offer a variety of physiological, safety, and financial benefits compared with other methods of specialized nutrition support.

Physiological Benefits

EN stimulates bile flow and prevents cholestasis (8). Nutrients are absorbed by the portal system, with subsequent delivery to the liver, which supports visceral protein synthesis and regulation of metabolic processes.

Animal studies indicate that enteral feeding may reduce the risk of bacterial translocation (9). Bacterial translocation, which is the passage of enteric flora and/or endotoxins through the epithelial mucosa to extraintestinal sites, may lead to sepsis and multisystem organ failure in the cancer patient (10–13). Research regarding the incidence of bacterial translocation in humans, however, is still under way (14,15).

Certain amino acids, such as glutamine, are provided by enteral formulas. Glutamine is the most abundant of the amino acids in the body and plays an important role in the metabolic processes of lymphocytes, macrophages, and enterocytes (16,17). During stress, glutamine may become conditionally essential (18). Glutamine is present in enteral formulas as intact protein, short-chain peptides, or free amino acids.

Immune-enhancing formulas are enriched with nutrients that have been shown to alter immune response, such as arginine, glutamine, n-3 fatty acids, and nucleotides (19). Studies indicate that these formulas can reduce the incidence of infectious complications in postsurgical GI cancer patients by 5% to 10% (20–22). Preoperative feeding may be particularly beneficial in reducing postsurgical complications (19).

EN can provide fiber, which is essential to gut function. Soy polysaccharide is the most common fiber additive in enteral formulas (23). Soy polysaccharide is inexpensive and easily suspended in liquid. Soy polysaccharide has been shown to increase stool weight and frequency and to decrease GI transit time in long-term tube-fed patients (24,25). Soluble fiber in the form of partially hydrolyzed guar has been shown to be beneficial in reducing the incidence of diarrhea in tube-fed septic patients, as well as in noncritically ill medical-surgical patients (26).

Fructo-oligosaccharides (FOS), which are nondigestible, short-chain simple sugars, are considered Prebiotics and are provided in some enteral formulas (27). Prebiotics are substances thought to promote the growth of beneficial bacteria in the colon (28,29). FOS are digested in the colon where they have been shown to selectively stimulate the growth of beneficial bifidobacteria while suppressing the growth of potentially harmful species, such as Clostridium perfringens (30). The bifidobacteria metabolize FOS by fermentation to the short-chain fatty acids (SCFA) acetate, propinate, and butyrate, enhancing water and electrolyte reabsorbtion (30,31). SCFA are the preferred fuel for the enterocytes; they also contribute to a slightly acidic colonic environment, which can inhibit the growth of Clostridium difficile (32,33). EN support is believed to decrease the catabolic response to sepsis and trauma (34).

Safety Benefits

Although EN is not without potential complications, it is generally associated with a lower risk for infectious complications than parenteral nutrition (PN) (35,36). One meta-analysis of 20 studies involving 1,033 patients found the risk of infection 13% lower for EN than for PN (37), whereas another meta-analysis found the risk of infection to be 36% lower for EN than for PN (38). EN has also been associated with 15% fewer postoperative complications and shortened postoperative length of stay (LOS) in malnourished cancer patients (38,39). EN avoids complications related to central venous catheters (eg, catheter sepsis, pneumothorax) in a patient population that is often immunosuppressed and at high risk for infectious complications (40). For a discussion of PN, see Chapter 14.

Economic Benefits

Formula, equipment, and personnel are less costly for EN than for PN (41,42). Depending on the formula, PN can be 4 to 25 times more costly than EN (41,43).

Although EN is less expensive than PN, EN can still present a substantial financial challenge to the cancer patient. Whether or not this therapy is a covered benefit under a patient's insurance policy depends on many factors, including the patient's diagnosis and treatment plans as well as the specific insurance policy.

INDICATIONS FOR ENTERAL NUTRITION

EN is indicated in the malnourished patient who is unable to consume sufficient nutrition orally, providing the GI tract is functional and enteral access can be safely obtained (20). Much of the literature indicates that severely malnourished patients (often defined as having 10% weight loss in 1 to 3 months) realize the greatest benefit from nutrition support (2,20,44–46). According to guidelines established by the American Society for Parenteral and Enteral Nutrition (ASPEN), candidates for nutrition support include (2) the following:

- Patients receiving anticancer treatment who are malnourished. (Tools, such as the Scored Patient-Generated Subjective Global Assessment [PG-SGA] and institution-specific guidelines, can help quantify nutrition risk [4].) For further discussion of nutrition screening and assessment, see Chapter 6.
- Patients receiving anticancer treatment who are expected to be unable to ingest sufficient nutrition for a prolonged period of time, 7 to 14 days.

DISEASE-SPECIFIC INDICATIONS FOR ENTERAL NUTRITION

Head and Neck Cancer

Patients with advanced head and neck cancer experience malnutrition due to the malignancy itself, often with an associated history of alcohol abuse and poor oral intake (46–48). In addition, treatment of head and neck cancer (eg, radiation therapy, chemotherapy, and surgery) significantly contributes to the severe malnutrition seen in these patients (49,50).

Head and neck cancer patients can be fed enterally, either into the stomach or into the jejunum (see Table 13.1). If placement by the endoscopic route is not available, surgical placement is an option. For patients receiving radiation therapy, gastrostomy tubes placed

Table 13.1 Enteral Access Based on Tumor Location

Tumor Site	*Enteral Access*	*Administration*
Head and neck	Gastrostomy (percutaneous or surgical)	Continuous, bolus, intermittent, or cycled
	Jejunostomy (percutaneous or surgical)	Continuous or cycled
Esophageal	Gastrostomy (percutaneous or surgical)	Continuous, bolus, intermittent, or cycled
	Jejunostomy (percutaneous or surgical)	Continuous or cycled
Gastric	Jejunostomy (percutaneous or surgical)	Continuous or cycled
Pancreatic	Jejunostomy (percutaneous or surgical)	Continuous or cycled

before initiation of radiation therapy have been shown to minimize weight loss and treatment interruptions and to decrease the incidence of dehydration requiring hospitalization (49,51).

Clinicians should consider the possibility of gastric metastasis when placing enteric feeding tubes in patients with head and neck cancer. Although estimates place incidence of this complication at approximately 1%, a 2001 literature review found that in all reported cases the tube had been placed by the "pull" method (52–54). Many experts recommend not using this method in head and neck cancer patients; some experts recommend laparoscopic tube placements instead of percutaneous (54–57).

Esophageal Cancer

Malnutrition associated with esophageal cancer is due in part to dysphagia from mechanical obstruction, but tumor-dependent metabolic alterations also contribute to the cachexia syndrome (58). Therapies associated with esophageal cancer (eg, radiation therapy, chemotherapy, and surgery) can further compromise the patient's status, making it difficult to meet nutrition needs through oral intake alone. Endoscopic or surgical placement of feeding tubes into the stomach or duodenum has been shown to be safe and is frequently successful in feeding this group of patients (59,60).

Gastric Cancer

Gastric resection for gastric cancer can cause early satiety, rapid transit, dumping syndrome, and hypoglycemia, as well as possible deficiencies of iron, calcium, vitamin B-12, and fat-soluble vitamins (3). It is important to review the surgical reports to clearly identify how much of the esophagus, stomach, and intestines are remaining. Percutaneous or surgical placement of feeding tubes into the jejunum may be used to feed this group of patients, if altered gastric emptying precludes sufficient oral intake (61).

Pancreatic Cancer

Pancreatic cancer is associated with a high incidence of malnutrition and weight loss (62). The four primary reasons are (*a*) gastric outlet obstruction from the tumor; (*b*) fat malabsorption and vitamin K deficiency due to biliary obstruction; (*c*) malabsorption secondary to pancreatic insufficiency; and (*d*) early satiety and delayed gastric emptying after gastric resection (63,64). EN in this group of patients may be administered through a jejunostomy tube. Also, pancreatic enzyme replacement, insulin therapy, and medium-chain triglycerides may be indicated if a total pancreatectomy is performed (65,66).

TREATMENT-SPECIFIC INDICATIONS FOR ENTERAL NUTRITION

Chemotherapy

Nausea, vomiting, mucositis, and GI dysfunction, experienced as a result of chemotherapeutic agents, may further compromise existing malnutrition in the cancer patient (67). Nutrition support is indicated for patients undergoing antineoplastic therapy who are malnourished and will be unable to ingest or absorb adequate nutrients for a prolonged period (2). Jejunal feedings may be the most appropriate EN route for patients experiencing chemotherapy-induced nausea and vomiting (2).

Radiation Therapy

Depending on the area of irradiation, nutrition alterations may result from nausea and vomiting, mucositis, dysphagia, diarrhea, enteritis, maldigestion, or malabsorption (68). Systemic side effects of radiation therapy include fatigue and anorexia, which can also contribute to nutritional depletion (69). Experimental evidence suggests enteral feeding with elemental formulas as a form of prophylaxis against radiation enteritis (70,71). For more information on radiation therapy, see Chapter 9.

Despite studies indicating that prophylactic placement of feeding tubes can prevent interruption in treatment schedules, studies have not shown that nutrition support during radiation improves tumor response or overall survival (3,49). However, prospective studies do indicate significant improvements in some aspects of quality of life, such as physical functioning and fatigue levels, in response to enteral feedings (72,73).

CONTRAINDICATIONS TO ENTERAL NUTRITION

EN is contraindicated if the GI tract is nonfunctional, enteral access cannot be safely obtained, or bowel rest is required (2,8). The following are examples of these situations (74,75):

- Intestinal obstruction distal to lowest enteral access
- Diffuse peritonitis
- Intractable vomiting
- Paralytic ileus
- Severe GI bleeding
- Uncorrectable diarrhea that complicates metabolic management
- High-output enterocutaneous fistula > 800 mL/day
- Intestinal ischemia
- Hemodynamic instability
- Prognosis not consistent with aggressive nutrition

SELECTING AN ENTERAL FORMULA

When selecting an enteral formula, registered dietitians (RDs) should consider the following key questions (76):

- Are the patient's digestive and absorptive capacities intact?
- Does the patient have significant organ dysfunction and how is it being managed?
- What are the patient's metabolic requirements?
- Are any of the formula components contraindicated by patient's clinical status (eg, high levels of amino acid in renal failure)?
- Does the patient require a fluid restriction?
- Does the patient's insurance policy cover the desired formula? If so, what documentation is required?
- If the insurance does not cover the formula, or will only cover a portion of the cost, is there a less expensive formula that will meet the patient's clinical needs?

Currently, there are more than 100 different formulas on the market. These can be categorized into polymeric, monomeric, and disease-specific formulas (see Table 13.2).

Polymeric Formulas

Polymeric formulas contain intact carbohydrate polymers, proteins, and triglycerides, so normal absorption and digestion are necessary (23). Most of these products are lactose- and gluten-free and are casein or soy protein isolate-based. Generally, these formulas provide 100% of the Recommended Daily Intake (RDI) for micronutrients in 2 L, although some meet these requirements in less volume (77). Polymeric formulas are available in the following varieties (23):

- *Standard.* General tube-feeding requirements: 1.0 to 1.2 kcal/mL caloric density; moderate protein density; isotonic or hypertonic osmolality (300 to 650 mOsm/kg water).
- *High nitrogen.* Indicated for patients with increased protein needs. Generally provides 40 to 66 g/L protein; 1 to 2 kcal/mL caloric density; high protein density; isotonic or hypertonic osmolality (300 to 650 mOsm/kg water).
- *Fiber supplemented.* Aids in normalizing bowel function and may help to promote blood glucose control for patients with glucose intolerance (78). Per liter, blenderized formulas contain 4.4 to 6 g fiber from fruits and vegetables. Semisynthetic formulas have 8 to 22 g fiber per liter in the form of soy polysaccharide, partially hydrolyzed guar gum, and/or soy fiber; 1 to 1.5 kcal/mL; moderate protein density; and isotonic or hypertonic osmolality (300 to 650 mOsm/kg water).

Table 13.2 Types of Enteral Formulas

Type of Product and Examples	*Energy Density*	*Protein Density*	*Osmolality*	*Characteristics*
Monomeric • Optimental (Ross) • Peptamen (Nestle) • Subdue (Novartis)	1.0–1.5 kcal/mL	Moderate to high	Hypertonic	Indicated for patients with impaired digestion or absorption. Generally low fat and/or fat is provided as MCT.
Disease-specific • Diabetisource AC (Novartis) • Glucerna (Ross) • Nutren Glytrol (Nestle)	1.0–2.0 kcal/mL	Low, moderate, or high	Isotonic or hypertonic	Indicated for specific disease states (eg, renal, hepatic, or respiratory failure, cancer, glucose intolerance, stress/trauma).
Polymeric				
Standard • Isocal (Novartis) • Nutren (Nestle) • Osmolite 1.0 (Ross)	1.0–1.2 kcal/mL	Moderate	Isotonic or hypertonic	General tube-feeding requirements.
High-nitrogen • Isocal HN (Novartis) • Nutren Replete (Ross) • Promote (Nestle)	1.0–1.5 kcal/mL	High	Isotonic or hypertonic	Indicated for patients with increased protein needs.
Fiber-supplemented • Fibersource (Novartis) • Jevity 1.0 (Ross) • Nutren 1.0 Fiber (Nestle)	1.0–1.5 kcal/mL	Moderate or high	Isotonic or hypertonic	Helps normalize bowel function. May improve blood glucose control.
Concentrated • Deliver 2.0 (Novartis) • Nutren 2.0 (Nestle) • TwoCal HN (Ross)	1.5–2.25 kcal/mL	Moderate to high	Hypertonic	Indicated for fluid restricted patients. Helpful in time-restricted patients.
Modular				
Carbohydrate polymer • Polycose (Ross)	2.0 kcal/mL	None	Hypertonic	Adds energy to formulas for patients who are fat-, protein-, or electrolyte-restricted.
Protein supplement • Beneprotein (Novartis) • Promod (Ross)	25–28 kcal/scoop	5–6 g/scoop	Hypotonic	Adds protein to formulas without significantly adding to volume.
Fiber supplement • Benefiber (Novartis)	16 kcal/Tbsp	None		Adds fiber to formula.

Manufacturers: Ross Products Division, Abbott Laboratories Inc, Columbus, OH; Nestle Clinical Nutrition, Glendale, CA; Novartis Medical Nutrition, Minneapolis, MN

- *Concentrated.* Indicated for fluid-restricted patients; may be helpful for patients whose daily treatment schedules leave them little time to infuse their feedings. Provides 1.5 to 2.25 kcal/mL or 2,000 kcal in 3¾ to 5½ 8-oz cans. If the patient is not on a fluid restriction, adequate water flushes are essential, because these formulas provide only 543 to 1,000 mL free water for every 2,000 kcal. In addition, some patients experience nausea on these formulas because the high fat content (up to 109 g/day) can delay gastric emptying.

Monomeric Formulas

Monomeric formulas contain nutrients that have been hydrolyzed for easier digestion and absorption (23). Proteins are present as short-chain peptides or free amino acids; carbohydrates as oligosaccharides or maltodextrin. Many of these formulas are low in fat, which is generally provided as a blend of long- and medium-chain triglycerides. Because of their hydrolyzed components, these formulas are usually hypertonic and more expensive than polymeric formulas (23). Despite the lack of data supporting use of monomeric formulas, anecdotal evidence demonstrates benefit in select patients (42). Monomeric formulas, such as Optimental (Ross Products Division, Abbott Laboratories, Columbus, OH), Subdue (Novartis Nutrition, Minneapolis, MN), or Peptamen (Nestle Clinical Nutrition, Glendale, CA), are a reasonable choice for patients thought to have impaired digestion from chemotherapy, radiation therapy, or GI surgery.

Disease-Specific Formulas

Disease-specific formulas are designed to meet the needs of patients with specific medical conditions, such as renal/hepatic/respiratory failure, glucose intolerance, and stress/trauma.

Additionally, there are cancer-specific formulas designed to help ameliorate tumor-induced cachexia and weight loss. Two 8-oz cans (the recommended daily usage) of formulas such as Promote (Ross Products Division, Abbott Laboratories, Columbus, OH) or Resource Support (Novartis Nutrition, Minneapolis, MN) contain 600 to 720 kcal, 2 g of eicosapentaenoic acid (EPA), and approximately 1 g of docosahexanoic acid (DHA). EPA and DHA are anti-inflammatory n-3 fatty acids and appear to interfere with the signaling pathways of proinflammatory cytokines and proteolysis-inducing factor (79–81). Use of these formulas has been associated with increases of approximately 1 kg during a course of 3 weeks (82,83). Pancreatic cancer patients have served as subjects for the research regarding n-3 fatty acids. More research in other cancer patient populations is needed to fully understand the role of n-3 fatty acids in changing the metabolic and hormonal milieu associated with cachexia.

Disease-specific formulas can be taken orally or as part of an enteral prescription. Additionally, it may be helpful to encourage the patient to view n-3 supplementation as medical intervention, to help encourage compliance. In one study of 200 pancreatic cancer patients, optimal gains of weight and lean body mass (LBM) were observed at intakes of 1.5 to 2 cans of supplement daily. However, mean intake was only 1.4 cans per day. Intakes at this level were not associated with any significant improvements in weight or LBM (83).

Modulars

Modulars supply a single nutrient or a combination of nutrients and consist primarily of intact macronutrient sources (77). They are used to increase either the carbohydrate, the protein, or the lipid content of an enteral prescription without significantly altering the amount of other nutrients or the volume of the formula itself.

Because commercially prepared formulas have become so readily available, modular components are not as widely used as they once were. When they are used, they are generally mixed with water and flushed into the tube, not mixed as part of the formula itself.

Addition of modulars does represent a "critical control point" from a food-safety standpoint. Diligent hand washing and sanitation practices must be observed to limit the opportunity for contamination.

Fluid

Most enteral formulas contain from 70% to 85% free water (23). The majority of patients who are solely supported by tube feeds require additional water to meet hydration requirements (eg, 150 mL water flushes every 4 to 6 hours). This is especially important for patients receiving high nitrogen or fiber-supplemented formulas or those who have increased losses due to fevers, diarrhea, chest tubes, fistula, ostomies, or gastric decompression tubes. For information regarding specific fluid calculations, see Chapter 7.

Table 13.3 Enteral Access Devices

Enteral Device	*Usual Tube Size*	*Aspiration Risk*	*Dumping Risk*	*Placement*	*Potential Longevity*
Nasoenteric Access					
Nasogastric	5–12 Fr	High	Low	Bedside	10–15 days
Nasoduodenal	5–12 Fr	Moderate	Moderate	Bedside Fluoroscopic Endoscopic	10–15 days
Nasojejeunal	5–12 Fr	Low	High	Bedside Fluoroscopic Endoscopic	10–15 days
Feeding enterostomies					
PEG	15–28 Fr	Moderate	Low	Endoscopic	1–2 years
JET-PEG	8–12 Fr tube threaded through a 20 Fr tube	Low	High	Endoscopic	Several months (often limited by occlusions or tube migration)
DPEJ	20 Fr	Low	High	Endoscopic	1–2 years
Gastrostomy	14–30 Fr	Moderate	Low	Surgical	1–2 years
Jejunostomy	8–24 Fr	Low	High	Surgical	1–2 years

Source: Data are from references 2, 20, 84, and 85.

TYPES OF ENTERAL ACCESS

There are two types of access for providing EN. Nasoenteric tubes are used for short-term access (< 4 wk). Feeding enterostomies are used for permanent or long-term access (≥ 4 wk). See Table 13.3 (2,20,84,85) for a review of nasoenteric access and feeding enterostomies.

NASOENTERIC ACCESS

Nasoenteric access is indicated when enteral support is expected to last less than 4 weeks. Small-bore tubing generally requires replacement after 10 to 15 days because of clogging, kinking, or dislodgment. If the patient is at high risk for aspiration, nasoduodenal access or nasojejunal access is indicated (86). For patients receiving radiation therapy to the head and neck area, the esophagus, or the mediastinum, nasoenteric tubes are not often used because they can irritate the area being radiated.

Feeding Enterostomies

Feeding enterostomies, or gastric access, is the generally preferred method because it allows formula to be delivered into the stomach and allows use of hypertonic solutions and bolus infusions. Feeding enterostomies include the following:

- Percutaneous endoscopic gastrostomy (PEG) is the most popular nonsurgical procedure for obtaining permanent access (87). PEG is formed by the placement of a tube through percutaneous hole that passes from the stomach through the anterior abdominal wall. Upper endoscopy is used to guide placement. Can be done on an outpatient basis.
- Open gastrostomy is a surgical incision with placement of a gastrostomy tube through the abdominal wall.
- Laparoscopic gastrostomy is a surgical incision with placement of a gastrostomy tube through

the abdominal wall. Laparoscopic gastrostomy is performed under general anesthesia, in conjunction with other laparoscopic procedures. This type of gastric access is associated with fewer complications than open surgical placement but bears similar cost (88).

- Cervical pharyngostomy is a surgical placement of a feeding tube into the pharynx or cervical esophagus and passed into the stomach. Adjunct to head and neck surgery (89).
- Jejunal access is indicated in the presence of gastroparesis, gastric outlet obstruction, or suspected aspiration. Studies indicate feeding beyond the ligament of Treitz is associated with decreased incidence of aspiration and pneumonia (90,91). Cyclic or continuous infusion via a feeding pump is generally required, and rates of up to 180 mL/h can be safely tolerated for most patients (20).
- In an endoscopic jejunostomy placed through a gastrostomy (JET-PEG or PEJ), a large-bore PEG is placed, then a smaller tube is threaded through the PEG and endoscopically guided into the jejunum. Small-bore extensions often migrate back to the stomach.
- Direct percutaneous endoscopic jejunostomy (DPEJ) is formed by the placement of a tube through percutaneous hole that passes from the jejunum through the anterior abdominal wall.
- Open jejunostomy is the surgical placement of a feeding tube through the abdominal wall into the jejunum. Usually placed at least 20 cm beyond the ligament of Treitz (92).
- Laparoscopic jejunostomy is a surgical incision, with placement of a tube through the abdominal wall into the jejunum. This type of jejunostomy is performed under general anesthesia, in conjunction with other laparoscopic procedures. Laparoscopic jejunostomy is associated with fewer complications than open surgical placement, but has a similar cost (88).

ADMINISTRATION

The method of administration depends on the location of the feeding tube, patient tolerance, and overall nutrition goals. Bolus, intermittent, continuous, and cyclic are the four methods of tube-feeding administration.

Bolus

Bolus feedings are administered with a catheter tip syringe to deliver 240 to 400 mL of formula in 20 minutes or less several times a day (93,94). This method is frequently used in home care or with rehabilitation patients because of minimal equipment needs and speed of delivery. Feedings administered too rapidly via this method can result in nausea, diarrhea, vomiting, distension, cramps, or aspiration (95).

Intermittent

Intermittent feedings deliver up to 300 to 600 mL of formula over a 30- to 60-minute period several times a day, usually by gravity drip (93,94). Many of the GI complaints associated with bolus feedings are lessened, but tolerance can still be poor in some patients (96). Equipment and time requirements are greater than for bolus feeding.

Continuous and Cyclic

Infusion pumps allow for slow infusion of formula, either continuously for 24 hours or cycled (eg, 6 to 8 hours during sleep, or, more commonly, 10 to 12 hours), to allow increased patient mobility when not connected to the feeding pump (93,94). These slow, controlled delivery methods have the best tolerance but the highest time and equipment requirements (96). Pump-assisted feedings are necessary for delivery of nutrients into the duodenum or jejunum.

INITIATION AND ADVANCEMENT

Early feeding (within 1 to 4 hours after placement) has been shown to be as safe as waiting 24 hours (8,97). Initiating feedings with full-strength isotonic formulas is recommended. Dilution of formula is not recommended because it offers an opportunity for contamination.

Continuous full-strength feedings can be initiated at 20 to 50 mL/h and increased by 10 to 20 mL/h every 4 to 6 hours until goal rate is achieved (93). Transition to bolus or intermittent feedings is best attempted once the patient demonstrates tolerance to continuous feedings.

COMPLICATIONS

Although generally considered to carry a lower risk of infectious complications than PN, EN is not completely innocuous (37–39). Complications related to the delivery of EN may be classified into three categories: mechanical, GI, and metabolic.

Mechanical Complications

Feeding-tube displacement and migration is a serious complication and may result in feedings being delivered to a location other than the one intended. This can result in aspiration, diarrhea, or peritonitis (85). Verification of tube placement by x-ray should be done before feedings are started or anytime tube malposition is suspected.

Feeding tube obstruction may occur because of viscous formulas, inappropriate medication administration, formula residue, and inadequate flushing (2). To reduce the risk of clogging, RDs should consider the following:

- Flush tubes with at least 20 mL of warm water every 4 hours during continuous infusion and before and after intermittent feedings and medications (2).
- Flush tubes before and after checking gastric residuals.
- Avoid acidic fluids, such as cranberry juice and cola, because they can degrade the tube, precipitate protein out of the formula, and cause clogging (2).
- Provide medications as elixirs rather than pills when possible.

If a tube does become clogged, irrigation with a syringe of warm water should be attempted first. If that is not successful, other options include the enzyme papain, activated pancreatic enzymes mixed with water and sodium bicarbonate, or declogging devices (generally, kits including thin plastic catheters and/or enzyme preparations to be used only by a trained professional) (2). When kinked or knotted tubing causes the obstruction, the tube must be either repositioned or replaced.

Pressure necrosis of the skin is caused by the feeding tube pressing against the mucosal surface. It may also result in mucosal ulceration, abscess formation, and perforation. The risk of pressure necrosis can be reduced by using small-bore polyurethane or silicon tubing, or by replacing nasoenteric access with a feeding enterostomy (86).

Leakage of the feeding tube contents can be the result of several problems. In the case of a dysfunctional tube, the tube should be replaced. If leakage is due to an infection, antibiotic therapy, debridement, and/or feeding tube removal may be necessary. Stomal enlargement is another reason for leakage and can be treated by decreasing the diameter of the stoma, and then replacing the tube. See Table 13.4.

Gastrointestinal Complications

Regurgitation occurs when the formula is not absorbed and consequently accumulates and refluxes back into the GI tract. This can occur when the formula is administered too rapidly or if the patient does not remain upright during or after feeding. The feedings should be held or decreased while establishing the cause of the problem. Aspiration may result as a complication of regurgitation. The risk of aspiration is reduced by elevating the head of the bed to 30 to 45 degrees, using the lowest level of sedation feasible, providing the feedings via continuous delivery, placing the feeding tube beyond the pyloric sphincter, and regularly checking gastric residuals (98). Residuals should be checked with a large syringe (at least 60 cc). The smaller the syringe, the greater the hydraulic pressure and the likelihood the tube will collapse. The recent North American Summit on Aspiration produced recommendations to hold tube feeding formula only if residuals are greater than 500 mL (98). In some instances, it may be desirable to feed into the small bowel, while decompressing the stomach with a temporary or permanent gastric tube.

Diarrhea is one of the most common GI complaints associated with EN. However, it is usually not caused by the feeding itself (99). If the GI tract is part of the field during radiation therapy, radiation enteritis may result (71). Also, surgery to various parts of the GI tract may contribute to diarrhea (eg, dumping syndrome after gastric resection). After small bowel resection, fat maldigestion and malabsorption may occur and can lead to diarrhea (67).

Broad-spectrum antibiotics may promote opportunistic proliferation of pathogenic organisms normally suppressed by competitive organisms in the GI tract (85). The result is diarrhea caused by the decreased absorption of fluid and electrolytes. Clostridium difficile, the organism most often associated with antibiotic-related diarrhea, accounts for 10% to 25% percent of all cases. Clostridium perfringens, Salmonella, Shigella, Campylobacter, Yersinia enterocolitica, and Escheria coli organisms have also been implicated (85). Production of the enzyme lactase can be

Table 13.4 Mechanical Complications in Enteral Nutrition

Complication	*Possible Causes*	*Prevention/Treatment*
Displacement/migration	• Coughing, vomiting, combative patient	• Replace tube and confirm placement
Obstruction	• Crushed medications	• Thoroughly crush medications; use liquid form when possible
	• Adhesion of formula to tube	• Flush after feeds; avoid acidic liquids that cause precipitation
	• Inadequate irrigation	• Flush adequately
Pressure necrosis	• Nasoenteric tube irritating mucosa	• Change to small-bore poly-urethane or silicon tube; change to feeding enterostomy
Leaking tube	• Dysfunctional tube	• Replace tube
	• Infection	• Consult with physician; antibiotics, debridement; lastly tube removal
	• Enlarged stoma	• Consult with physician on surgically decreasing size of stoma

decreased during pelvic irradiation, with lactose intake causing diarrhea. Currently, most enteral formulas are lactose free.

Overfeeding, hypoalbuminemia, osmotically active medication, sorbitol-containing medication, and microbial contamination of the formula also can cause diarrhea (85). Immune-compromised patients are particularly susceptible to diarrhea, pneumonia, and septicemia, from infusion of contaminated product.

Constipation also may occur during EN. Certain types of chemotherapeutic agents, decreased activity, inadequate free water, and pain medications may contribute to constipation (4). A nutritional remedy for this problem can be the use of fiber-containing formulas. Adequate free water is essential in preventing constipation in any patient, especially when using a fiber-containing formula. For a summary of GI complications and possible treatments, see Table 13.5 (85,98).

Metabolic Complications

Refeeding syndrome is a potential metabolic complication of nutrition support. It is caused by the rapid serum depletion of potassium, phosphorous, and magnesium. This occurs in response to feeding; as insulin moves, these minerals are moved intracellularly, for use in metabolic pathways (100,101). The electrolyte abnormalities created by refeeding may result in generalized muscle weakness, tetany, cardiac dysfunction, seizures, arrhythmias, excess sodium and water retention, hemolytic anemia, phagocyte dysfunction, and death from cardiac or respiratory failure (102,103).

Careful screening to identify patients at risk is crucial. The following conditions can put patients at risk of developing refeeding syndrome (100,101):

- Weight < 70% ideal body weight
- Classic kwashiorkor (malnutrition associated with inadequate protein intake)
- Classic marasmus (malnutrition associated with inadequate energy intake)
- Chronic alcoholism
- NPO for 7 to 10 days with evidence of stress and depletion
- Morbid obesity with massive weight loss
- Prolonged IV hydration of fluid only, without energy-containing macronutrients

Other recommendations to decrease the likelihood of refeeding syndrome include (*a*) correcting electrolyte, vitamin, and trace element disorders before feeding (104); (*b*) slowly increasing the calories provided over 2 to 3 days (101); and (*c*) carefully monitoring electrolytes, vital signs, and fluid volume throughout therapy (101,104).

Dehydration, hypernatremia, and azotemia may occur during EN. These complications often occur in noncommunicative patients who cannot express or alleviate thirst. It is important to closely monitor the fluid status of tube-fed patients. See Table 13.6 for a

Table 13.5 Gastrointestinal Complications in Enteral Nutrition

Complication	*Possible Causes*	*Prevention/Treatment*
High residuals	• Decreased gastric motility	• Elevate head of bed 30°–45°; metoclopramide, erythromycin 200–500 cc bedside algorithm; > 500 cc hold feeding; small bowel feedings
Aspiration, reflux, gastric retention	• Impaired gag reflex, altered gastric motility • Patient laying flat • Displaced tube	• Continuous infusion, check residuals • Elevate head of bed • Monitor tube placement, position distal to ligament of Treitz
Nausea/vomiting, cramping, distension, bloating, hypermotility	• Rapid formula administration • High fat content of formula • Cold formula	• Advance rate gradually • Evaluate for change to lower-fat formula • Administer at room temperature
Diarrhea	• Fiber-free formula	• Use formula with soluble fiber (partially hydrogenated guar gum)
	• Formula administration	• Advance rate gradually; continuous infusion; decrease rate temporarily
	• Overfeeding	• Reduce energy intake
	• Hypoalbuminemia	• Elemental or semi-elemental diet initially
	• Malabsorption	• Consult with physician on prescribing pancreatic enzymes
	• Bacterial contamination	• Clean technique; change tubing frequently; observe appropriate hang-time; select formula with fructo-oligosaccharides (FOS)
	• Medications (antibiotics, sorbitol-containing liquids, H_2 blockers, lactulose, magnesium-containing antacids, potassium and phosphorus supplements)	• Consult with physician to change medications or add antimotility medication
Constipation	• Inadequate fluid • Decreased gastric motility • Inadequate bulk • Medications • Inactivity	• Increase free water • Provide stool softener • Increase fiber (soy polysaccharide) • Provide prune juice • Increase activity

Source: Data are from references 85 and 98.

review of metabolic complications and possible treatments (94,105).

Medication Interactions With Enteral Feeding

A thorough review of medications is important when initiating EN and on an ongoing basis, to lessen the chance of an interaction. Medications of concern for this patient population include the following:

- *Phenytoin.* Concurrent administration of phenytoin and EN decreases serum concentrations of phenytoin, possibly because of protein binding magnesium and calcium cations (106).
- *Warfarin.* Vitamin K intake can affect drug action; warfarin may sequester enteral formula protein, causing decreased bioavailability.
- *Theophylline.* Concurrent administration with EN decreases absorption of theophylline (106).

Table 13.6 Metabolic Complications in Enteral Nutrition

Complication	*Possible Causes*	*Prevention/Treatment*
Dehydration	• Inadequate free water; high fluid output; hypertonic feeds	• Monitor fluid status; monitor weight daily (1 kg change = 1 L fluid); increase free water to meet fluid needs as assessed
Overhydration	• Excess fluid intake	• Select concentrated formula
Elevated glucose	• Insulin resistance • Metabolic stress	• Change to fiber-containing formula • Insulin
Hypercapnia	• Excess carbohydrate • Overfeeding	• Limit carbohydrate to ≤ 50% total energy; monitor carbon dioxide • Consider decreasing total calories provided
Hypernatremia	• Inadequate free water, excess sodium	• Assess fluid and electrolytes status; increase free water to meet fluid needs as assessed
Hyponatremia	• Fluid overload • Syndrome of inappropriate antidiuretic hormone (SIADH) • Excess gastrointestinal losses	• Use more concentrated formulas • Diurese if necessary, fluid restriction • Provide sodium supplement
Hyperkalemia	• Excess potassium; decreased excretion	• Monitor serum levels; consult with physician to treat with kayexalate; consider low-potassium formula
Hypokalemia	• Aggressive refeeding • Potassium-wasting diuretics; insulin therapy; overhydration	• Decrease formula rate by half; consult with physician to replace potassium • Supplement with potassium
Hyperphosphatemia	• Renal insufficiency, phosphate-containing antacid	• Provide phosphate binders, low-phosphorus formula; consult with physician to change medications
Hypophosphatemia	• Aggressive refeeding; insulin therapy; phosphate-binding antacids	• Monitor and correct serum levels; consult with physician to change medications
Hypomagnesemia	• Decreased potassium • Increased gastrointestinal losses • Decreased serum carrier proteins	• Correct potassium • Supplement magnesium • To correct for low plasma protein levels (albumin), use the following calculation*: Corrected Magnesium (Mg) = Actual Serum Mg + 0.08 × (4 – Serum Albumin), where Mg is measured in mEq/L and Albumin is measured in g/L

*This calculation should *not* be used in patients with renal impairment nor in transplant patients receiving cyclosporine, which can cause magnesium wasting.

Source: Data are from references 94 and 105.

High osmolality and sorbitol content of elixir can cause diarrhea (107).

- *Antacids and H2 blockers.* Antacids and H2 blockers increase the pH of the stomach, which has been linked to bacterial colonization and migration from the stomach (108). Magnesium-containing antacids can cause diarrhea, but changing to one that contains calcium or aluminum can alleviate the problem. Antacids used in conjunction with sucralfate therapy have been associated with bezoar formation in tube-fed patients (108).
- *Furosemide.* Diarrhea secondary to sorbitol content of oral solution.
- *Ciprofloxacin.* Concurrent administration with EN has been found to decrease the bioavailability of ciprofloxacin by 27% to 67% (109). This is attributed to chelation with divalent cations in the formula.

TRANSITION TO ORAL INTAKE

Resuming oral feedings often requires a team approach. If the patient has had dysphagia, a swallowing evaluation by a speech-language pathologist is recommended, to verify safety of oral intake. If the patient can eat safely, calorie counts should be conducted to quantify oral intake.

Once the patient is consuming 50% of needs orally, the tube feeding can be decreased. Nocturnal tube feeding during the transition to oral intake should be encouraged, to help promote appetite (110,111).

Tube feeds can be discontinued when the patient is meeting 75% of nutrition needs orally. Oral nutrition supplements can be used to make up any deficit (110,111).

TRANSITION TO HOME

Discharge plans should be considered at the initiation of enteral therapy. A teachable and motivated patient or caregiver is essential for a successful home experience. Education should begin in the hospital and continue in the home setting. The amount of time and education required before a patient is independent with feeding will vary with the therapy used and the patient's ability to learn. A reputable home care provider who communicates with the health care team is crucial.

Discharge needs include formula, equipment (syringe, pump, pole, etc), other supplies (dressings, etc), and visits from an in-home clinician if the patient is homebound. Cost of formula used is another consideration. Medicare and Medicaid cover most of the expenses if the patient has a qualifying diagnosis (112). However, some payers will only cover the cost of supplies, and the patient will be responsible for the cost of the formula.

PALLIATIVE CARE

For patients electing palliative care, EN may still be provided as a supportive measure providing nourishment, fluid, and electrolytes. The goal of palliative care is to promote patient comfort. The literature has been divided as to whether or not artificial nutrition and hydration play a helpful role in palliative care (113,114).

The decision to withhold or withdraw nutrition and hydration from someone who is actively dying is a complex ethical, legal, and emotional issue (115,116). Open communication between patients, physicians, and family members can help avoid unnecessary pain and suffering (117). Discussions about the patient's wishes and plan of care, weighing risks and benefits of enteral feeding and examining personal beliefs and biases, are necessary (118).

REFERENCES

1. Ollenschlager G, Viell B, Thomas W, Konkol K, Burger B. Tumor anorexia: causes, assessment, treatment. *Cancer Res.* 1991;121:249–259.
2. ASPEN Board of Directors and the Clinical Guidelines Task Force. Guidelines for the use of parenteral and enteral nutrition in adult and pediatric patients. *JPEN J Parenter Enteral Nutr.* 2002;26(suppl 1): SA1-SA138.
3. Harrison LE, Fong Y. Enteral nutrition in the cancer patient. In: Rombeau JL, Rolandelli RH, eds. *Enteral and Tube Feeding*. Philadelphia, Pa: WB Saunders; 1997:300–323.
4. Bloch AS. Cancer. In: Matarese LE, Gottschlich MM, eds. *Contemporary Nutrition Support Practice.* Philadelphia, Pa: WB Saunders; 1998:475–495.
5. Peltz G. Nutrition support in cancer patients: a brief review and suggestion for standard indications criteria. *Nutr J.* 2002;1:1.

6. Kitchen P, Forbes A. Parenteral nutrition. *Curr Opin Gastroenterol.* 2003;19:144–147.
7. Abou-Assi S, Khurana V, Schubert M. Gastric and postpyloric total enteral nutrition. *Curr Treat Options Gastroenterol.* 2005;8:145–152.
8. Gopalan S, Khanna S. Enteral nutrition delivery technique: pharmaceutical aspects, devices and techniques. *Curr Opin Clin Nutr Metab Care.* 2003;6: 313–317.
9. Wildhaber BE, Yang H, Spencer AU, Drongowski RA, Teitelbaum DH. Lack of enteral nutrition effects on the intestinal immune system. *J Surg Res.* 2005; 123:8–16.
10. Schattner M, Shike M. Nutrition support of the patient with cancer. In: Shils ME, Shike M, Ross CA, Caballero B, Cousins RJ, eds. *Modern Nutrition in Health and Disease.* 10th ed. Philadelphia, Pa: Lippincott Williams and Wilkins; 2006:1291–1313.
11. Moore FA, Feliciano DV, Andrassy RJ, McArdle AH, Booth FV, Morgenstein-Wagner TB, Kellum JM Jr, Welling RE, Moore EE. Early enteral feeding, compared with parenteral, reduces postoperative septic complications. The results of a meta-analysis. *Ann Surg.* 1992;216:172–183.
12. Kudsk KA. Gut mucosal nutrition support-enteral nutrition as primary therapy after multiple system trauma. *Gut.* 1994;35(suppl):S52-S54.
13. Suchner V, Senftleben U, Eckart T, Scholz MR, Beck K, Murr R, Enzenbach R, Peter K. Enteral versus parenteral nutrition: effects on gastrointestinal function and metabolism. *Nutrition.* 1996;12:13–22.
14. Alverdy JC, Laughlin RS, Wu L. Influence of the critically ill state on host-pathogen interactions within the intestine: gut-derived sepsis redefined. *Crit Care Med.* 2003;31:598–607.
15. Lipman TO. Bacterial translocation and enteral nutrition in humans: an outsider looks in. *JPEN J Parenter Enteral Nutr.* 1995;19:156–165.
16. Van Der Hulst R, Van Kreel B, Meyenfeldt M, Brummer R, Arends J, Deutz N, Soiters P. Glutamine and the preservation of gut function. *Lancet.* 1993;341: 1363–1365.
17. Saito H, Furukawa S, Matsuda T. Glutamine as an immunoenhancing nutrient. *JPEN J Parenter Enteral Nutr.* 1999;23(suppl 5):S59-S61.
18. Waters B, Kudsk KA, Jarvi EJ, Brown RO, Fabian TC, Wood GC. Effect of route of nutrition on recovery of hepatic organic anion clearance after fasting. *Surgery.* 1994;115:370–374.
19. McCowen KC, Bistrian BR. Immunonutrition: problematic or problem solving? *Am J Clin Nutr.* 2003;77:764–770.
20. Schattner M. Enteral nutrition support of the patient with cancer: route and role. *J Clin Gastroenterol.* 2003;36:297–302.
21. de Luis DA, Izaola O, Cuellar L, Terroba MC, Aller R. Randomized clinical trial with an enteral arginine-enhanced formula in early post surgical head and neck cancer patients. *Euro J Clin Nutr.* 2004;58: 1505–1508.
22. Montejo JC, Zarazaga A, Lopez-Martinez J, Urrutia G, Roque M, Blesa AL, Celaya S, Conejero R, Galban C, Garcia de Lorenzo A, Grau T, Mesejo A, Ortiz-Leyba C, Planas M, Ordonez J, Jimenez FJ; Spanish Society of Intensive Care Medicine and Coronary Units. Immunonutrition in the intensive care unit: a systematic review and consensus statement. *Clin Nutr.* 2003;22:221–233.
23. Olree K, Vitello J, Sullivan J, Kohn-Keeth C. Enteral formulations. In: Merritt RM, Souba WW, Kohn-Keeth C, eds. *The A.S.P.E.N. Nutrition Support Practice Manual.* Silver Springs, Md: American Society for Parenteral and Enteral Nutrition; 1998:4.1–4.9.
24. Evans MA, Shronts EP. Intestinal fuels: glutamine, short chain fatty acids and dietary fiber. *J Am Diet Assoc.* 1992;92:1239–1246.
25. Heymsfield SB, Roongspisuthipong C, Evert M, Casper K, Heller P, Akrabawi SS. Fiber supplementation of enteral formulas: effect on the bioavailability of major nutrients and gastrointestinal tolerance. *JPEN J Parenter Enteral Nutr.* 1998;12:265–273.
26. Spapen H, Diltoer M, Van Malderen C, Opdenacker G, Suys E, Huyghens L. Soluble fiber reduces the incidence of diarrhea in septic patients receiving total enteral nutrition: a prospective, double-blind, randomized, and controlled trial. *Clin Nutr.* 2001;20: 301–305.
27. Whelan K, Judd P, Preddy V, Taylor M. Enteral feeding: the effect on faecal output and short chain fatty acid concentrations. *Proc Nutr Soc.* 2004;63:105–113.
28. Broussard E, Surawicz C. Probiotics and prebiotics in clinical practice. *Nutr Clin Care.* 2004;7:104–113.
29. Langlands S, Hopkins M, Coleman N, Cummings J. Prebiotic carbohydrates modify the mucosa associated with microflora of the human large bowel. *Gut.* 2004;53:1610–1616.
30. Bornet FR, Brouns F, Tashiro Y, Duvillier V. Nutritional aspects of short-chain fructooligosaccharides:

natural occurrence, chemistry, physiology and health implications. *Dig Liver Dis*. 2002;34(suppl 2):S111-S120.

31. Slavin JL, Nelson NL, McNamara EA, Cashmere K. Bowel function of healthy men consuming liquid diets with and without dietary fiber. *JPEN J Parenter Enteral Nutr.* 1985;9:317–321.
32. Kripke SA, Fox AD, Berman JM, Settle RG, Rombeau JL. Stimulation of intestinal mucosal growth with intracolonic infusion of short-chain fatty acids. *JPEN J Parenter Enteral Nutr*. 1989;13:109–116.
33. Scheppach W, Bartram P, Richter A, Richter F, Liepold H, Dussel G, Hofstetter G, Kasper H. Effect of short-chain fatty acids on human colonic mucosa in vitro. *JPEN J Parenter Enteral Nutr*. 1992;16: 43–48.
34. Wray CJ, Mammen JM, Hasselgren PO. Catabolic response to stress and potential benefits of nutrition support. *Nutrition*. 2002;18:971–977.
35. Simpson S, Doig G. Parenteral versus enteral nutrition in critically ill patients: a meta-analysis of trials using the intention to treat principle. *Intensive Care Med.* 2005;31:12–23.
36. Gramlich L, Kichian K, Pinilla J, Rodych N, Dhaliwal R, Heyland D. Does enteral nutrition compared to parenteral nutrition result in better outcomes in critically ill adult patients? A systematic review of the literature. *Nutrition.* 2004;20:843–848.
37. Braunschweig C, Levy P, Sheean PM, Wang X. Enteral compared with parenteral nutrition: a meta-analysis. *Am J Clin Nutr.* 2001;74:534–542.
38. Bozzetti F, Braga M, Gianotti L, Gavazzi C, Mariani L. Postoperative enteral versus parenteral nutrition in malnourished patients with gastrointestinal cancer: a randomized multicentre trial. *Lancet.* 2001;358: 1487–1492.
39. Bertrand PC, Piquet MA, Bordier I, Monnier P, Roulet M. Preoperative nutritional support at home in head and neck cancer patients: from nutritional benefits to the prevention of the alcohol withdrawal syndrome. *Curr Opin Clin Nutr Metab Care.* 2002;5: 435–440.
40. Rolstonk V. Challenges in the treatment of infection caused by gram positive and gram negative bacteria in patients with cancer and neutropenia. *Clin Infect Dis.* 2005;40(Suppl 4):S246-S252.
41. Tchekmedyian NS. Costs and benefits of nutrition support in cancer. *Oncology.* 1995;9(Suppl 11): 79–84.
42. Tchekmedyian NS. Pharmacoeconomics of nutritional support in cancer. *Semin Oncol.* 1998;25(2 Suppl 6):62–69.
43. Braga M, Gianotti L, Gentilini O, Parisi V, Salis C, Di Carlo V. Early postoperative enteral nutrition improves gut oxygenation and reduces costs compared with total parenteral nutrition. *Crit Care Med.* 2001;29:242–248.
44. Van Way CW. Perioperative nutrition support as an adjunct to surgical therapy for cancer. *Nutr Clin Pract.* 2002;17:214–217.
45. Ravasco P, Monteiro-Grillo I, Vidal PM, Camilo ME. Nutritional deterioration in cancer: the role of disease and diet. *Clin Oncol.* 2003;15:443–450.
46. Thun M, Peto R, Lopez A, Monaco J, Henley S, Heath C, Doll R. Alcohol consumption and mortality among middle-aged and elderly U.S. adults. *N Engl J Med.* 1997;337:1705–1714.
47. Tanable H, Yokota K, Shibata N, Satoh T, Watari J, Kohoyo Y. Alcohol consumption as a major risk factor in development of early esophageal cancer in patients with head and neck cancer. *Intern Med.* 2001;40:692–696.
48. Enziger P, Mayer R. Medical progress: esophageal cancer. *N Engl J Med.* 2003;349:2241–2252.
49. Lee JH, Machtay M, Unger LD, Weinstein GS, Weber RS, Chalian AA, Rosenthal DI. Prophylactic gastrostomy tubes in patients undergoing intensive irradiation for cancer of the head and neck. *Arch Otolaryngol Head Neck Surg.* 1998;124:871–875.
50. Riccardi D, Allen K. Nutritional management of patients with esophageal and esophagogastric junction cancer. *Cancer Control.* 1999;6:64–72.
51. Scolpio JS, Spangler PR, Romano MM, McLaughlin MP, Salassa JR. Prophylactic placement of gastrostomy feeding tubes before radiotherapy in patients with head and neck cancer: is it worthwhile? *J Clin Gastroenterol.* 2001;33:215–217.
52. Lin HS, Ibrahim HZ, Keng JW, Fee WE, Terris DJ. Percutaneous endoscopic gastrostomy: strategies for prevention and management of complications. *Laryngoscope.* 2001;11:1847–1852.
53. Maccabee D, Sheppard BC. Prevention of percutaneous endoscopic gastrostomy stoma metastases in patients with active oropharyngeal malignancy. *Surg Endosc.* 2003;17:1678.
54. Sinclair JJ, Scolapio JS, Stark ME, Hindr RA. Metastasis of head and neck carcinoma to the site of percutaneous endoscopic gastrostomy: a case report and

literature review. *JPEN J Parenter Enteral Nutr.* 2001;25:282–285.

55. Thakore JN, Mustafa M, Suryaprasad S, Agraval S. Percutaneous endoscopic gastrostomy associated gastric metastasis. *J Clin Gastroenterol.* 2003; 37:307–311.
56. Meurer MF, Kenady DE. Metastatic head and neck carcinoma in a percutaneous gastrostomy site. *Head Neck.* 1993;15:70–73.
57. Bhama JK, Haas MK, Fisher WE. Spread of pharyngeal cancer to the abdominal wall after percutaneous endoscopic gastrostomy. *Surg Laparosc Endosc Percutan Tech.* 2001;11:375–378.
58. Burt ME, Brennan MF. Nutritional support of the patient with esophageal cancer. *Semin Oncol.* 1984; 11:127–135.
59. Margolis M, Alexander P, Trachiotis GD, Gharagozloo F, Lipman T. Percutaneous endoscopic gastrostomy before multimodality therapy in patients with esophageal cancer. *Ann Thorac Surg.* 2003;76: 1694–1698.
60. Angus F, Burakoff R. The percutaneous endoscopic gastrostomy tube. Medical and ethical issues in placement. *Am J Gastroenterol.* 2003;98:272–277.
61. Herrman V, Fuhrman M, Borum P. Wasting diseases. In: Merritt RM, Souba WW, Kohn-Keeth C, eds. *The A.S.P.E.N. Nutrition Support Practice Manual.* Silver Springs, Md: American Society for Parenteral and Enteral Nutrition; 1998:11.1–11.15.
62. US Cancer Statistics Working Group. *United States Cancer Statistics, 2000 Incidence*. Atlanta, Ga: Department of Health and Human Services, Centers for Disease Control and Prevention, and National Cancer Institute; 2003.
63. Wakasugi H, Hara Y, Abe M. A study of malabsorption in pancreatic cancer. *J Gastroenterol.* 1996;31:81–85.
64. Thor P, Poplela T, Sobocki J, Herman R, Matyja A, Huszno B. Pancreatic carcinoma-induced changes in gastric myoelectric activity and emptying. *Hepatogastroenterology.* 2002;49:268–270.
65. Braga M, Cristallo M, De Franchis R, Mangiagalli A, Zerbi A, Agape D, Primignani M, Di Carlo V. Pancreatic enzyme replacement therapy in post-pancreatectomy patients. *Int J Pancreatol.* 1989;5(suppl): 37–44.
66. Robert A. Adequate enzyme replacement after total pancreatectomy. *JAMA.* 1989;261:2638–2639.
67. Kokal WA. The impact of antitumor therapy on nutrition. *Cancer.* 1985;55:273–278.
68. Henriksson R, Bergstrom P, Franzen L, Lewin F, Wagenius G. Aspects on reducing gastrointestinal adverse effects associated with radiotherapy. *Acta Oncol.* 1999;38:159–164.
69. Capra S, Ferguson M, Reid K. Cancer: impact of nutrition intervention outcome—nutrition issues for patients. *Nutrition.* 2001;17:769–772.
70. McArdle AH, Reid EC, Laplante MP, Freeman CR. Prophylaxis against radiation injury. The use of elemental diet prior to and during radiotherapy for invasive bladder cancer and in early postoperative feeding following radical cystectomy and ileal conduit. *Arch Surg.* 1986;121:879–885.
71. Craighead PS, Young S. Phase II study assessing the feasibility of using elemental supplements to reduce acute enteritis in patients receiving radical pelvic radiotherapy. *Am J Clin Oncol.* 1998;21:573–578.
72. Roberge C, Tran M, Massoud C, Poiree B, Duval N, Damecour E, Frout D, Malvy D, Joly F, Lebailly P, Henry-Amar M. Quality of life and home enteral tube feeding: a French prospective study in patients with head and neck or oesophageal cancer. *Br J Cancer.* 2000;82:263–269.
73. Loeser C, von Herz U, Kuchler T, Rzehak P, Muller MJ. Quality of life and nutritional state in patients on home enteral tube feeding. *Nutrition.* 2003;19: 605–611.
74. Cresci GA. Enteral access: the role of the nutrition support dietetics professional. *Support Line.* 2002; 24:12–18.
75. Trujillo EB, Robinson M. Nutrition feeding critically ill patients: current concepts. *Crit Care Nurs.* 2001;21:60–66.
76. Trujillo EB. Enteral nutrition: a comprehensive overview. In: Matarese LE, Gottschlich MM, eds, *Contemporary Nutrition Support Practice.* Philadelphia, Pa: WB Saunders; 1998:192–201.
77. Gottschlich MM, Shronts EP, Hutchins AM. Defined formula diets. In: Rombeau JL, Rolandelli RH, eds. *Enteral and Tube Feeding.* Philadelphia, Pa: WB Saunders; 1997:207–239.
78. Coulston AM. Clinical experience with modified enteral formulas for patients with diabetes. *Clin Nutr.* 1998;17(Suppl 2):46–56.
79. Jho D, Babcock TA, Helton WS, Espat NJ. Omega-3 fatty acids: implications for the treatment of tumor-associated inflammation. *Am Surg.* 2003;69:32–36.
80. Tisdale MJ. The "cancer cachectic factor." *Support Care Cancer.* 2003;11:73–78.

81. Barber MD. The pathophysiology and treatment of cancer cachexia. *Nutr Clin Pract.* 2002;17:203–209.
82. Barber MD, Fearon KC, Tisdale MJ, McMillan DC, Ross JA. Effect of a fish oil-enriched nutritional supplement on metabolic mediators in patients with pancreatic cancer cachexia. *Nutr Cancer.* 2001;40:118–124.
83. Fearon KCH, von Meyenfeldt MF, Moses AGW, van Geenen R, Roy A, Gouma DJ, Giacosa A, Van Gossum A, Bauer J, Barber MD, Aaronson NK, Voss AC, Tisdale MJ. Effect of a protein- and energy-dense n-3 fatty acid enriched oral supplement on loss of weight and lean tissue in cancer cachexia: a randomized double blind trial. *Gut.* 2003;52:1479–1486.
84. DeChicco RS, Matarese LE. Determining the nutrition support regimen. In: Matarese LE, Gottschlich MM, eds. *Contemporary Nutrition Support Practice.* Philadelphia, Pa: WB Saunders; 1998:185–191.
85. Beyer PL. Complications of enteral nutrition In: Matarese LE, Gottschlich MM, eds. *Contemporary Nutrition Support Practice.* Philadelphia, Pa: WB Saunders; 1998:216–226.
86. Minard G, Lysen L. Enteral access. In: Gottschlich M, Furhman M, Hammond K, Holcombe B, Seider D, eds. *The Science and Practice of Nutrition Support: A Case-Based Core Curriculum.* Dubuque, Iowa: ASPEN; 2001:167–188.
87. Minard G. Enteral access. *Nutr Clin Pract.* 1994;9:172–182.
88. Nagle AP, Murayama KM. Laparoscopic gastrostomy and jejunostomy. *J Long Term Eff Med Implants.* 200414:1–12.
89. Clevenger FW, Rodriguez DJ. Decision-making for enteral feeding administration: the why behind the where and how. *Nutr Clin Pract.* 1995;10:104–113.
90. Rombeau JL, Caldwell MD. *Enteral and Tube Feeding.* Philadelphia, Pa: WB Saunders; 1984.
91. Heyland DK, Drover JW, MacDonald S, Nocak F, Lam M. Effect of postpyloric feeding on gastroesophageal regurgitation and pulmonary microaspiration: results of a randomized controlled trial. *Crit Care Med.* 2001;29:1495–1501.
92. Heyland DK, Drover JW, Dhaliwal R, Greenwood J. Optimizing the benefits and minimizing the risks of enteral nutrition in the critically ill: role of small bowel feeding. *JPEN J Parenter Enteral Nutr.* 2002;26(6 Suppl):S51-S57.
93. Skipper A. *A Dietitian's Handbook of Enteral and Parenteral Nutrition.* 2nd ed. Gaithersburg, Md: ASPEN; 1998.
94. Lord L, Trumbore L, Zaloga G. Enteral nutrition implementation and management. In: Merritt RM, Souba WW, Kohn-Keeth C, eds. *The A.S.P.E.N. Nutrition Support Practice Manual.* Silver Springs, Md: American Society for Parenteral and Enteral Nutrition; 1998:5.10–5.14.
95. Metheny NA. Risk factors for aspiration. *JPEN J Parenter Enteral Nutr.* 2002;26(6 Suppl):S26-S31.
96. Shang E, Geiger N, Sturm JW, Post S. Pump-assisted versus gravity-controlled enteral nutrition in long-term percutaneous endoscopic gastrostomy patients: a prospective controlled trial. *JPEN J Parenter Enteral Nutr.* 2003;27:216–219.
97. Stein J, Schulte-Bockholt A, Sabin M, Keymling M. A randomized prospective trial of immediate vs. next-day feeding after percutaneous endoscopic gastrostomy in intensive care patients. *Intensive Care Med.* 2002;28:1656–1660.
98. McClave SA, De Meo MT, De Legge MH, Di Sario JA, Heyland DK, Maloney JP, Metheny NA, Moore FA, Scolapio JS, Spain DA, Zaloga GP. North American summit on aspiration in the critically ill patient: consensus statement. *JPEN J Parenter Enteral Nutr.* 2002;26(6 Suppl):S80-S85.
99. Hamaoui E, Kodsi R. Complications of enteral feeding and their prevention. In: Rombeau JL, Rolandelli RH, eds. *Enteral and Tube Feeding.* Philadelphia, Pa: WB Saunders; 1997:554–574.
100. Alpers D, Klein S. Refeeding the malnourished patient. *Curr Opin Gastroenterol.* 1999;15:151–155.
101. Solomon S, Kirby D. The refeeding syndrome: a review. *JPEN J Parenter Enteral Nutr.* 1990;14:90–96.
102. Afzal NA, Addai S, Fagbemi A, Murch S, Thomson M, Heuschkel R. Refeeding syndrome with enteral nutrition in children: a case report, literature review and clinical guidelines. *Clin Nutr.* 2002;21:515–520.
103. Marinella MA. Refeeding syndrome: implications for the inpatient rehabilitation unit. *Am J Phys Med Rehabil.* 2004;83:65–68.
104. Crook MA, Hally V, Pantelli JV. The importance of the refeeding syndrome. *Nutrition.* 2001;17:632–637.
105. Russell M, Cromer M, Grant J. Complications of enteral nutrition therapy. In: Matarese LE, Gottschlich MM, eds. *The Science and Practice of Nutrition Support: A Case-Based Core Curriculum.* Silver Spring, Md: American Society for Parenteral and Enteral Nutrition; 2001:189–209.
106. Rollins CJ. General pharmacological issues. In: Matarese LE, Gottschlich MM, eds. *Contemporary*

Nutrition Support Practice. Philadelphia, Pa; WB Saunders; 1998:303–323.

107. Holtz L, Milton J, Sturek JK. Compatibility of medications with enteral feeding. *JPEN J Parenter Enteral Nutr.* 1987;11:183–186.
108. Thomson FC, Naysmith M, Lindasy A. Managing drug therapy in patients receiving enteral and parenteral nutrition. *Hosp Pharm.* 2000;7:155–164.
109. Healy D, Brodbeck M, Clendening C. Ciprofloxacin absorption is impaired in patients given enteral feedings orally and via gastrostomy and jejunostomy tubes. *Antimicrobial Agents Chemo.* 1996;40:6–10.
110. Guenter P, Silkrowski M. *Tubefeeding: Practical Guidelines and Nursing Protocols.* Gaithersburg, Md: ASPEN; 2001.
111. Dietary Department, the University of Iowa Hospital and Clinics. *Enteral Nutrition: A Handbook for Dietitians and Health Professionals.* Iowa City, Iowa: Iowa State Press; 1990.
112. Roman M. Home enteral nutrition: what the hospital-based dietitian needs to know. *Support Line.* 2003; 25(5):17–20.
113. Printz LA. Terminal dehydration, a compassionate treatment. *Arch Intern Med.* 1992;152:697–700.
114. Fainsinger RL, Bruera E. The management of dehydration in terminally ill patients. *J Palliat Care.* 1994;10:55–59.
115. Welk TA. Clinical and ethical considerations of fluid and electrolyte management in the terminally ill client. *J Intraven Nurs.* 1999;22:43–47.
116. Schwarte AM. Withdrawal of nutrition support from the terminally ill. *Crit Care Nurs Clin N Am.* 2002; 14:193–196.
117. McClement SE, Denger LF, Harlos MS. Family beliefs regarding the nutritional care of a terminally ill relative: a qualitative study. *J Palliat Med.* 2003;6:737–748.
118. Slomka J. Withholding nutrition at the end of life: clinical and ethical issues. *Cleve Clin J Med.* 2003; 70:548–552.

Chapter 14

Parenteral Nutrition in Medical or Surgical Oncology

ROBERT S. DECHICCO, MS, RD, CNSD, AND EZRA STEIGER, MD, FACS, CNSP

OVERVIEW

Parenteral nutrition (PN) is administered to oncology patients with the intent of improving nutritional status in order to increase the response rate to therapy and decrease morbidity and mortality. This chapter examines the indications for PN, components of PN, and PN administration techniques. This chapter also examines the potential benefits of PN, which must be balanced against the cost of the therapy and potential adverse consequences.

EFFECT OF PARENTERAL NUTRITION ON NUTRITIONAL STATUS AND OUTCOMES

PN is effective in improving nutritional indexes in patients with cancer, but its effect on clinical outcome is not clear. PN has been associated with increases in weight, body fat, and visceral proteins in patients receiving chemotherapy (1–4) or radiation therapy (5–7). However, most studies have been unable to demonstrate a consistent increase in lean body mass (2,8–10).

Several investigations have demonstrated a significant reduction in postoperative complications, such as wound infections in moderately-to-severely malnourished patients receiving preoperative PN for at least 7 days (11,12). PN may also improve long-term survival in patients undergoing bone marrow transplantation (13). In other cases, PN either had no effect (14,15) or has been associated with an increased incidence of complications (11,16), decreased survival (9,17), and decreased duration of remission (1) in patients receiving chemotherapy, radiation therapy, or surgery.

PN has also been administered in an attempt to decrease antineoplastic therapy-related toxicities, such as leukopenia, thereby allowing more aggressive treatment and improved response rates, but the data are not conclusive regarding whether PN truly improves outcomes (17,18). PN can stimulate tumor growth in animals (19,20), but this has not been supported by in vivo studies in humans (9,21).

INDICATIONS FOR PARENTERAL NUTRITION

The decision to administer PN should be determined by the patient's disease status, gastrointestinal (GI) function, level of stress, and degree of malnutrition. Enteral nutrition (EN) support is preferable to PN because EN provides nutrients in a less invasive, more cost-efficient manner and helps to preserve nutritional status and gut integrity with less risk of infectious complications (22,23). However, PN is a viable therapy in patients who are unable to tolerate nutrition via the gut.

Indications for PN in patients with cancer include the following (24):

- Nonfunctional GI tract
- The need for bowel rest whether caused by the patient's underlying disease or as a consequence of antineoplastic therapy
- Severe diarrhea/malabsorption
- Radiation enteritis
- Short bowel syndrome
- Intractable nausea/vomiting
- Bowel obstruction
- Ileus
- Severe pancreatitis
- Enterocutaneous fistula
- Graft-versus-host disease (GVHD) of the gut

PN should *not* be routinely administered to patients undergoing chemotherapy, radiation therapy, or surgery. Rather, PN should be reserved for patients who are moderately to severely malnourished and who are unable to be fed enterally for at least 1 week. Preoperative PN is indicated for moderately to severely malnourished patients who are able to safely delay surgery for 7 to 14 days (24).

Contraindications for PN include a functional GI tract, inability to obtain intravenous (IV) access, and when therapy is needed for fewer than 5 days in patients without severe stress or malnutrition. PN is not indicated in patients with a poor prognosis and short life expectancy who are not actively being treated for their underlying disease.

PRACTICAL ASPECTS OF PARENTERAL NUTRITION ADMINISTRATION

The goal of PN is to provide nutrients safely and effectively. The clinician must understand the components of the PN solution and techniques of administration, to maximize the benefits while minimizing the potential adverse consequences of the therapy.

Macronutrients

Macronutrients used in PN solutions are carbohydrate in the form of dextrose, protein in the form of amino acids, and fat in the form of lipid emulsions (Table 14.1). The amounts of these macronutrients that should be administered to patients are based on their clinical and nutritional status, type and duration of therapy, and nutritional requirements.

Dextrose is generally well tolerated and the least expensive source of IV calories. The optimal intake of carbohydrate should be adequate to support brain and nerve tissue function and to prevent gluconeogenesis without causing adverse consequences, such as excess carbon dioxide production or hyperglycemia. The minimum carbohydrate requirement for an adult is 100 to 150 g/day, whereas the dextrose infusion rate should not exceed 4 mg/kg/min in critically ill patients and 7 mg/kg/min in stable patients (25).

Table 14.1 Macronutrients in Parenteral Nutrition Solutions

Macronutrient	*Energy, kcal/g*	*Availability, %*
Carbohydrate	3.4	5–70
Amino acids	4.0	3–20
Lipids	9.0	10–30

Lipids are not only a source of calories but also provide essential fatty acids (EFAs). The optimal intake of IV lipid is not known. Current guidelines suggest that fat intake should be limited to 1 g/kg/day, especially in critically ill patients (25). Minimum requirements for EFAs can be met by providing at least 4% to 8% of total calories as IV lipids. This can be accomplished by admixing fat with the PN solution or by infusing 250 mL of 20% fat emulsion 3 times per week. Lipids should be infused slowly to avoid reduced lipid clearance and impaired reticuloendothelial function (26,27).

Amino acid solutions are available as a standard mixture of essential and nonessential amino acids. They are also available in disease-specific formulas for patients in acute renal failure or for those with hepatic encephalopathy who are not responsive to standard treatment.

Electrolytes

Electrolytes are added daily to the PN solution to maintain electrolyte homeostasis and acid-base balance. Electrolyte requirements vary among individuals and are based on clinical status, renal function, and pharmacotherapy. For a summary of IV electrolyte requirements for adults with normal renal function, see Table 14.2 (24). In addition to maintenance requirements, it is necessary to replace electrolytes lost via the GI tract due to fistulas, high-output ostomies, or persistent vomiting or diarrhea. Reviewing the

Table 14.2 Daily Intravenous Electrolyte Requirements for Adults with Normal Renal Function

Electrolytes	*Usual Adult IV Dose*
Sodium	1–2 mEq/kg
Potassium	1–2 mEq/kg
Chloride	As needed to maintain acid-base balance
Acetate	As needed to maintain acid-base balance
Magnesium	8–20 mEq
Phosphorus	20–40 mM
Calcium	10–15 mEq

Source: Data are from reference 24.

patient's maintenance IV fluids before starting PN may help to estimate electrolyte requirements. However, it is important to understand that, in general, PN will increase electrolyte requirements, particularly potassium, magnesium, and phosphorus, in order to support anabolism.

Fluid

The volume of a PN solution is based on a patient's fluid requirements while also accounting for other sources of oral and IV fluid intake, such as diet, medications, and blood products. The volume of a PN solution can be minimized to a degree, if necessary, primarily based on the nutritional composition of the formula and concentration of the base solutions used in the admixture. A patient's hydration status should be monitored daily by physical assessment and by reviewing input/output records and laboratory values.

Vitamins and Trace Elements

Vitamins and trace elements are essential for normal metabolism and cellular function and should be added to PN solutions daily. Intravenous dosing requirements for vitamins and trace elements are generally higher than enteral requirements, because they are intended to address the increased needs of malnourished critically ill patients (Table 14.3) (24).

It is important to be aware of the content of multivitamin and trace element solutions. Some multivitamin solutions do not contain vitamin K, because it may interfere with anticoagulation therapy. Multitrace element solutions can contain anywhere from four to six components. Most trace elements and some vitamins can be added as single entities if needed.

Table 14.3 Daily Parenteral Vitamin and Trace Element Requirements for Adults

Micronutrient	*Amount*
Vitamins	
Vitamin A	700–900 μg
Vitamin D	5–15 μg
Vitamin E	15 μg
Vitamin K	90–120 μg
Vitamin C	75–90 mg
Folic acid	400 μg
Niacin	14–16 mg
Riboflavin	1.1–1.3 mg
Thiamin	1.1–1.2 mg
B-6	1.3–1.7 mg
B-12	2.4 μg
Pantothenic acid	5 mg
Biotin	30 μg
Trace elements	
Chromium	10–15 μg
Copper	0.3–0.5 mg
Manganese	60–100 μg
Zinc	2.5–5.0 mg*
Selenium	20–60 μg

*Add 2.0 mg for catabolism, 12.2 mg/L small bowel fluid loss, 17.1 mg/kg stool loss.

Source: Data are from reference 24.

Medications

The use of PN as a vehicle for administering medications is generally not recommended because of potential incompatibility between the drug and components of the solution, the inability to titrate the drug or discontinue the dose without discontinuing the solution, and the necessity to infuse medications continuously rather than intermittently. Potential advantages of using PN solutions to deliver medications include cost savings due to decreased use of materials and labor, fluid savings due to a decrease in IVs, and a lower risk of contamination due to decreased manipulation of the IV lines. Examples of common medications that can be added to a PN solution include heparin, famotidine, octreotide, methylprednisilone, and regular insulin. A pharmacist should be consulted before adding any medication to a PN solution.

Formula Selection

Central vs Peripheral PN

The type of PN formula and route of administration is determined by the clinical and nutritional status of the patient, along with the type of IV access. Central PN is usually preferred in patients who are stressed and hypermetabolic or who require a fluid restriction, because the formula can be concentrated since it is infused via a large vein. Central PN is also preferred if it is anticipated that therapy will be needed more than 1 week or if central IV access is already in place.

A central venous access device (CVAD) can be categorized as temporary or long-term. A temporary catheter is usually placed at bedside in hospitalized patients and is intended to remain in place for a few days to a few weeks. A long-term CVAD is usually placed surgically or radiographically and can remain in place for weeks to months for use both inside and outside an acute care setting. An example of a long-term CVAD is a Hickman, Broviac, Groshong, peripherally inserted central catheter (PICC), or implanted port. Many patients with long-term CVADs require multiple lumens to be able to accommodate more than one IV therapy, such as PN, chemotherapy, blood products, antibiotics, or pain medications simultaneously.

Peripheral PN can be infused via a peripheral catheter when central IV access is not in place and therapy is expected to be needed for less than 1 week. Peripheral PN requires a formula that is modest in osmolarity and periodic changing of IV sites, to prevent thrombophlebitis. Peripheral PN solutions with a final dextrose concentration of 10% or less and an osmolarity less than 900 mOsm/kg are generally well tolerated by peripheral veins (28). Since peripheral PN may be limited in dextrose and protein, it is appropriate for patients who are mildly stressed or malnourished. Indications for peripheral PN include the following:

- Short term (ie, < 5 to 7 days)
- Mild-to-moderate malnutrition
- Normal to mildly increased metabolic rate
- No fluid restriction
- No allergy to IV lipids
- No central access in place

Lipid-Based vs Dextrose-Based Formula

Peripheral formulas are generally lipid-based, because dextrose and amino acids are more osmotically active than fat. In addition, lipid-based solutions are appropriate when minimizing carbohydrate intake is desirable, such as in patients with diabetes or glucose intolerance or when trying to wean patients with excess carbon dioxide retention from ventilators. Central solutions can be either lipid- or dextrose-based. Dextrose-based solutions are preferred for patients who can tolerate the carbohydrate load, thereby avoiding concerns with compatibility and immunosuppression associated with IV lipids (27).

Administration Techniques

In the hospital, PN is usually administered continuously because this requires less effort and manipulation of the IV lines, and management of fluid and electrolytes is easier. Because PN has the potential to induce or exacerbate metabolic disturbances, correction of electrolytes and glucose abnormalities should be done before initiating PN when possible.

When initiating PN, the patient should receive one half the desired dextrose calories for the first 24 hours, to assess tolerance to the carbohydrate load. If the patient tolerates the half-calorie regimen without hyperglycemia, the carbohydrate calories can be increased.

For patients on long-term therapy or for those being discharged to home or an extended care facility, PN is usually cycled over 12 hours, to allow freedom from the infusion pump and IV pole. Cycling may also help prevent cholestasis and elevated liver function tests (29). The usual method used to cycle PN is to subtract 4 hours each day from the administration time until the desired cycle length is achieved without

Box 14.1
Calculation of Parenteral Nutrition Cycle Rates

1-hour taper down

Main rate = Total volume/(cycle hours—½ hour)
1st-hour taper rate = Main rate/2

2-hour taper down

Main rate = Total volume/[(cycle hours—2 hours) + 0.75]
1st-hour taper rate = Main rate/2
2nd-hour taper rate = 1st hour taper rate/2

1-hour taper up, 1-hour taper down

Main rate = Total volume/(Cycle hours—1 hour)
Taper rates = Main rate/2

1-hour taper up, 2-hour taper down

Main rate = Total volume/[(Cycle hours—2 hours) + 0.25]
1st-hour taper-up and 1st-hour taper-down rates = Main rate/2
2nd-hour taper-down rate = 1st-hour taper rate/2

2-hour taper up, 2-hour taper down

Main rate = Total volume/[(Cycle hours—3 hours) + 0.50]
2nd-hour taper-up rate and 1st-hour taper-down rate = Main rate/2
1st-hour taper-up rate and 2nd-hour taper-down rate = 2nd hour taper-up rate/2

Source: Data are from reference 30.

hyperglycemia or other complications. See Box 14.1 (30) for formulas to calculate PN cycling rates.

Tapering (ie, gradually increasing or decreasing the infusion rate at the beginning or end of the cycle) is used to prevent sudden changes in blood glucose caused by the abrupt infusion or discontinuation of carbohydrate. The purpose of tapering is to help the patient avoid hyperglycemia at the beginning of the cycle and rebound hypoglycemia at the end of the cycle.

Monitoring

Monitoring patients during PN infusion will help prevent PN-associated complications and assess nutritional status and the efficacy of therapy. As shown in Table 14.4 (31), serum levels of electrolytes, blood urea nitrogen, and creatinine should be monitored daily for the first several days after the initiation of PN and then less frequently once the patient is stable. Blood glucose should be checked every 6 hours until the patient is stable on PN providing full calories. The patient's weight, fluid intake and output, and vital signs should be reviewed daily. Nutritional parameters, such as visceral proteins, nitrogen balance, and anthropometrics, can be assessed at baseline and then checked weekly because there is little change from day to day.

Complications

Complications associated with PN can be categorized as mechanical, infectious, or metabolic, and as acute or long-term. These complications generally arise from nutrient deficiencies/excesses or problems with the delivery system. Box 14.2 (32) lists some of the long-term complications of PN. Careful patient monitoring, catheter care, and formula preparation and administration will help prevent complications.

Table 14.4 Monitoring Guidelines for Patients Receiving Parenteral Nutrition*

Parameter	*Frequency*
Serum glucose, serum electrolytes, BUN, creatinine	Before initiation of PN, daily for at least the first 3 days of PN administration, then weekly if stable
Serum magnesium, serum phosphorus	Before initiation of PN, daily for at least the first 3 days of PN administration if baseline abnormal or at risk for refeeding syndrome, then weekly if stable
Serum calcium, LFTs, CBC, PT/INR	Before initiation of PN
Serum triglycerides	Before initiation of PN. Repeat if baseline abnormal or if receiving lipid-based PN or medications

Abbreviations: BUN, blood urea nitrogen; CBC, complete blood cell count; INR, international normalized ratio; LFT, liver function tests PN, parenteral nutrition; PT, prothrombin time.

*Assumes abnormal tests are repeated and patients are treated as clinically indicated.

Source: Data are from reference 31.

Hyperglycemia

Hyperglycemia is the most common metabolic complication of PN. Evidence suggests that strict blood glucose control decreases morbidity and mortality in critically ill patients (33). Because of the availability of intravenous insulin infusions drips, safe achievement of tight blood glucose control without increasing the risk of hypoglycemia is often more feasible in the intensive care unit (ICU) setting than in the regular nursing units. Therefore, a reasonable blood glucose goal is 80 to 120 mg/dL for critically ill patients in an ICU setting and 100 to 150 mg/dL for noncritically ill patients on regular nursing wards (34).

The risk of hyperglycemia can be reduced by limiting the amount of dextrose to 200 g/day when starting a patient on PN. For patients with a history of diabetes and for those who have demonstrated glucose intolerance, dextrose should be limited to 150 g/day initially and regular insulin added to the solution. The amount of insulin added to the initial formula should be based on the patient's home regimen if the patient is insulin dependent or can be estimated at 0.1 unit regular insulin per gram dextrose to start (35).

If hyperglycemia occurs during PN infusion, it can be treated in the short term by administering regular insulin subcutaneously, using a sliding scale based on the blood glucose level (Table 14.5) (34). Because of the constant infusion of dextrose, the amount of subcutaneous insulin required is generally higher in patients receiving PN than in patients consuming an oral diet. The total amount of subcutaneous insulin administered in the past 24-hour period should then be calculated, and a portion (usually one-half to two-thirds) added to the subsequent PN bag. Hyperglycemia can also be treated by limiting total energy intake, which decreases carbohydrate content, or by replacing dextrose with fat calories.

Hypoglycemia

Hypoglycemia is usually caused by excess insulin or by abrupt discontinuation of a central PN solution. To prevent hypoglycemia, central PN should be decreased to half rate for 1 hour before discontinuing. Blood glucose should be checked 1 hour after discontinuation of the PN solution, until a stable pattern is noted. If the PN is stopped abruptly, a 10% dextrose solution should be infused in its place for 1 hour. Peripheral PN can be discontinued without tapering, because the dextrose content is generally below 10%. If hypoglycemia occurs, it can be treated by giving the patient carbohydrate orally, if possible, or by administering an ampule of D_{50} IV. If the cause of hypoglycemia is excessive insulin in the PN solution, the bag should be discontinued.

Refeeding Syndrome

Refeeding syndrome is a less common but potentially more serious complication of PN. Refeeding

Box 14.2

Complications of Long-Term Parenteral Nutrition

Mechanical

- Venous thrombosis
- Catheter occlusion

Infectious

- Catheter sepsis
- Tunnel infection
- Exit site/cuff infection
- Bloodstream infection

Metabolic

- Metabolic bone disease: osteomalacia, osteoporosis
- Hepatic disease: hepatic steatosis, cholestasis
- Biliary disease: biliary sludge, gallstones
- Renal: decreased glomerular filtration rate, tubular dysfunction
- Gastrointestinal: gastroparesis, intestinal hypoplasia

Source: Data are from reference 32.

syndrome is of particular concern in oncology patients because of the prevalence of protein-energy malnutrition in this population. The risk of refeeding syndrome can be decreased by repletion of electrolytes before initiating PN and by limiting the amount of dextrose in the PN solution to 150 g/day to start (25). Fluid status and electrolytes, especially phosphorus, magnesium, and potassium, should be monitored closely for at least the first several days and replaced as necessary. Energy intake should be advanced cautiously during several days, provided that the patient's fluid and electrolyte levels are acceptable.

HOME PARENTERAL NUTRITION

Cancer is the most common diagnosis for patients on home PN in the United States (36), although the effect of PN on length and quality of life in these patients remains controversial. In select cancer patients, home PN can improve quality of life and survival (37–39). However, a diagnosis of cancer is associated with poorer outcomes than is a diagnosis of other primary diseases. The 5-year survival rate for home PN patients at one institution was 38% for cancer patients compared with 48% for those with motility disorders, 54% for those with radiation enteritis, 60% for those with ischemic bowel, and 92% for those with inflammatory bowel disease (40).

Indications for home PN are the same as those used in an acute care setting. However, because of the length and complexity of home PN, a patient must also meet additional criteria to be considered a candidate. A patient should be medically and emotionally stable and have a reasonable life expectancy. A patient should be able to perform the tasks associated with home PN or have a primary caregiver who is available during the time the solution is infusing. A patient should have a long-term CVAD in place and be on a stable PN formula before discharge. There should be a program in place to monitor the patient and to deal with complications after discharge. The patient's need for home PN should be reviewed periodically.

TRANSITION TO ENTERAL FEEDINGS

One of the primary goals for patients on PN, whenever possible, is to transition from IV nutrition to nutrition via the GI tract. EN should be started as soon as the patient has adequate GI function. However, PN should not be discontinued until the patient has demonstrated the ability to digest, absorb, and utilize enteral nutrients in adequate amounts either orally, via a feeding tube, or in combination. As a general rule, when transitioning patients from PN to EN, PN should be

Table 14.5 Subcutaneous Sliding Scale Insulin for Patients Receiving Parenteral Nutrition

Blood Glucose, mg/dL	*Regular Humulin Insulin, Units*
150–199	1–2
200–249	2–4
250–299	3–6
300–350	4–8
> 350	5–10

Source: Data are from reference 34.

decreased once intake equals 500 kcal/day and discontinued once the patient is meeting 60% of his or her energy and protein goals (25).

REFERENCES

1. Shamberger RC, Brennan MF, Goodgame JT Jr, Lowry SF, Maher MM, Wesley RA, Pizzo PA. A prospective, randomized study of adjuvant parenteral nutrition in the treatment of sarcomas: results of metabolic and survival studies. *Surgery.* 1984;96:1–13.
2. Shike M, Russell D, Detsky AS, Harrison JE, McNeill KG, Shepherd FA, Feld R, Evans WK, Jeejeebhoy KN. Changes in body composition in patients with small-cell lung cancer. *Ann Intern Med.* 1984;101:303–309.
3. Smith RC, Hartemink R. Improvement of nutritional measures during preoperative parenteral nutrition in patients selected by the prognostic nutritional index: a randomized controlled trial. *JPEN J Parenter Enteral Nutr.* 1988;12:587–591.
4. De Cicco M, Panarello G, Fantin D, Veronesi A, Pinto A, Zagonel V, Monfardini S, Testa V. Parenteral nutrition in cancer patients receiving chemotherapy: effects on toxicity and nutritional status. *JPEN J Parenter Enteral Nutr.* 1993;17:513–518.
5. Kinsella TJ, Malcolm AW, Bothe A, Valerio D, Blackburn GL. Prospective study of nutritional support during pelvic irradiation. *Int J Radiat Oncol Biol Phys.* 1981;7:543–548.
6. Burt ME, Gorschboth CM, Brennan MF. A controlled, prospective, randomized trial evaluating the metabolic effects of enteral and parenteral nutrition in the cancer patient. *Cancer.* 1982;49:1092–1105.
7. Burt ME, Stein TP, Brennan MF. A controlled randomized trial evaluating the effects of enteral and parenteral nutrition on protein metabolism in cancer-bearing man. *J Surg Res.* 1983;34:303–314.
8. Nixon DW, Lawson DH, Kutner M, Ansley J, Schwarz M, Heymsfield S, Chawla R, Cartwright TH, Rudman D. Hyperalimentation of the cancer patient with protein-calorie undernutrition. *Cancer Res.* 1981;41:2038–2045.
9. Nixon DW, Moffitt S, Lawson DH, Ansley J, Lynn MJ, Kutner MH, Heymsfield SB, Wesley M, Chawla R, Rudman D. Total parenteral nutrition as an adjunct to chemotherapy of metastatic colorectal cancer. *Cancer Treat Rep.* 1981;65:121–128.
10. Drott C, Unsgaard B, Schersten T, Lundholm K. Total parenteral nutrition as an adjuvant to patients undergoing chemotherapy for testicular carcinoma: protection of body composition—a randomized, prospective study. *Surgery.* 1988;103:499–506.
11. Perioperative total parenteral nutrition in surgical patients. The Veterans Affairs Total Parenteral Nutrition Cooperative Study Group. *N Engl J Med.* 1991; 325:525–532.
12. Bozzetti F, Gavazzi C, Miceli R. Perioperative total parenteral nutrition in malnourished, gastrointestinal cancer patients: a randomized, clinical trial. *JPEN J Parenter Enteral Nutr.* 2000;24:7–14.
13. Weisdorf SA, Lysne J, Wind D, Haake RJ, Sharp HL, Goldman A, Schissel K, McGlave PB, Ramsay NK, Kersey JH. Positive effect of prophylactic total parenteral nutrition on long-term outcome of bone marrow transplantation. *Transplantation.* 1987;43: 833–838.
14. Holter AR, Fischer JE. The effects of perioperative hyperalimentation on complications in patients with carcinoma and weight loss. *J Surg Res.* 1977;23 :31–34.
15. Thompson BR, Julian TB, Stremple JF. Perioperative total parenteral nutrition in patients with gastrointestinal cancer. *J Surg Res.* 1981;30:497–500.
16. Brennan MF, Pisters P, Rosner M, Quesada O, Shike M. A prospective randomized trial of total parenteral nutrition after major pancreatic resection for malignancy. *Ann Surg.* 1994;220:436–444.
17. Jordan WM, Valdivieso M, Frankmann C, Gillespie M, Issell BF, Bodey GP, Freireich EJ. Treatment of advanced adenocarcinoma of the lung with ftorafur, doxorubicin, cyclophosphamide, and cisplatin (FACP) and intensive IV hyperalimentation. *Cancer Treat Rep.* 1981;65:197–205.
18. Weiner RS, Kromer BS, Clamon GH, Feld R, Evans W, Moran EM, Blum R, Weisenthal LM, Pee D, Hoffman FA, DeWys WD. Effects of intravenous hyperalimentation during treatment in patients with small cell lung cancer. *J Clin Oncol.* 1985;3:949–957.
19. Steiger E, Oram-Smith J, Miller E, Kuo L, Vars HM. Effects of nutrition on tumor growth and tolerance to chemotherapy. *J Surg Res.* 1975;18:455–461.
20. Daly JM, Copeland EM, Dudrick SJ. Effect of intravenous nutrition on tumor growth and host immunocompetence in malnourished animals. *Surgery.* 1978; 84:655–658.
21. Mullen JL, Buzby GP, Matthews DC, Smale BF, Rosato EF. Reduction of operative morbidity and mortality by combined preoperative and postoperative nutritional support. *Ann Surg.* 1980;192:604–613.
22. Moore FA, Moore EE, Jones TN, McCroskey BL,

Peterson VM. TEN versus TPN following major abdominal trauma—reduced septic morbidity. *J Trauma.* 1989;29:916–922.

23. Kudsk KA, Croce MA, Fabian TC, Minard G, Tolley E, Poret A, Kuhl MR, Brown RO. Enteral versus parenteral feeding. Effects on septic morbidity after blunt and penetrating abdominal trauma. *Ann Surg.* 1992; 215:503–511.
24. ASPEN Board of Directors and the Clinical Guidelines Task Force. Guidelines for the use of parenteral and enteral nutrition in adults and pediatric patients. *JPEN J Parenter Enteral Nutr.* 2002;26:SA1–SA138.
25. Skipper A, Millikan KW. Parenteral nutrition implementation and management. In: *The ASPEN Nutrition Support Practice Manual.* Silver Spring, Md: American Society of Parenteral and Enteral Nutrition; 1998:9–12.
26. Jensen GL, Mascioli EA, Seidner DL, Istfan NW, Domnitch AM, Selleck K, Babayan VK, Blackburn GL, Bistrian BR. Parenteral infusion of long- and medium-chain triglycerides and reticuloendothelial system function in man. *JPEN J Parenter Enteral Nutr.* 1990;14:467–471.
27. Seidner DL, Mascioli EA, Istfau NW, Porter KA, Selleck K, Blackburn GL, Bistrian BR. Effects of long-chain triglyceride emulsions on reticulothelial system function in humans. *JPEN J Parenter Enteral Nutr.* 1989;13:614–619.
28. Krzywda EA, Edmiston CE. Parenteral access and equipment. In: *The ASPEN Nutrition Support Practice Manual.* Silver Spring, Md: American Society of Parenteral and Enteral Nutrition; 1998:7–8.
29. Maini B, Blackburn GL, Bistrian BR, Flatt JP, Page JG, Bothe A, Benotti P, Reinhoff HY. Cyclic hyperalimentation: an optimal technique for preservation of visceral protein. *J Surg Res.* 1976;20:515–525.
30. Hamilton C, Lennon E, Saylor K, Sladky H. Home nutrition support. In: Parekh N, DeChicco R, eds. *The Cleveland Clinic Foundation Nutrition Support Handbook.* Cleveland, Ohio: Cleveland Clinic Foundation; 2004:174.
31. ASPEN. *Clinical Pathways and Algorithms for Delivery of Parenteral and Enteral Nutrition Support in Adults.* Silver Spring, Md: American Society of Parenteral and Enteral Nutrition; 1998.
32. Buchman AL. Complications of long-term home total parenteral nutrition: their identification, prevention, and treatment. *Dig Dis Sci.* 2001;46:1–18.
33. van den Berghe G, Wouters P, Weekers F, Verwaest C, Bruyninckx F, Schetz M, Vlasselaers D, Ferdinande P, Lauwers P, Bouillon R. Intensive insulin therapy in the critically ill patients. *N Engl J Med.* 2001;345: 1359–1367.
34. McMahon MM. Management of parenteral nutrition in acutely ill patients with hyperglycemia. *Nutr Clin Pract.* 2004;19:120–128.
35. Romanski SA, McMahon MM. Diabetes mellitus. In: *The ASPEN Nutrition Support Practice Manual.* Silver Spring, Md: American Society of Parenteral and Enteral Nutrition; 1998:22–26.
36. Howard L, Ament M, Fleming CR, Shike M, Steiger E. Current use and clinical outcome of home parenteral and enteral nutrition therapies in the United States. *Gastroenterology.* 1995;109:355–365.
37. Cozzaglio L, Balzola F, Cosentino F, DeCicco M, Fellagara P, Gaggiotti G, Gallitelli L, Giacosa A, Orban A, Fadda M, Gavazzi C, Pirovano F, Bozzetti F. Outcome of cancer patients receiving home parenteral nutrition. Italian Society of Parenteral and Enteral Nutrition (S.I.N.P.E.). *JPEN J Parenter Enteral Nutr.* 1997; 21:339–342.
38. August DA, Thorn D, Fisher RL, Welchek CM. Home parenteral nutrition for patients with inoperable malignant bowel obstruction. *JPEN J Parenter Enteral Nutr.* 1991;15:323–327.
39. Hoda D, Jatoi A, Burnes J, Loprinzi C, Kelly D. Should patients with advanced, incurable cancer ever be sent home with total parenteral nutrition? A single institution's 20-year experience. *Cancer.* 2005;103: 863–868.
40. Scolapio JS, Fleming CR, Kelly DG, Wick DM, Zinsmeister AR. Survival of home parenteral nutrition-treated patients: 20 years of experience at the Mayo Clinic. *Mayo Clinic Proc.* 1999;74:217–222.

Chapter 15

Pharmacological Management of Nutrition Impact Symptoms Associated With Cancer

JAMIE H. VON ROENN, MD

INTRODUCTION

Cancer and its treatment may result in a number of nutrition impact symptoms, including anorexia, cachexia, nausea and vomiting, constipation, mucositis, diarrhea, xerostomia, and malabsorption. This chapter examines the pharmacological management of these nutrition impact symptoms and explains when clinicians should consider pharmacological intervention. Specific pharmacological agents are discussed, including their mechanism of action and side effects. For nutrition recommendations on managing these symptoms, see Appendix A.

ANOREXIA AND CACHEXIA

Anorexia and cachexia are frequent clinical problems associated with cancer and ultimately affect most patients with advanced disease (1). Cachexia refers to a multifactorial syndrome that is characterized by loss of appetite, generalized wasting, muscle atrophy, and a variety of metabolic abnormalities (2). Diagnosing and correcting nutrition impact symptoms that may contribute to involuntary weight loss are the first steps in the management of anorexia (loss of appetite) and cachexia. Unfortunately, many patients experience weight loss without easily identifiable and/or reversible causes.

The medical management of anorexia and cachexia requires a careful evaluation of symptoms and medications that may interfere with the ability to consume adequate intake. If specific symptoms (eg, nausea, mucositis) cannot be identified and managed with nutrition recommendations, then pharmacological agents should be considered.

Pharmacological agents used in the treatment and management of anorexia and cachexia include dronabinol, megestrol acetate, dronabinol plus megestrol acetate (MA), corticosteroids, anabolic agents, and metoclopramide. An intervention should be chosen based on the patient's treatment goals and his or her prognosis. For patients with very limited survival (< 3 months) whose primary goal is to increase enjoyment of eating, megestrol acetate or corticosteroids may be useful (1). For most patients, treatment is intended to improve oral intake, weight, and, ideally, function. To achieve this, an approach that combines an appetite-enhancing agent (eg, dronabinol, megestrol acetate, corticosteroids, metoclopramide) with exercise and an anabolic medication (see section on "Oxandrolone") may be ideal.

Dronabinol

Dronabinol, the primary orexigenic component of marijuana, has been shown to stimulate appetite in patients with acquired immunodeficiency syndrome (AIDS) and cancer-related anorexia (3–7). Results of studies conducted in cancer patients with weight loss and AIDS patients are highlighted in Table 15.1 (4,7).

Table 15.1 Dronabinol Trials

Patient Population (reference)	*No. of Subjects*	*Treatment*	*Appetite*	*Weight*
Advanced cancer (4)	30	Dose ranging study: 2.5 mg/day; 2.5 mg twice a day; 5 mg/day	Improved in patients in 2 higher dose groups	Decreased rate of weight loss
Advanced cancer (4)	18	2.5 mg 3 times a day	Improved in 13/18	No weight change
AIDS (7)	89	Dronabinol 2.5 mg PO twice a day vs placebo	Improved in 19/50	No weight change

Source: Data are from references 4 and 7.

The only prospective, randomized study of dronabinol for the treatment of cachexia enrolled patients with AIDS-related weight loss. Patients were randomly assigned to either placebo or dronabinol 2.5 mg orally twice daily for 6 weeks. Patients treated with dronabinol had greater improvement in appetite and mood than placebo-treated patients. There was no significant difference in weight between the treatment groups. After the 6-week study period, patients were offered treatment with dronabinol for up to 1 year. Available data from the 90 patients in the study extension demonstrate continued appetite stimulation for at least 6 months and body weight gain of 2 kg or more in 38% of patients (7).

Dizziness, euphoria, somnolence (drowsiness), and poor concentration have been reported as the most common side effects (4,5,7). Its use is contraindicated in patients that have sensitivity to sesame oil and should be used with caution when given concomitantly with sedatives and other psychoactive medications (8). Decreasing the dose may eliminate or lessen adverse effects. Initiating Dronabinol at the lower dose range and increasing the dose gradually to the higher dose range has also been shown to help manage side effects and to provide maximum therapeutic effect (8).

In sum, Dronabinol 2.5 mg PO BID has been shown to be effective for improving appetite as well as for decreasing nausea in patients with advanced cancer (3–5).

Megestrol Acetate

Megestrol acetate, a synthetic, orally active progestational agent used widely for the treatment of metastatic breast cancer, has been reported to stimulate appetite and weight gain. Treatment with conventional doses of megestrol acetate (160 mg/day) produces appetite stimulation and weight gain in about 30% of patients with advanced breast cancer (9). Several placebo-controlled, randomized studies have demonstrated the benefit of megestrol acetate for cancer-related cachexia (see Table 15.2) (10–12).

Across the studies, patients treated with megestrol acetate reported improved appetite, increased caloric intake and body weight, and improved sense of well-being. The beneficial effects of megestrol acetate on appetite and weight are dose dependent, with greater benefit at higher doses. However, recent trials evaluating the impact of megestrol acetate on body composition demonstrate that most of the increased weight is due to increased fat mass (10–12).

Megestrol acetate, which has glucocorticoid effects, can interfere with normal endocrine activities, resulting in impotence in men and adrenal insufficiency or decreased glucose tolerance. Most randomized trials (10–12) have failed to show a significant increase in either edema or deep vein thrombosis with megestrol acetate therapy.

For patients experiencing cancer-related anorexia, megestrol acetate 800 mg (20 mL oral suspension) PO every morning can provide significant weight gain and increased appetite. Megestrol acetate, available in 20- and 40-mg tablets or as an oral suspension (40 mg/mL), is the most potent appetite stimulant (5,13).

Dronabinol Plus Megestrol Acetate (MA)

Recently, a randomized, placebo-controlled trial compared the efficacy of combination dronabinol and

Table 15.2 Cancer Cachexia Placebo-Controlled Trials of Megestrol Acetate (MA)

Authors (reference)	*No. of Subjects*	*MA Dose*	*Appetite*	*Weight*
Loprinzi et al (10)	133	800 mg vs placebo	Improved	Gain (mean = 1.4 kg for MA group)
Bruera et al (11)	40	480 mg (crossover trial)	Improved	Gain
Tchekmedyian et al (12)	89	600 mg	Improved	Gain

Source: Data are from references 10–12.

megestrol acetate to each agent individually for advanced cancer patients (see Table 15.3) (14). In the dose and schedules, MA is superior to dronabinol in the treatment of cancer-related anorexia, and the addition of dronabinol does not confer additional benefit to treatment with MA alone (14).

Corticosteroids

Numerous uncontrolled studies have advocated the use of corticosteroids for the treatment of cancer-related anorexia and cachexia. Multiple randomized, placebo-controlled trials have demonstrated appetite enhancement with corticosteroid treatment (15–19). Table 15.4 (15–19) highlights the results of these trials. In all of the studies, appetite improvement was short lived (often < 8 weeks) and did not translate into weight gain. In general, these trials enrolled patients with advanced cancer who were, as a result, treated with short courses (< 3 months) of treatment. In this advanced cancer population, improvement in appetite was associated with a self-reported improvement in quality of life.

The efficacy of dexamethasone, megestrol acetate, and fluoxymesterone (an anabolic agent) was compared in patients with advanced cancer and weight loss (20). Four-hundred-eighty patients were stratified on the basis of primary tumor site, weight loss in the preceding 2 months, planned concurrent therapy, performance status, and predicted survival (< 4 months, 4 to 6 months, > 6 months). Patients were randomly assigned to receive megestrol acetate 800 mg/day, dexamethasone 0.75 mg PO four times per day, or fluoxymesterone 10 mg PO twice per day. Patient characteristics were well balanced across the treatment groups. Median time on study was about 2 months. Over the relatively brief period of treatment, appetite stimulation and weight gain were not significantly different for patients treated with megestrol acetate or dexamethasone but were significantly better than in those treated with fluoxymesterone (20). All three drugs were reasonably well tolerated.

Prolonged use of corticosteroids may result in proximal muscle weakness, osteoporosis, delirium, fluid retention, adrenal suppression, glucose intolerance, hyperglycemia, and electrolyte disturbances (1,21,22).

For patients with very advanced cancer and limited survival (< 8 weeks), corticosteroids may provide palliation of anorexia. For bedridden patients, in particular, corticosteroids may be useful, as exacerbation of muscle wasting is not of particular concern. Corticosteroids may be a particularly good treatment choice for patients who require co-analgesia with an anti-inflammatory agent (eg, the patient with painful bone metastases) (1,21). Although clear dosing guidelines are not available from the published trials, dexamethasone 4 mg every morning is a reasonable initial dose (1,21). A proton pump inhibitor should be given concomitantly, to avoid gastric irritation. Use of corticosteroids after 12:00 pm should be avoided, because of the potential for insomnia (1,21).

Oxandrolone

Oxandrolone is a synthetic, oral anabolic agent approved for treatment of weight loss after extensive surgery, chronic infection, or severe trauma and to offset the protein catabolism associated with the prolonged administration of steroids. In patients with cancer-related weight loss, a phase II trial of oxandrolone 10 mg orally twice daily, in combination with standardized nutrition recommendations and a progressive resistance exercise program (Thera-bands),

Table 15.3 Dronabinol plus Megestrol Acetate (MA) Treatments

Treatment	*No. of Subjects*	*Subjects with Improved Appetite (%)*	*Subjects With Weight Gain ≥ 10% (%)*
MA 800 mg/day + placebo	159	75	11
Dronabinol 2.5 mg twice a day + placebo	152	49	3
MA 800 mg/day + dronabinol 2.5 mg twice a day	150	66	8

Source: Data are from reference 14.

Table 15.4 Corticosteroid Trials

Authors (reference)	*Steroid, Dose*	*Appetite*	*Weight*
Moertel et al (15)	Dexamethasone, .75-1.5 mg orally 4 times a day	Improved	No change
Wilcox et al (16)	Prednisolone, 5 mg PO 3 times a day	Improved	No change
Bruera et al (17)	Methylprednisolone, 16 mg twice/day	Improved	No change
Della Cuna GR et al (18)	Methylprednisolone, 125 mg/day intravenously	Improved	No change
Popiela et al (19)	Methylprednisolone, 125 mg/day intravenously	Improved	No change

Source: Data are from references 15–19.

demonstrated an increase in total and lean tissue weight with treatment (23). Of the first 37 patients treated, weight increased by 3.5% and lean tissue mass by 7.5%. Improvement in weight and lean body mass correlated with improvements in quality-of-life scores as well as with performance status.

A prospective, randomized trial of oxandrolone in patients with advanced cancers of the upper aerodigestive tract demonstrated similar results (24). Sixty-four patients with aerodigestive tract cancers were randomized to oxandrolone 10 mg orally twice daily or placebo. Oxandrolone-treated patients significantly increased their weight and lean body mass compared to placebo-treated patients. Although final results from this study have not yet been published, the increase in lean body mass associated with oxandrolone and the associated improvement in performance status and quality of life are of significant interest.

Registered dietitians should note that, although a number of anabolic agents (growth hormone, oxandrolone, nandrolone) are either approved or currently being evaluated for the treatment of AIDS-associated weight loss, data regarding their use in cancer-associated cachexia are only available with oxandrolone.

The only adverse effect noted in the previously mentioned study (23,24) was a transient increase in transaminases, reversible with discontinuation of the drug. Its use is contraindicated in patients that have been diagnosed with breast and prostate cancer with hypercalcemia, severe hepatic dysfunction, and nephrosis (8). It should be used with caution in patients receiving concomitant warfarin therapy and existing cardiac, renal, or hepatic disease (8).

Oxandrolone is a well-tolerated anabolic agent. The phase III study has not yet been published, but the preliminary data are encouraging.

β-hydroxy β-methylbutyrate (Juven)

β-hydroxy β-methylbutyrate (HMB) is a dietary supplement made up of a combination of three nutrients—a metabolite of leucine, L-glutamine, and L-arginine—each of which has been shown to decrease protein breakdown. HMB has been evaluated as a dietary supplement in both patients with wasting secondary to cancer and HIV infection. A 24-week randomized, prospective study of HMB vs a nonessential amino acid supplement evaluated patients with advanced cancer and at least a 5% weight loss. Thirty-two patients were available for evaluation at the 4-week visit, at which point a significant increase in fat-free mass in the HMB supplemented group was noted, compared to the control group (+1.12 ± 0.68 kg vs –1.34 ± –0.78 kg, respectively). The response to the 24 weeks of supplementation was evaluated by an intent-to-treat analysis, and the effect was maintained during the 24 weeks without any adverse effects on quality of life (25).

In a similar study in patients with HIV-related weight loss, 68 patients with weight loss of at least 5% were randomly assigned to receive either a placebo-nutrient mixture or HMB 3 g/day in two divided doses during an 8-week period. Forty-three subjects completed the 8-week protocol. HMB-treated patients gained 3 ± 0.5 kg of body weight, whereas those receiving the placebo supplement gained 0.37 kg ± 0.84 kg. This gain in weight was predominantly lean body mass, with no significant toxicities reported (26). A meta-analysis of dietary supplements evaluated to augment lean mass and strength gain during resistance training has similarly reported only two to be of benefit: creatine and HMB (27). HMB is supplied in powdered packets, with two packets taken daily.

No significant toxicities have been reported from this supplement. Although limited data are available, there is early evidence to suggest that supplementation with β-hydroxy β-methylbutyrate may be of benefit, particularly in concert with a resistance exercise program.

Metoclopramide

Early satiety as a result of delayed gastric emptying and gastroparesis may occur in up to 60% of patients with anorexia and cancer-related weight loss (28). It is frequently reported by patients with ascites or hepatomegaly. Metoclopramide, an antiemetic and prokinetic agent, may relieve cancer-related anorexia, particularly when associated with dysmotility. In a small, phase II study in advanced cancer patients with anorexia, metoclopramide 10 mg four times per day improved anorexia in 17 of 20 patients (29).

Diarrhea occurs infrequently at this dose. Hyperactivity is common and responds to dose reduction or treatment with diphenhydramine (21).

Delayed gastric emptying is common in patients with advanced cancer and may be exacerbated by the decrease in gut motility associated with opioid analgesic use. This agent should be considered for any patient who complains of early satiety and anorexia.

NAUSEA AND VOMITING

Oncology patients experience nausea and vomiting secondary to treatment (chemotherapy, radiation therapy) as well as from the underlying disease. Prolonged emesis can lead to dehydration, weight loss, metabolic abnormalities, and electrolyte imbalance (30). Prolonged nausea and vomiting are complex symptoms that adversely affect quality of life and are treatment-related toxicities most feared by patients.

Understanding the etiology of nausea and vomiting for a particular patient allows selection of pathogenesis-based treatment. Complex neural pathways interact to produce nausea and vomiting (21). The final common pathway is in the emetic center, located in the brain stem. Stimulation of the emetic center comes from the chemoreceptor trigger zone, located adjacent to the fourth ventricle. Stimulation of the vomiting center may occur as a result of vagal and sympathetic afferents secondary to both visceral and cardiac symptoms. The chemoreceptor trigger zone is stimulated by a variety of chemicals, whereas direct stimulation of the vomiting center may occur secondary to increased intracranial pressure or direct stimulation of the center from metastatic or primary tumors. Motion sickness and some medications (aspirin, opioids) may stimulate the vestibular apparatus and cause vertigo in addition to nausea and vomiting.

To assist clinicians with managing nausea and vomiting associated with chemotherapy, a classification system developed by Hesketh and Ettinger outlines the emetogenic potential of commonly used chemotherapeutic agents (31,32). For more information, see Chapter 8 on chemotherapy.

There are many causes of nausea and vomiting in addition to those secondary to treatment. Other medications (eg, opioids) may cause nausea. Brain metastases, peptic ulcers, bowel obstruction, infection, and heart disease are just a few causes of nausea and vomiting in the patient with cancer (30). Relief of symptoms is best achieved when therapy is directed at the underlying etiology.

Pharmacological agents used to treat nausea and vomiting include antiemetics, butyrophenones, substituted benzamides, serotonin receptor antagonists, benzodiazepines, corticosteroids, anticholinergics, and cannabinoids. For example, combining two or more drugs from different classes is often essential for control of chemotherapy-related nausea and vomiting (not a focus of this discussion). The serotonin antagonists, in combination with corticosteroids, are effective for prevention of the acute nausea and vomiting seen with highly or moderately emetogenic chemotherapy. For delayed nausea and vomiting (emesis 24 to 96 hours posttreatment) associated with highly emetogenic chemotherapy agents, the new NK-1 antagonists show promise as the most effective available agents (33).

Visceral Causes of Nausea

Mechanical problems in the gut secondary to tumor obstruction or peritoneal carcinomatosis will lead to distension of viscera and produce nausea, with or without emesis. Nausea secondary to visceral distension is mediated through dopamine and serotonin receptors in the gut and, as a result, is likely to respond to dopamine antagonists and serotonergic antagonists (21). For the patient without obstruction, prokinetic agents also may be of benefit.

Constipation is a common cause of nausea related to visceral distension, as is the "squashed stomach" syndrome, seen in patients with bulky hepatomegaly or high-volume ascites.

Chemical Causes of Nausea and Vomiting

A variety of medications, most notably opioids and alcohol, stimulate the chemoreceptor trigger zone through both dopamine and serotonergic receptors. Additionally, the nausea and vomiting seen with hypercalcemia, uremia, and hyponatremia are all mediated through this same mechanism. Again, a combination of dopamine antagonists, with or without prokinetic agents, and serotonergic antagonists are likely to be of benefit.

Central Nervous System Causes of Vomiting

Increased intracranial pressure secondary to edema related to intraparenchymal brain lesions directly stimulate the vomiting center, leading to nausea and vomiting. Corticosteroids, by reducing edema, are the most effective treatment. In addition, antihistamines may be beneficial, as increased intracranial pressure results in stimulation of histamine receptors.

Vestibular Causes of Vomiting

Vestibular nausea and vomiting are characterized by increased nausea with motion, with or without ringing in the ears, change in hearing, or skull tenderness. Both opioids and aspirin may cause vestibular nausea. An acoustic neuroma (a tumor of the eighth cranial nerve) or bone metastases, similarly, may cause these symptoms.

If possible, the offending medication should be removed. Antihistamines or anticholinergic agents should be initiated.

Antiemetics

Antiemetics offer relief of symptoms and are most effective when used prophylactically rather than to treat existing nausea and/or vomiting (1,30,33). As with the treatment of pain, preventive approaches are more likely to provide the best control of nausea and vomiting. Whenever possible, the antiemetic choice should be based on the understanding of its mechanism of action and the physiological basis of the patient's symptoms.

See Table 15.5 for a list of drugs and classes used as antiemetics. For disease-related emesis, a single agent may provide effective control of symptoms.

Phenothiazines

Phenothiazines block dopamine receptors in the chemoreceptor trigger zone (CTZ) (1). Extrapyramidal symptoms (EPS) (which are uncommon), sedation, hypersensitivity, and hypotension are the most common side effects (1). The phenothiazines are relatively inexpensive antiemetics, which are often effective for prevention of opioid-related nausea and nonchemotherapy-related nausea of unclear etiology. These agents may produce sedation for some patients (1,30).

Butyrophenones

Butyrophenones are dopamine receptor antagonists. Their major side effects are sedation and dystonic reactions (1,30). In general, these agents are more sedating than the phenothiazines. They are an excellent choice for patients who have only mild nausea and for those patients with neuropsychological symptoms, like delirium, hallucinations, or irritability (1,30).

Substituted Benzamides

Substituted benzamides (like metoclopramide) block dopamine receptors in the CTZ and, peripherally, increase esophageal sphincter tone, improve gastric emptying, and increase transit through the small bowel (1,30). Metoclopramide is primarily used for its prokinetic effects. The major side effects are EPS (3% to 31%), restlessness, drowsiness, fatigue, nausea, and diarrhea (1,30).

The major use of metoclopramide is for the treatment of delayed gastric emptying, which may be secondary to autonomic dysfunction, ascites, extensive intra-abdominal tumor, or opioid-induced decreases in GI tract peristalsis (1,29,30). It also is used with the hope of lessening constipation as well.

Serotonin Receptor Antagonists

Serotonin receptor antagonists block serotonin receptors peripherally in the upper gastrointestinal tract or in the area postrema located in the CTZ. They are prescribed primarily for acute, chemotherapy-induced nausea and vomiting. These agents also are effective for prevention of nausea and vomiting from upper abdominal radiation therapy. They are effective and safe in single doses prechemotherapy for the prevention of acute, chemotherapy-induced nausea and vomiting (33). There is no difference in efficacy between the oral and intravenous routes (33). Their primary side effects are headache, constipation, somnolence, and EKG changes (30).

The major difference between the available agents is the significantly longer half life of palonosetron, compared with the other agents, which translates into a greater percentage of patients with control of their delayed nausea and vomiting, compared to treatment with the other serotonin receptor antagonists (33).

Benzodiazepines

Benzodiazepines are a potentially useful class of drugs for patients with anxiety related to prior or anticipated nausea or vomiting. The major side effects are sedation, confusion, amnesia, and slurred speech (22).

Corticosteroids

Corticosteroids are effective for treating nausea and vomiting from a variety of causes used alone or in combination (33). The method of action is unknown, but they exhibit central and peripheral effects. Corticosteroids (generally dexamethasone) are the drugs of choice for the nausea and vomiting due to increased intracranial pressure and gastrointestinal obstruction. Their side effects include increased appetite, mood changes, anxiety, euphoria, headache, metallic taste, abdominal discomfort, and hyperglycemia (22).

Anticholinergics

Anticholinergics are primarily used for the nausea associated with motion sickness. These agents block acetylcholine in the emetic center (30). They are used most often when nausea is refractory and/or related to motion. The primary side effects are urinary retention, dry eyes, and constipation (30).

Cannabinoids

Cannabinoids are used to prevent nausea and vomiting with a level of efficacy similar to that of prochlorperazine. The most common side effects are mood changes, increased appetite, hypotension, tachycardia, and blurred vision (3,30,33).

CONSTIPATION

Constipation is a frequent problem for patients with cancer. Constipation refers to the infrequent or difficult passage of stool. It may be characterized by infrequent stools, discomfort passing stool, abnormally hard stool, or a sense of incomplete rectal emptying (1,34). Constipation is an exceedingly common problem, occurring in about 40% of patients referred to a palliative care clinic (1). Common causes of constipation include medications (eg, opioids and antidepressants), decreased mobility, dehydration, bowel obstruction, spinal cord compression, decreased physical activity, and other neurologic disorders (1). If left untreated, constipation causes significant distress (1,30).

The first step in managing constipation is to eliminate contributing factors and to increase fluid intake and activity level, if possible. Ideally, these measures, with stool softeners and laxatives, as appropriate, should be initiated *before* constipation occurs.

Table 15.5 Antiemetics

Drug Class	*Drug (Brand Name*)*	*Route(s)*	*Mechanism*	*Site of Action*	*Side Effects*	*Comments*
Phenothiazines	Perphenazine (Trilafon)	Oral, injection	DA	CTZ	EPS, sedation, hypotension	Prochlorperazine is the most effective agent in this class; perphenazine may be effective with high IV doses; prochlorperazine is available in sustained-release capsule, which should not be crushed.
	Prochlorperazine (Compazine)	Oral, rectal, injection				
	Promethazine (Phenergan)	Oral, rectal, injection				
	Thiethylperazine (Torecan)	Oral, rectal, injection				
Butyrophenone	Droperidol (Inapsine)	Oral, injection	DA	CTZ	EPS, sedation	EPS is seen rarely because this is a result of long-term exposure; droperidol is more sedating than haloperidol.
	Haloperidol (Haldol)	Oral, rectal, injection				
Benzamide	Metoclopramide (Reglan)	Oral, rectal, injection	DA or $5HT_3$ in high doses	CTZ	EPS, sedation, fatigue, diarrhea, nausea	Also used in early satiety and anorexia.
Serotonin antagonist	Dolasetron (Anzemet)	Oral, injection	$5HT_3$	CTZ, PGSEC	Headache, diarrhea, constipation, EKG changes, somnolence	Increased effect with corticosteroids.
	Granisetron (Kytril)	Oral, injection			Headache, diarrhea, constipation, somnolence	
	Ondansetron (Zofran)	Oral, injection				

Benzodiazepines	Lorazepam (Ativan)	Oral, injection	BDZ	Unknown	Sedation, confusion, amnesia, slurred speech	Effective for anticipatory nausea/anxiety; lorazepam may be placed under the tongue.
	Diazepam (Valium)	Oral, injection				
Corticosteroids	Dexamethasone (Decadron)	Oral, injection	Unknown	Unknown	Increased appetite, anxiety, mood changes, euphoria, headache, metallic taste, hyperglycemia	Most effective when used with $5HT_3$.
Anticholinergic	Scopolamine (Transderm)	Patch	ACH	Emetic center	Urinary retention, dry eyes, constipation	Effective for nausea related to motion.
Cannabinoid	Dronabinol (Marinol)	Oral	Unknown	CNS	Mood changes, increased appetite, hypotension, tachycardia	Well tolerated in younger patients; may be crushed.

Abbreviations: ACH, anticholinergic; BDZ, benzodiazepine; CNS, central nervous system; CTZ, chemoreceptor trigger zone; DA, dopamine antagonist; EKG, electrocardiogram; EPS, extrapyramidal side effects; $5HT_3$, serotonin antagonist; PGSEC, peripheral gastrointestinal stimulation to emetic center.

*Trilafon (Schering, Kenilworth, NJ 07033); Compazine (Glaxo Smith Kline, Research Triangle Park, NC 27709); Phenergan (Wyeth, Madison, NJ 07940); Torecan (Novartis Summit, NJ 07901; Roxane, Columbus, OH 43228; and Boehringer Ingelheim, Ridgefield, CT 06877-0368); Inapsine oral injection (Akorn Inc, Buffalo Grove, IL 60089 and Taylor Pharmaceuticals, San Clemente, CA 92673-6232); Haldol (Ortho McNeil, Raritan, NJ 08869-0602); Reglan (Wyeth, Madison, NJ 07940 and Schwarz Pharma, Mequon WI 53092); Anzemet (Aventis, Kansas City, MO 64137-1405); Kytril (Roche Laboratories, Nutley, NJ 07110); Zofran (GlaxoSmithKline, Research Triangle Park, NC 27709); Ativan oral injectible (Wyeth, Madison, NJ 07940 and Baxter Healthcare, Round Lake, IL 60073); Valium (Roche Laboratories, Nutley, NJ 07110); Decadron, Merck (White House Station, NJ 08889-1000); Transderm (Sandoz, Princeton, NJ 08540 and Mylan Pharmaceuticals, Morgantown, WV 26504-4310); Marinol (Roxane, Columbus, OH 43228).

Table 15.6 Antidiarrheals and Laxatives

Drug Class	*Drug (Brand Name*)*	*Route(s)*	*Mechanism of Action*	*Side Effects*
Antidiarrheals				
Bulk forming agent	Psyllium (Metamucil, Citrucel)	Powder, chewable wafer, liquid	Absorbs water from intestine	Bowel obstruction, diarrhea, abdominal cramps, constipation
	Calcium polycarbophil (FiberCon)	Chewable tablet		
	Attapulgite (Kaopectate)	Chewable tablet, liquid		
Antimotility agent	Loperamide (Imodium)	Tablet capsule, liquid	Inhibits peristalsis, prolongs transit time	Rash, nausea, vomiting, dry mouth, abdominal cramps, constipation
	Diphenoxylate/atropine (Lomotil)	Tablet capsule, liquid		
Miscellaneous antidiarrheal	Octreotide (Sandostatin)	IV	Mimics somatostatin, decreases fluid	Rash, flushing, edema, fatigue, headache, dizziness, increased LFT
Laxatives				
Stool softener	Docusate (Colace)	Capsule, liquid	Reduces surface tension of the stool to allow softening	Diarrhea, abdominal cramping
Stimulant	Senna (Senokot)	Tablet	Stimulates myenteric plexus	Diarrhea, abdominal cramping
	Biscodyl (Dulcolax)	Tablet, suppository, rectal solution		
Bulk-forming agent	Psyllium (Metamucil, Citrucel, Perdiem)	Granules, powder, chewable squares, chewable wafers	Holds water in stool	Diarrhea, abdominal cramping, constipation, bowel obstruction
Hyperosmotic laxative	Glycerine	Suppository, oral solution	Local irritation	Headache, vomiting, dizziness, confusion, diarrhea
Lubricant	Mineral oil	Rectal solution	Local irritation	Headache, vomiting, dizziness, confusion, diarrhea
Saline laxative	Magnesium hydroxide (Milk of Magnesia)	Tablet, liquid	Retains water in intestinal lumen	Dizziness, visual disturbances, dyspnea, nausea, constipation
Osmotic cathartic	Dibasic sodium phosphate (Fleet)	Tablet	Unknown	Mood changes, increased appetite, hypotension, tachycardia

*Metamucil (Proctor & Gamble, Cincinnati, OH 45241); Citrucel (GlaxoSmithKline, Research Triangle Park, NC 27709); FiberCon (Lederle Laboratories, Philadelphia, PA 19101-1245); Kaopectate (Pfizer, New York, NY 10017-5755); Imodium (Ortho McNeil, Raritan, NJ 08869-0602); Lomotil (Searle, Skokie, IL 60077); Sandostatin (Novartis, Summit, NJ 07901); Colace (Purdue, Samford, CT 06901-3431); Senokot (Purdue, Samford, CT 06901-3431); Dulcolax (GlaxoSmithKline, Research Triangle Park, NC 27709); Perdiem (many manufacturers); Milk of Magnesia (many manufacturers); Fleet (CB Fleet Company, Lynchburg, VA 24506).

Intervention for constipation requires careful titration of laxatives. Once constipation is relieved, a preventive strategy should be implemented to maintain daily spontaneous bowel movements. For a review of both oral and rectal interventions, see Table 15.6.

The bulk-forming agents, such as psyllium (Metamucil, Procter and Gamble, Cincinnati, OH; Citrucel, GlaxoSmithKline, Middlesex, UK; Perdiem, Novartis Consumer Healthcare, Parsippany, NJ; Benefiber, Novartis Consumer Healthcare, Parsippany, NJ) must be taken with adequate amounts of fluid and used cautiously in patients at risk for bowel obstruction. Furthermore, they are not very effective for patients who have limited physical activity. These agents work by increasing stool bulk and increasing water content in the colon. They are usually effective after 2 to 4 days. Bloating, abdominal cramping, and distension are the major side effects (1).

Lubricant laxatives allow easier passage of stool. Mineral oil is usually effective within 6 to 8 hours of administration. It is not recommended for chronic constipation. It is useful for acute treatment of fecal impaction (1).

Magnesium and sodium salts are osmatic cathartics that promote fluid movement into the gut. These agents generally work quickly, within 3 hours. The most common side effects are abdominal bloating and cramping (1). Examples of these agents include magnesium hydroxide (Phillips's Milk of Magnesia, Bayer HealthCare, Morristown, NJ) and dibasic sodium phosphate (Fleet, CB Fleet Company, Lynchburg, VA), as an enema or oral solution, and magnesium citrate.

Lactulose and sorbitol are examples of osmotic cathartics that are not absorbed or degraded in the small intestine. They are usually effective within 24 to 48 hours. Their primary side effect is flatulence (about 20% of patients), and their sweet taste makes them unpalatable for some patients (1).

The contact cathartics are the most widely used group of laxatives. They work primarily by increasing colon peristalsis and by reducing net absorption of water and electrolytes. The classes of agents, their onset of action, and their side effects are summarized in Table 15.7.

Opioid antagonists specific for the μ-opioid receptor, such as naloxone, can reverse opioid-induced constipation (35). Naloxone can provide relief of opioid-induced constipation without reversal of opioid analgesia. The initial dose of naloxone should be low (≤ 5 mg), to prevent withdrawal (35). A newer μ-opioid receptor antagonist, methylnaltrexone, does not cross the blood brain barrier and, as a result, does not produce withdrawal symptoms. An initial report noted that 80% of patients with chronic opioid-induced constipation have a bowel movement within 4 hours of receiving intravenous methylnaltrexone (36).

MUCOSITIS

Mucositis is a frequent complication of chemotherapy and radiation therapy (1). Mouth care is important to prevent possible infection and/or further irritation. Mucositis is painful, and the use of topical anesthetic agents and healing agents may be beneficial. Oral candidiasis is the most common infectious cause of mucositis, especially in patients receiving antibiotic therapy or high-dose steroids (1).

Although there are anecdotal reports suggesting a variety of agents as prophylaxis for mucositis, very few have shown benefit in randomized trials (1). Sucking on ice chips (cryotherapy) for 35 minutes beginning 5 minutes before administration of 5-fluorouracil-based chemotherapy reduces oral mucositis by 50% (37). The ice produces temporary vasoconstriction of the oral mucosa and reduces local drug delivery.

Effective oral care uses dietary alterations, general good oral hygiene, topical local anesthetics, and systemic analgesics as needed. Patients with mucositis should be offered a diet that requires limited contact with the oral mucosa (ie, little chewing required). Patients should avoid salty, acidic, coarse, dry, or spicy foods (1).

Cleansing agents, like chlorhexidine (Peridex, Zila Pharmaceuticals, Phoenix, AZ), should not be used because they may increase local discomfort. Healing/coating agents, such as sucralfate (Carafate, Axcan Scandipharm, Birmingham, AL), have been widely used, but most studies suggest no benefit for mucositis from this agent (38). Topical anesthetics, such as viscous lidocaine, provide some local pain relief, but the effect is of short duration.

Mucositis mouthwashes/preparations are institution specific, usually containing some combination of nystatin, Maalox (Novartis Consumer Healthcare, Parsippany, NJ) or Mylanta (Johnson & Johnson, Merck Consumer Pharmaceuticals, Fort Washington, PA), diphenhydramine, hydrocortisone, tetracycline,

Table 15.7 Contact Cathartics

Drug	*Time to Effect, hours*	*Side Effects*	*Comments*
Cascara senna	6–12	May cause red urine	Useful for opioid-related constipation
Bisacodyl	Oral: 6–12 Suppository: 1	Allergy to these agents may occur	Overuse carries risk of dehydration
Ducosate	24–72	May facilitate intestinal absorption or hepatic uptake of other drugs	Functions as determents, allowing water and fats to mix with stool; especially useful in patients with hard stools
Ducosate sodium	24–72	Dyspepsia with liquid formation	Indicated for prevention of opioid-induced constipation

and viscous lidocaine. Antifungal agents, such as fluconazole (Diflucan, Pfizer, New York, NY) (tablets, suspension, injection), nystatin (Mycostatin, Bristol-Myers Squibb, New York, NY) suspension, or clotrimazole (Mycelex, Ortho McNeil Pharmaceutical, Raritan, NJ) troches, may be used prophylactically or as treatment for oral candidiasis.

DIARRHEA

Both cancer and its treatment may cause diarrhea. Chemotherapy, particularly antimetabolites, causes diarrhea, with severity related to dose and schedule (1). Diarrhea is the most common acute toxicity of pelvic irradiation (1). Both nonpharmacological and pharmacological measures are recommended to control diarrhea. Nonpharmacological measures include rehydration, frequent small meals, and avoidance of foods or medications that might worsen diarrhea.

The antimotility agents loperamide and diphenoxylate/atropine are most commonly used to treat acute diarrhea. Potential side effects include rash, nausea, vomiting, constipation, abdominal cramps, dry mouth, abdominal distension, and fatigue (22).

For chemotherapy-related diarrhea, octreotide has been shown to be more effective than loperamide in multiple randomized trials (39). Octreotide (Sandostatin, Novartis Consumer Healthcare, Parsippany, NJ) mimics natural somatostatin and decreases gastric fluid. It is indicated for treatment-related diarrhea refractory to other antidiarrheals. It can be given intravenously or subcutaneously, generally at a starting dose of 0.1 mg twice to three times daily (1). The dose can be titrated to effect. Potential side effects include flushing, edema, fatigue, headache, anorexia, nausea, vomiting, and increased liver function tests (22).

Opioids decrease gastrointestinal motility and increase oral-cecal transit time, resulting in fewer bowel movements (21). Tincture of opium has not been prospectively evaluated for treatment-related diarrhea but is another useful antidiarrheal agent.

XEROSTOMIA AND MALABSORPTION

Therapy, particularly radiation of the head and neck, may cause xerostomia requiring saliva stimulants or artificial saliva. Pilocarpine (Salagen, MGI Pharma, Bloomington, MN) is a saliva stimulant that stimulates cholinergic receptors in the mouth to produce saliva. The recommended dose is a 5-mg tablet three times a day (1). Amifostine (Ethyol, MedImmune Oncology, Gaithersburg, MD) is a cytoprotective agent that has been shown to reduce the incidence of acute and late xerostomia in previously untreated squamous-cell head and neck cancer patients receiving radiotherapy (40). The recommended dose of 200 mg/m^2 is administered 15 to 30 minutes before each radiotherapy treatment. Potential side effects of administration include nausea, vomiting, hypotension, allergic reaction, and venous catheter complications (8).

Malabsorption and associated steatorrhea from pancreatic insufficiency can be improved with pancreatic enzymes. (See Table 15.8 for a list of available pancreatic enzymes.) Side effects include nausea, abdominal cramps, constipation, and diarrhea (22).

Table 15.8 Pancreatic Enzyme Preparations

*Product(s)**	*Dosage Form*	*Do Not Crush*	*Lipase, USP Units*	*Amylase, USP Units*	*Protease, USP Units*
Cotazym, Ku-Zyme HP	Capsule		8,000	30,000	30,000
Cotazym-S	Capsule, enteric-coated spheres	X	5,000	20,000	20,000
Creon	Enteric-coated microspheres	X	8,000	30,000	13,000
Entolase, Pancrease, Protilase	Capsule, delayed release	X	4,000	20,000	25,000
Entolase HP	Enteric-coated microbeads	X	8,000	40,000	50,000
Festal II	Tablet, delayed release	X	6,000	30,000	20,000
Ilozyme	Tablet		11,000	30,000	30,000
Pancrease MT	Tablet				
Pancrease MT 4	Capsule, enteric-coated microtablets	X	4,000	12,000	12,000
Pancrease MT 10	Capsule, enteric-coated microtablets	X	10,000	30,000	30,000
Pancrease MT 16	Capsule, enteric-coated microtablets	X	16,000	48,000	48,000
Viokase	Powder		16,800 per 0.7 g	70,000 per 0.7 g	70,000 per 0.7 g
	Tablet		8,000	30,000	30,000
Zymase	Capsule, enteric-coated spheres	X	12,000	24,000	24,000

*Cotazym (Organon, West Orange, NJ 07052); Ku-Zyme HP (Schwarz Pharma, Mequon WI 53092); Cotazym-S (Organon, West Orange, NJ 07052); Creon (Solvay Pharmaceuticals, Marietta, GA 30062); Entolase (Wyeth, Madison, NJ 07940); Pancrease (Ortho McNeil, USA, Raritan, NJ 08869-0602); Protilase (Rugby Watson Pharmaceuticals, Corona, CA 91720); Entolase HP (Wyeth, Madison, NJ 07940); Festal II (Aventis Pharmaceuticals, Kansas City, MO 64137-1405); Ilozyme (Adria, Kalamazoo, MI 49001 and Savage Laboratories, Melville, NY 11747); Pancrease MT 4 (Ortho McNeil, USA, Raritan, NJ 08869-0602); Pancrease MT 10 (Ortho McNeil, USA, Raritan, NJ 08869-0602); Pancrease MT 16 (Ortho McNeil, USA, Raritan, NJ 08869-0602); Viokase (Axcan Scandifarm, Birmingham, AL 35242 and Paddock Laboratories, Minneapolis, MN 55427); Zymase (Organon, West Orange, NJ 07052).

REFERENCES

1. American Society of Clinical Oncology. *Optimizing Cancer Care—The Importance of Symptom Management. Volumes I and II.* Alexandria, Va: American Society of Clinical Oncology; 2003.
2. Tisdale MJ. Pathogenesis of cancer cachexia. *J Support Oncol.* 2003;1:159–168.
3. Sallan SE, Cronin C, Zelan M, Zinberg NE. Antiemetics in patients receiving chemotherapy for cancer: a randomized comparison of delta-9-tetrahydrocannabinol and prochlorperazine. *N Engl J Med.* 1976;302: 135–138.
4. Wadleigh R, Spaulding M, Lembersky B, Zimmer M, Shepard K, Plasse T. Dronabinol enhancement of appetite in cancer patients [Abstract 1280]. *Proc Am Soc Clin Oncol.* 1990;9:331.

5. Nelson K, Walsh D, Deeter P, Sheehan F. A phase II study of delta-9-tetrahydrocannabinol for appetite stimulation in cancer-associated anorexia. *J Palliat Care.* 1994;10:14–18.
6. Gorter R, Seefrid M, Volberding P. Dronabinol effects on weight in patients with HIV infection. *AIDS.* 1992; 6:127–128.
7. Beal JE, Olson R, Laubernstein L, Morales JO, Bellman P, Yangco B, Lefkowitz L, Plasse TF, Shepard KV. Dronabinol as a treatment for anorexia associated with weight loss in patients with AIDS. *J Pain Symptom Manage.* 1995;10:89–97.
8. Micromedex Healthcare Series: Thomson Micromedex, Greenwood Village, Colorado (Vol 125 expires 9/2005).
9. Gregory EJ, Cohen SC, Oives DW. Megestrol acetate therapy for advanced breast cancer. *J Clin Oncol.* 1985;3:155–160.
10. Loprinzi CL, Ellison NM, Schaid DJ, Krook JE, Athmann LU, Dose AM, Mailliard JA, Johnson PA, Ebbert LP, Geeraerts LA. Controlled trial of megestrol acetate for the treatment of cancer anorexia and cachexia. *J Natl Cancer Inst.* 1990;82:1127–1132.
11. Bruera E, MacMillan K, Kuehn N, Hanson J, MacDonald RN. A controlled trial of megestrol acetate on appetite, calorie intake, nutritional status and other symptoms in patients with advanced cancer. *Cancer.* 1990;66:1279–1282.
12. Tchekmedyian NS, Tait N, Moody M, Greco FA, Aisner J. Appetite stimulation with megestrol acetate in cachectic cancer patients. *Semin Oncol.* 1986;13:37–43.
13. Tchekmedyian NS, Tait A, Mandy M, Aisner J. High dose megestrol acetate: a possible treatment for cachexia. *JAMA.* 1987;9:1195–1198.
14. Jatoi A, Windschitl HE, Loprinzi CL, Sloan JA, Dakhil SR, Mailliard JA, Pundaleeka S, Kardinal CG, Fitch TF, Krook JE, Novotny PJ, Christensen B. Dronabinol versus megestrol acetate versus combination therapy for cancer-associated anorexia: a North Central Cancer Treatment Group study. *J Clin Oncol.* 2002;20: 567–573.
15. Moertel C, Schulte A, Reitemeier R. Corticosteroid therapy of preterminal gastrointestinal cancer. *Cancer.* 1974;33:1607–1609.
16. Wilcox J, Corr J, Shaw J. Prednisone as an appetite stimulant in patients with cancer. *Br Med J.* 1984; 200:37.
17. Bruera E, Roca E, Cedaro L, Carraro S, Chacon R. Action of oral methylprednisolone in terminal cancer patients: a prospective randomized double-blind study. *Cancer Treat Rep.* 1985;69:751–754.
18. Della Cuna GR, Pellegrini A, Piazzi M. Effect of methylprednisolone sodium succinate on quality of life in pre-terminal cancer patients: a placebo controlled, multi-center study. *Eur J Cancer Clin Oncol.* 1989;25:1817–1821.
19. Popiela T, Lucchi R, Giongo F. Methylprednisolone as palliative therapy for female terminal cancer patients. *Eur J Cancer Clin Oncol.* 1989;25:1923–1929.
20. Loprinzi CL, Kugler J, Slvon J, Maillaid J, Krook J, Wilwerding M, Rowland K. Phase II randomized comparison of megestrol acetate, dexamethasone and fluoxymesterone for the treatment of cancer anorexia/ cachexia [Abstract 167]. *Proc Am Soc Clin Oncol.* 1997;16:48a.
21. Doyle D, Hanks G, MacDonald N, eds. *Oxford Textbook of Palliative Medicine.* London, England: Oxford Medical Publications; 1993.
22. *2005 Physicians' Desk Reference.* Montvale, NJ: Thomson Healthcare; 2005.
23. Von Roenn JH, Tchekmedyian S, Sheng K-N, Ottery FD. Oxandrolone in cancer-related weight loss: improvement in weight, body cell mass (BCM), performance status, and quality of life (QOL) [Abstract 1450]. *Proc Am Soc Clin Oncol.* 2002;363a.
24. Tchekmedyian S, Fesen M, Price LM, Ottery FD. Ongoing placebo-controlled study of oxandrolone in cancer-related weight loss. Poster presentation at 45th Annual Meeting of the American Society of Therapeutic Radiology and Oncology, Salt Lake City, Utah, October 19–23, 2003, Poster 1039.
25. May PE, Barber A, D'Olimpio JT, Hourihane A, Abumrad NN. Reversal of cancer-related wasting using oral supplementation with a combination of beta-hydroxy-beta-methylbutyrate, arginine, and glutamine. *Am J Surg.* 2002;183:471–479.
26. Clark RH, Feleke G, Din M, Yasmin T, Singh G, Khan FA, Rathmacher JA. Nutritional treatment for acquired immunodeficiency virus-associated wasting using beta-hydroxy beta-methylbutyrate, glutamine, and arginine: a randomized, double-blind, placebo-controlled study. *JPEN J Parenter Enteral Nutr.* 2000;24:133–139.
27. Nissen SL, Sharp RL. Effect of dietary supplements on lean mass and strength gains with resistance exercise: a meta-analysis. *J Appl Physiol.* 2003;94:651–659.
28. Curtis EB, Krech R, Walsh TD. Common symptoms in patients with advanced cancer. *J Palliat Care.* 1991; 7:25–29.

29. Kris MG, Yeh SDJ, Gralla RJ. Symptomatic gastroparesis in cancer patients—a possible cause of cancer-associated anorexia that can be improved with oral metoclopramide [Abstract]. *Proc Am Soc Clin Oncol.* 1985;4:1038A.
30. Mannix KA. Gastrointestinal symptoms: palliation of nausea and vomiting. In Doyle D, Hanks G, MacDonald N, eds. *Oxford Textbook of Palliative Medicine.* London, England: Oxford Medical Publications; 1993:489–499.
31. Hesketh PJ, Kris MG, Grunberg SM, Beck T, Hainsworth JD, Harker G, Aapro MS, Gandara D, Lindley CM. Proposal for classifying the acute emetogenicity of cancer chemotherapy. *J Clin Oncol.* 1997; 15:103–109.
32. Ettinger DS. Preventing chemotherapy-induced nausea and vomiting: an update and review of emesis. *Semin Oncol.* 1995;23(Suppl 10):6–18.
33. Ettinger DS, Bierman PJ, Bradbury B, Ellis G, Ignoffo RJ, Kirkegaard S, Kloth DD, Krauss A, Kris MG, Lim D, Markiewicz MA, McNulty R, Noonan K, Stucky-Marshall L, Todaro B, Urba S, Yowell S [NCCN Antiemesis Panel Members]. NCCN Practice Guidelines: Antiemesis. National Comprehensive Cancer Network Clinical Practice Guidelines in Oncology—v.1.2004. Available at: http://www.nccn.org. Accessed March 10, 2005.
34. Mancini I, Bruera E. Constipation in advanced cancer patients. *Support Care Cancer.* 1998;6:356–364.
35. Sykes NP. An investigation of the ability of oral naloxone to correct opioid-related constipation in patients with advanced cancer. *Palliat Med.* 1996;10:135–144.
36. Yuan CS, Foss JF, O'Connor M, Toledano A, Roizen MF, Moss J. Methylnaltrexone prevents morphine-induced delay in oral-cecal transit time without affecting analgesia: a double-blind randomized placebo-controlled trial. *Clin Pharmacol Ther.* 1996;59:469–475.
37. Rocke LK, Loprinzi CL, Lee JK, Kunselman SJ, Iverson RK, Finck G, Lifsey D, Glaw KC, Stevens BA, Hatfield AK. A randomized clinical trial of two different durations of oral cryotherapy for prevention of 5-fluorouracil-related stomatitis. *Cancer.* 1993;72: 2234–2238.
38. McGinnis WL, Loprinzi CL, Buskirk SJ, Sloan JA, Drummond RG, Frank AR, Shanahan TG, Kahanic SP, Moore RL, Schild SE, Humphrey SL. Placebo-controlled trial of sucralfate for inhibiting radiation-induced esophagitis. *J Clin Oncol.* 1997;15:1239–1243.
39. Cascinu S, Fedeli A, Fedeli SL, Catalano G. Octreotide versus loperamide in the treatment of fluorouracil-induced diarrhea: a randomized trial. *J Clin Oncol.* 1993;11:148–151.
40. Brizel DM, Wasserman TH, Henke M, Strnad V, Rudat V, Monnier A, Eschwege F, Zhang J, Russell L, Oster W, Sauer R. Phase III randomized trial of amifostine as a radioprotector in head and neck cancer [erratum in *J Clin Oncol.* 2000;18:4110–4111]. *J Clin Oncol.* 2000;18:3339–3345.

Chapter 16

Complementary and Alternative Medicine

LAURA L. MOLSEED, MS, RD
CONSULTING EDITOR: KATHRYN HAMILTON, MA, RD

INTRODUCTION

Complementary and alternative medicine (CAM) describes a variety of medical, health, and lifestyle practices and therapies that are not traditionally part of conventional medicine; however, many medical practices, including oncology, are evaluating and integrating CAM therapies into their practices. "Complementary" implies that these therapies are used in addition to conventional treatment and can be used for supportive care and to improve quality of life (1). "Alternative" implies that practices and therapies are used in place of conventional medicine.

Many health care practitioners are concerned that patients will use these therapies in lieu of more conventional therapies with better safety and efficacy records; in fact, this happens much less often than predicted (2). Most individuals choose CAM therapies as an adjunct to their traditional medical treatments (2); therefore, the potential for interactions with conventional medicine exists. This chapter describes the use of CAM and categories of CAM practices. In particular, it explores the nutritional implications of CAM encountered in oncology settings and examines common diet therapies, phytochemicals, dietary supplements, herbs and botanicals, and metabolic therapies. This chapter also provides suggestions for communication and education on this emerging practice.

APPEAL OF CAM

In a health care climate where clinicians often cannot provide promises of definitive cancer cures, where adverse side effects from conventional cancer treatment can be substantial, and where the cancer treatment process can be overwhelming and sometimes less than personal, CAM practices have an appeal to individuals diagnosed with cancer and their caregivers. Research studies (3,4) have shown benefit of CAM therapies in the areas of symptom relief and improved quality of life. For many individuals, participating in a therapy that is considered safe and possibly efficacious can result in feelings of empowerment, wellness, and hope, regardless of whether the individual's outcome is symptom management or treatment.

PREVALENCE OF CAM

The prevalence of CAM has steadily increased in the last several decades, but it really started to draw attention from the scientific community in the early 1990s. According to telephone surveys conducted between 1990 and 1997 by Eisenberg et al (5), the general use of CAM treatments increased by 8%, from 34% in 1990 to 42% in the 1997. This study also highlighted a need for increased communication between the health care practitioners and clients—results showed that fewer than 40% of CAM therapies used were discussed with the physician or health care provider. Another telephone survey, conducted by Kessler et al in 1997 (6), found 67.6% of individuals polled had used at least one CAM therapy in their lifetime. That study also confirmed the consistent rise in use of CAM therapies during the past 4 decades.

The National Center for Complementary and Alternative Medicine (NCCAM) and the National Center for Health Statistics (NCHS) released results of the most comprehensive CAM survey in 2004 (7). This survey concurred with Eisenberg and Kessler's findings and reported that more than 60% of adults surveyed use some form of CAM.

Although these studies were not specific to the use of CAM in cancer treatment, the data are compelling. Individuals reporting the highest use in all three surveys are female, younger, well educated, have higher incomes, have recently been hospitalized, and are former smokers (5–7). The types of CAM treatments varied greatly, as did the purposes and settings in which they were used. In the general population, however, the most popular CAM therapies from these studies included the following (5–7):

- Relaxation therapy
- Lifestyle diets
- Herbal medications
- Homeopathy
- High-dose vitamin therapy
- Energy healing
- Biofeedback
- Chiropractic medicine
- Massage therapy
- Imagery
- Spiritual healing
- Self-help groups
- Commercial weight loss programs
- Hypnosis
- Acupuncture
- Folk remedies

More specific to the oncology population, a study published in 2005 by researchers at the James P. Wilmot Cancer Center, in Rochester, New York, reviewed the use of CAM therapies in cancer treatment (8). The researchers reported the following:

- More than 90% of patients surveyed reported using at least one form of CAM.
- Prayer, relaxation, and exercise were the most widely used forms of CAM.
- Of the patients using CAM, the majority discussed the use of CAM modalities with at least one physician. The most frequent CAM modalities discussed were diets, massage, and herbal medicine.

CAM PRACTICES

NCCAM classifies CAM into five major domains (7):

1. *Whole medical systems.* According to NCCAM, whole medical systems involve "complete systems of theory and practice that have evolved independently from or parallel to conventional medicine." Examples of whole medical systems include traditional Chinese medicine (TCM), Ayurvedic medicine, homeopathy, and naturopathy.
2. *Mind-body interventions.* Mind-body interventions examine the interactions between an individual's brain, mind, body, and behaviors. According to NCAAM, mind-body interventions also examine the ways in which "emotional, mental, social, spiritual, and behavioral factors can directly affect health." Examples of mind-body interventions include meditation, yoga, and tai chi.
3. *Biologically based therapies.* Biologically based therapies involve the use of natural and biologically based practices and products. According to NCAAM, examples of biologically based therapies include, but are not limited to the following: botanicals, animal-derived extracts, vitamins, minerals, fatty acids, amino acids, proteins, prebiotics and probiotics, whole diets, functional foods.
4. *Manipulative and body-based methods.* Manipulative and body-based methods concentrate on bodily structures and systems, including bones and joints, soft tissues, and the circulatory and lymphatic systems. Examples include chiropractic and osteopathic manipulation, massage therapy, Tui Na, reflexology, rolfing, Bowen technique, Trager bodywork, Alexander technique, Feldenkrais method, and others. Some of these practices come from traditional systems of medicine; others were

developed within the last 2 centuries (eg, chiropractic medicine).

5. *Energy therapies.* Energy therapies are based on the concept that imbalances in an individual's energies cause illness. According to NCCAM, energy therapies examine energy fields of two types: (*a*) veritable energy, which is measurable, and (*b*) putative energy, which has not yet been measurable by reproducible means. Examples of treatment modalities using veritable energies include magnetic therapy, sound energy therapy, and light therapy. Examples of treatment modalities using putative energies include acupuncture, qi gong, homeopathy, and therapeutic touch. Some of the terms used to describe an individual's energy or life force include *qi* in TCM, *ki* in the Japanese Kampo system, and *doshas* in Ayurvedic medicine.

The following sections provide a more in-depth look at biologically based therapies, including diet therapies, phytochemicals, dietary supplements, vitamins and minerals, herbs and botanicals, and metabolic therapies.

COMMON DIET THERAPIES

Diet therapies are some of the oldest and most commonly used CAM practices in the treatment of disease. Although diet and nutrition modification have a better researched role in primary cancer prevention, the role of diet in secondary cancer prevention is less defined. Recent studies (Women's Interventional Nutrition Study and Dean Ornish Study) (9,10) have demonstrated a positive relationship between diet and cancer prognosis, but more research is needed. Using diet therapy as the sole treatment for cancer is not scientifically warranted at this time; however, diet and nutrition modification should be encouraged as a means to improve quality of life and to maintain health.

Vegetarian Diets

The American Cancer Society (11) and a number of other health-oriented agencies recommend a plant-based diet for better health and possibly cancer prevention. Vegetarian-type diets can range from plant-based diets to vegan diets (Table 16.1). In CAM, vegetarian diets can be used in a number of ways. They can be part of a "detoxification" program (12), or they may be used alone as an adjuvant program to conventional cancer treatment.

Proponents of vegetarian diets often also encourage the use of "natural" or organic foods (12). Of note, the US Department of Agriculture (USDA) established the National Organic Program (13), as the result of the Organic Foods Production Act of 1990 (14). It is not necessary to consume only organic foods while following a vegetarian diet; however, if people are interested in incorporating more organic foods in their diet, it is now easier to identify which foods are produced to organic specifications, because they carry the USDA Organic Seal. To date, however, using strictly organic foods, or not using them, is a choice, and although proponents feel strongly that organic food is more nutritious, this has yet to be definitively documented.

When coupled with proper education and careful meal planning, a vegetarian diet can be a healthy, nutrient-complete diet. Vegetarian diets are rich in whole grains, fruit, vegetable fiber, and phytochemicals and are low in total dietary fat, saturated fat, and animal fat. A wide variety of vegetarian and organic foods are readily available in many supermarkets and specialty food stores. Vegetarian diets that are not balanced may be lacking in specific nutrients, including protein, vitamin B-12, calcium, magnesium, zinc, and iron. It may be difficult for individuals who are experiencing treatment-related side effects or who have very particular tastes to obtain adequate nutrition following a strict vegetarian diet. Those individuals may explore the lacto-ovo vegetarian or plant-based diets as alternatives. If needed, dietetics professionals can encourage the use of alternate protein sources and vitamin and mineral supplements for individuals who are undergoing active cancer treatment and who adopt a vegetarian or vegan diet.

Vegetarian diets have been under investigation by the medical community as an adjuvant therapy to conventional therapies in the treatment of some cancers (15). Reductions in the incidence of nonmelanoma skin cancer (MNSC) and actinic keratosis have been found in individuals following a low-fat, low-saturated fat, and low-animal fat diet (15).

Macrobiotic Diet

Macrobiotic diet guidelines, as outlined in Box 16.1 (16), are very similar to a strict vegetarian diet. The term "macrobiotic" is derived from Greek and means

Table 16.1 Vegetarian Diets

Diet	*Description*	*Comments*
Plant-based	Diets that are primarily based on plant foods and include very little or no animal products such as meat	Recommended as a means to obtain a nutrient-rich diet that is generally low in fat and high in fiber
Lacto-ovo vegetarian	Predominantly vegetarian diet that includes milk/milk products and eggs	
Vegan	Strict vegetarian diet that avoids all animal products	Requires good menu/meal planning to ensure adequate nutrient content

big or great life. Around the turn of the 20th century, the diet was promoted by George Ohsawa, as "a natural way of living leading to health and happiness" (17). It incorporates a number of elements from TCM.

Today, the Kushi Institute (18) is one of the leading proponents of the macrobiotic philosophy and the macrobiotic lifestyle. According to the Michio Kushi, the Kushi Institute's founder, most physical ailments experienced today result from poor nutrition and an unhealthy, unnatural lifestyle (19). The Kushi Institute's macrobiotic philosophy also proposes that the development of cancers (which are categorized as *yin* or *yang* cancers) can result from an overconsumption of either *yin* foods or *yang* foods in one's diet and/or an overaccumulation of waste products in the body (18). *Yin* and *yang* are principles in TCM and represent opposing forces, such as light and dark. These principles are often characterized in the popular *yin/yang* symbol.

Individuals who follow the macrobiotic principles are encouraged to achieve a balance between *yin* and *yang* with the foods that they eat and with the environment in which they live (18,19). This balance is called *chi,* which, according to TCM, is the balance of negative and positive forms in the body and is believed to be essential for good health.

These restrictions, however, can make it very difficult for individuals with cancer to follow this diet and lifestyle philosophy when they are experiencing side effects from treatment. It also can be a very labor-intensive dietary regimen, requiring special cooking techniques, specific pots and pans, and the use of conventional ovens rather than microwaves. Eating in a peaceful, relaxing environment and additional relaxation exercises are encouraged.

Typically, the foods to be consumed are customized to the individual. Depending on the type of cancer, the part of the body affected, age and gender of the individual, and the climate in which the individual lives, the specific foods included may vary, and other foods may be limited or allowed in greater quantities (19). Strict adherence is recommended when individuals have active disease, but once they are disease free, they can gradually reintroduce select foods.

Because food choices can be so restrictive, there is potential for weight loss and for protein, vitamin B-12, and calcium deficiencies. It is imperative that individuals who decide to follow this diet regimen be monitored closely (19).

Currently, there is no scientific evidence indicating that this diet, used alone or as a complement to conventional therapy, cures cancer. Further research on the efficacy of macrobiotic diet regimens is clearly needed because macrobiotics remains a commonly used therapy in the cancer community (19).

Four attempts to substantiate the claims of persons who adopted the Kushi Institute macrobiotic diet were made in the 1980s and 1990s. However, each attempt has resulted in a poor investigation, with little supporting evidence (19).

PHYTOCHEMICALS

Phytochemicals, the biologically active, naturally occurring chemical components in plant foods, are receiving increasing support from the medical and nutrition communities for their role in health and disease prevention (20). For example, there is moderate evidence to correlate consumption of foods rich in lutein and zeaxanthin with a reduction in age-related

Box 16.1

Guidelines for Individuals Consuming a Macrobiotic Diet

Choose Often

- *Whole grains.* Should comprise 50%-60% of each meal. Examples are brown rice, whole wheat berries, barley, and millet.
- *Regionally grown fruit.* Should be consumed several times a week.
- *Vegetables.* Should comprise 25%–30% of daily food intake. Raw vegetables can comprise up to one-third of the total vegetable intake. The rest can be prepared by a variety of methods, including steaming, boiling, baking, and sautéing.
- *Beans.* Should comprise 10% of daily food intake. Examples include cooked beans or bean products such as tofu, tempeh, and natto.
- *Soup.* 1 to 2 cups or bowls per day should be consumed. Common choices are miso and shoyu, which are made from fermented soybeans.

Choose Less Often

- *Fish or seafood.* A small amount may be consumed several times per week. Condiments such as horseradish, wasabi, ginger, mustard, or grated daikon help cleanse the body from the effects of fish and seafood.
- *Seeds and nuts.* Should be consumed in moderation. May be eaten raw or lightly roasted and salted.
- *Flour products.* Can be eaten occasionally. Examples are noodles, pasta, bread, and baked goods.
- *Desserts.* Can be eaten by individuals in good health in moderation, 2–3 times per week. Desserts prepared with naturally sweet foods, such as apples, squashes, adzuki beans, and dried fruit, or with natural sweeteners, such as rice syrup, barley malt, and amazake, are preferred.

Avoid

- *Meat, eggs, poultry, and dairy.*
- *Sweeteners.* Examples are sugar, honey, molasses, chocolate, and carob.
- *Tropical fruit.* Examples are mango, pineapple, and papaya.

Other Recommendations

- *Unrefined vegetable oil.* The preferred oil for cooking. The most common is dark sesame oil. Light sesame oil, corn oil, and mustard seed oil are also recommended.
- *Condiments and seasonings.* Commonly used seasonings include natural sea salt, shoyu, brown rice vinegar, umeboshi vinegar, umeboshi plums, grated ginger root, fermented pickles, gomashio (roasted sesame seeds), roasted seaweed, and sliced scallions.

Note: Diet guidelines should be individualized on the basis of age, gender, activity levels, and health needs. Climate and season are also considerations.

Source: Data are from reference 16.

macular degeneration (21). There is also evidence that correlates the consumption of glucosinolates and indoles via cruciferous vegetables with reduced risk of certain types of cancer (22–24).

Epidemiological findings of lower incidence of breast, prostate, and endometrial cancer in populations that have high intakes of phytoestrogen-rich foods have sparked interest and investigation to determine their protective effects (20,25). Isoflavones and lignans are precursors of the two main classes of phytoestrogens. Soy products, whole grain cereals, seeds, berries and nuts are examples of phytoestrogens in the food supply (25).

Researchers in breast cancer have been studying the effect of phytoestrogens in the proliferation of breast cancer cells. In vitro studies of some ER-

Table 16.2 Protein and Isoflavone Content of Selected Soy Foods

Soy Product	*Serving Size*	*Total Protein, g*	*Isoflavone, mg*
Soy milk, unfortified	1 cup	7	10
Tofu	½ cup	10	25
Soybean, green cooked	½ cup	11	50
Texturized soy protein	¼ cup	11	33
Soy flour, low-fat	½ cup	11	50

Source: Data are from reference 30.

positive breast cancer cells have shown proliferation of cancer cells with low levels of genistein, a very weak estrogen-like compound found in isoflavones (26,27). The growth of ER-positive breast cancer cells seems to diminish as the amount of genistein increases (28); however, ER-negative cells have shown reduced growth in the presence of even low levels of genistein. Adding to the confusion of patients and the health care community, other in vitro studies have contradicted these findings (28). Concerns that soy proteins may interact with tamoxifen are well founded; however; some recent studies have shown that the use of soy may enhance tamoxifen's effect (27).

The evidence on phytoestrogens and cancer treatment is inconclusive; therefore, the current recommendation is to discourage soy supplementation in women with breast cancer. Conversely, there are indications that soy may be beneficial to men with prostate cancer (10,29). Food remains the best source of these phytoestrogens; supplements are less reliable and consistent (see Table 16.2) (27,30).

Because of a lack of conclusive scientific evidence, there is no specific recommendation for flaxseed consumption, except to make it part of a healthy plant-based diet. Of note, if the flaxseeds are not ground, the lignan and n-3 fatty acid components are not readily available for absorption, and the flax serves primarily as a good source of fiber.

DIETARY SUPPLEMENTS

Dietary supplement consumption is a common CAM practice among individuals with cancer (5,6). As defined by Congress in the Dietary Supplement Health and Education Act (31), dietary supplements are substances that are intended to supplement the diet; contain one or more dietary ingredients (including vitamins, minerals, herbs, or other botanicals; amino acids; and other substances) or their constituents; are intended to be taken by mouth as a pill, capsule, tablet, or liquid; and are labeled on the front panel as being a dietary supplement. Table 16.3 compares the manufacturing, regulation, and standardization of drugs and supplements (32).

A 2004 Institute of Medicine (IOM) report (33) on the safety of dietary supplements recommends a framework for cost-effective and science-based evaluation by the Food and Drug Administration (FDA). Under proposed FDA regulation (34), manufacturers would be required to evaluate the identity, purity, quality, strength, and composition of their dietary supplements. In the meantime, although some companies are still manufacturing their products according to

Table 16.3 Regulation of Marketing Claims for Medications and Dietary Supplements

Prescriptions and Over-the-Counter Medications	*Dietary Supplements*
Manufacturers must follow GMPs.	FDA is currently developing some guidelines for manufacturers.
Must be proven safe and efficacious before marketing.	Manufacturers are responsible for ensuring safety, not efficacy.
Manufacturers must submit scientific data to substantiate claims of benefit to FDA.	Manufacturers are not required to submit substantiation data for claims of benefit to FDA. Manufacturers can cite existing literature. FTC monitors truth in labeling.

Abbreviations: FDA, Food and Drug Administration; FTC, Federal Trade Commission; GMPs, Good Manufacturing Practices.

Source: Data are from reference 32.

their own established standards, many more are starting to submit for certification from the US Pharmacopeia (USP), Consumer Labs, or NSF International Dietary Supplement Certification Program. If a product has a seal from one of these organization, consumers can be assured that the product in the body is correctly identified and described, and that it was manufactured under regulated guidelines.

These organizations do not, however, evaluate efficacy (34). Although a number of dietary supplements have been shown to be of benefit during cancer therapy, others can be of little value or may even be harmful. Some dietary supplements can interfere with conventional medications and produce detrimental effects. For example, St. John's wort, a proven therapy for mild depression, interferes with the cytochrome in the metabolic pathway for drug metabolism (35). Taken in addition to a number of common cancer medications and other health-related medications, St. John's wort can alter the anticipated effect of the prescribed medication. For a review of commonly used dietary supplements in the oncology practice, and for their implications for nutrition, health, safety, and efficacy, see Table 16.4 (36–56).

Vitamins and Minerals

Vitamin and mineral supplementation is probably the most popular biologically based CAM practice. According to recent estimates, 50% of all Americans take some kind of nutrient supplement (57). Many individuals simply take a standard multiple vitamin-mineral combination. However, high-dose vitamin and mineral therapy (referred to as orthomolecular medicine) has become common complementary practice for individuals with cancer.

Antioxidant vitamins, such as vitamins E and C and beta carotene, are popular single-agent supplements used by many people, including individuals undergoing active anticancer treatments, such as chemotherapy and radiation therapy (37,57). Because antioxidant vitamins and minerals neutralize free radicals and have potential for enhancing immune function, many individuals view them as supportive therapies. In addition, antioxidants inhibit oxidative stress and have the potential for improved response to chemotherapy (37).

Questions and concerns remain regarding the usefulness of antioxidant supplements. Some studies show decreases in the effectiveness of chemotherapy and radiation therapy when antioxidant supplements are taken; other studies show an ability to enhance chemotherapy and reduce tumor growth (34–37,57). Antioxidants inactivate free radicals and decrease chemotherapy and radiation therapy damage on normal cells (34,37), but large doses may also prevent the same damage on cancer cells, rendering the chemotherapy less effective (37). Although antioxidant therapy may reduce side effects associated with chemotherapy, they may also reduce the effectiveness of the cancer therapy (3,21,37). It is for this reason, a lack of clear-cut benefit or determinant, that the American Cancer Society has decided to conservatively recommend that people get antioxidants through food sources rather than from supplements (58). For a review of commonly used vitamins and minerals, see Table 16.4. For a list of resources regarding CAM, including vitamins and minerals, see Appendix B.

Herbs and Botanicals

Herbal and botanical medicines have been used for well over 3,000 years in Asia and by Native Americans to treat a variety of ailments, including cancer. Today, herbs and botanicals are still used by many for symptom management and improved quality of life. They are sold in a variety of different forms, such as the natural herb/botanical, pills/capsules, powders, tinctures, and even poultices.

The concentration of the active ingredients in the herbs/botanicals will vary depending on the plant, species, conditions in which the plant is grown and stored, what part of the plant is used, and the preparation method used (59,60). All of these factors will affect potency and, consequently, medicinal benefit.

Before the early 1990s, herbal and botanical therapies were largely ignored by Western medical practices. However, growing interest in the public and professional communities has propelled research efforts and monies. Table 16.5 (59–63) reviews some common herbal and botanical products used by individuals with cancer.

METABOLIC THERAPIES

Metabolic therapies are much less popular than the vegetarian or macrobiotic diet therapies; however, they are still practiced, in part or in entirety, throughout the United States. Metabolic therapies are based, at least in part, on the assumption that cancer and other disease

Table 16.4 Vitamins, Minerals, and Selected Dietary Supplements

Supplement (references)	*Adult DRI*	*Adult UL*	*Nutrition and Health Implications*	*Efficacy*
Vitamin A (retinoic acid) (36,37)	Men: 900 µg. Nonpregnant, nonlactating women: 700 µg Pregnant women: 770 µg Lactating women: 1300 µg	3000 µg	Intakes > UL can cause nausea, vomiting, diminished appetite, weight loss, joint pain, abdominal discomfort, irritability, bone deformities, and hepatomegaly.	• Some forms of Vitamin A are being investigated as anticancer agents. • Dietary supplementation is not effective as a cancer treatment.
Beta carotene (38–40)	No DRI established	No UL established	There are no known toxicities. Recent clinical trials revealed that high-risk populations who received beta carotene supplementation had higher cancer rates.	• May inhibit the growth of abnormal cells, strengthen immune response, fortify cell membranes, and alter abnormal cell production. • Works in concert with other antioxidants. Used alone, suppresses uptake of other carotenoids.
Vitamin C (37–41)	Men: 90 mg Nonpregnant, nonlactating women: 75 mg Pregnant women: 85 mg Lactating women: 120 mg	2000 mg	Megadoses (2,000–10,000 mg/day) may cause diarrhea, dental erosion, clotting abnormalities, kidney stones, infertility, vitamin B-12 destruction, and low copper and selenium levels.	• Increased activity of doxorubicin, cisplatin, and paclitaxel. • Increased effects when used in combination with vitamins E and K.
Vitamin E (37–39,42)	Men and nonlactating women: 15 mg alpha-tocopherol Lactating women: 19 mg alpha-tocopherol	1000 mg	Megadoses have the potential to interfere with the absorption of vitamin K. Little other toxicity has been noted.	• There is currently no evidence to support megadoses as a cancer treatment. Vitamin E is an antioxidant and may have a role in cancer prevention.
Selenium (38,40,43)	Men and nonpregnant, non-lactating women: 55 µg Pregnant women: 60 µg Lactating women: 70 µg	400 µg	Prolonged intakes > 750 µg/day may cause slowed growth, eye damage, hair loss, tooth decay, and compromised bone function.	• Protects cell membranes from free radical damage. Effects seem to be enhanced with vitamin E. • Potential role in cancer prevention in areas with low soil levels of selenium. • Currently, there is no evidence to support its use as a treatment for cancer.

(continued)

Table 16.4 Vitamins, Minerals, and Selected Dietary Supplements (*continued*)

Supplement (references)	*Adult DRI*	*Adult UL*	*Nutrition and Health Implications*	*Efficacy*
Zinc (36,37)	Men: 11 mg Nonpregnant, nonlactating women: 8 mg Pregnant women: 11 mg Lactating women: 12 mg	40 mg	Intakes > 150 mg/day may suppress immune function. Intakes > 25 mg/day may impede copper absorption. High doses may cause nausea and vomiting.	• Assists in immune enhancement and wound healing. • May improve taste perception during radiation therapy. • There is no evidence to suggest that megadoses will be of benefit in cancer treatment.
L-Glutamine (44–56)	Not applicable	Not applicable	Questionable for high doses to enhance tumor growth. More research is required to determine mechanisms of action.	• There is strong evidence that glutamine does not prevent or reduce chemotherapy-induced oral mucositis/stomatitis. • There is mixed evidence regarding the ability of glutamine to reduce chemotherapy-induced diarrhea. • There is mixed evidence regarding the ability of glutamine to reduce nutritional impact symptoms associated with bone marrow transplant. • There is no evidence available that directly supports that oral glutamine can reduce mucositis associated with radiation therapy. • Glutamine has not been shown to reduce radiation-induced mucositis.
Coenzyme Q10 (ubiquinone) (39,40)	Not applicable	Not applicable	There have been no toxic effects reported from CoQ10.	• Proponents claim that cancer patients lack CoQ10 in their blood and that it has a profound effect on the human immune system. • Currently, there is no clinical evidence to support this and some studies indicate that it may enhance breast cancer cell growth.

Abbreviations: DRI, Dietary Reference Intake; UL, Tolerable Upper Limit.

Source: Data are from references 36–56.

Table 16.5 Herbs and Herbal Products

Herb or Herbal Product	*Claim(s)*	*Efficacy*	*Safety*	*Current Recommendations*
Black cohosh	• Alleviates menopausal symptoms, including hot flashes, depression, mood swings, and sleep disturbances.	• Considered German Commission E—safe, no contraindications. • Conflicting data on effectiveness compared with placebo and HRT.	• Potentiates antihypertensive drugs. • May potentiate HRT. • Headaches, vertigo, impaired vision and impaired circulation have been reported.	• No evidence that black cohosh is better than standard therapy in treating menopausal symptoms. • Individuals should take for 6 months or less. • Estrogenic effects are questionable. • Does not appear to bind to estrogen receptors or stimulate estrogen-dependent tumors in animals. More studies are needed.
Chaparrel	• Alleviates pain. • Reduces congestion. • Increases urine excretion. • Induces vomiting. • Reduces inflammation. • Serves as an antioxidant.	• No anticancer effect in animal studies. • May actually stimulate some malignancies, including renal cell carcinoma.	• Long-term use in rats increased lesions in mesentery lymph nodes and kidneys. • Hepatotoxic causing cholestatic hepatitis typically resolves with discontinuation of use, but has progressed to cirrhosis and acute liver failure.	• Not recommended. Chaparrel was removed from GRAS list.
Echinacea	• Stimulates the immune system. • Treats wounds.	• Widely used in Germany to treat the common cold and respiratory and urinary tract infections. Scientific evidence in United States is lacking.	• Substantial side effects have not been observed. Allergies may occur in individuals allergic to plants from the daisy family. • Counteracts with immunosuppressant agents.	• May be used with caution. • Not recommended for use for > 8 consecutive weeks. • Not recommended during pregnancy or lactation.
Essiac	• Strengthens the immune system. • Reduces tumor size.	• No documented anticancer effects for essiac.	• Not safe for consumption and illegal to distribute in the United States.	• Not recommended.
Evening primrose oil/GLA*	• Reduces inflammation. • Reduces the risk of breast cancer. • Reduces pain associated with rheumatoid arthritis. • Reduces symptoms of PMS.	• One study, which was neither randomized nor blind, in breast cancer patients, indicated GLA may enhance the effects of tamoxifen.	• Side effects of nausea, bloating, and soft stools have been reported. • May lower seizure threshold when used with tricyclic antidepressants and anticonvulsant medications.	• Seems to be safe in doses ≥ 2.8 g/day. • Not recommended for women who are pregnant or breast-feeding.

(continued)

Table 16.5 Herbs and Herbal Products (*continued*)

Herb or Herbal Product	*Claim(s)*	*Efficacy*	*Safety*	*Current Recommendations*
Garlic	• Reduces the risk of stomach and colon cancers. • Has a protective effect on cancer cell lines. • Reduces infection.	• Potentially decreases nitrosamine and nitrite accumulation. There are conflicting reports in epidemiological studies about the protective effects of garlic in cancer. Strongest association appears with stomach and colorectal cancer prevention. • The active ingredient in garlic is allicin.	• Well tolerated except for the strong body odor associated with high intakes. Increased bleeding time associated with 10 g/day raw garlic for 2 months.	• May affect platelet aggregation. Patients undergoing surgery or taking blood-thinning agents should not take garlic supplements.
Ginger	• Reduces nausea. • Aids digestion. • Increases urine excretion.	• Has been found to be useful in treating motion sickness. Antiemetic properties are due to the local action on the stomach, not the central nervous system. However, there is no evidence directly supporting the relationship between an intake of ginger and the reduction of cancer-related symptoms.	• No toxicities have been reported. Very large overdoses may cause central nervous system depression and cardiac arrhythmias. Thrombocytopenia has been reported in people taking large doses. • Note that ginger interferes with warfarin. Ginger may alter calcium channel blocker effects.	• May be used for temporary relief of nausea.
Ginseng (*Panax*)	• Provides energy to those who experience fatigue. • Helps the body fight cancer. • Immunomodulatory effects. • Radioprotective effects.	• Positive immuno- and radioprotective effects in animal models. Human studies are needed.	• High doses of ginseng are associated with estrogenic effects, insomnia, irritability and anxiety, diarrhea, headache • Long-term studies are needed.	• Not recommended for use beyond 6 wk.

(*continued*)

Table 16.5 Herbs and Herbal Products (*continued*)

Herb or Herbal Product	*Claim(s)*	*Efficacy*	*Safety*	*Current Recommendations*
Green tea extract	• Helps prevent cancer. • Serves as an antioxidant.	• Polyphenols, epigallocatechin, and epigallocatechin-3 gallate inhibit cell proliferation and tumor promotion in animal models. Leaf contains flavonoids with antioxidant properties.	• 6 to 10 cups/day of tea appear to be safe. • Individuals who are sensitive to caffeine should be made aware that green tea contains caffeine. • May enhance antitumor activity of doxyrubicin. • May interfere with iron absorption.	• Research is needed to clarify the use of green tea as an anticancer agent.
Hoxey herbs (a formula consisting of poke root, burdock root, barberry root, buckthorne bark, and stillinga root)	• Help the body fight cancer.	• No documented benefit.	• Not recommended.	• Not recommended.
Kombucha tea (Manchurian tea or kargasok tea)	• Stimulates the immune system.	• Antitumor activity claims are unsubstantiated.	• Kombucha tea is susceptible to microbial contamination. • Acidosis, aspergillosis, nausea, vomiting, and jaundice have been reported.	• Not recommended.
Milk thistle	• Protects the liver.	• Seems to protect undamaged liver cells from toxins. May be helpful in cirrhosis and hepatitis.	• No adverse effects have been noted. • Active ingredient is silymarin.	• Considered safe for use. May have beneficial effects.
Mistletoe (American and European)	• American mistletoe is said to stimulate smooth muscle, increase blood pressure, and increase uterine and intestinal contractions. • European mistletoe is said to decrease blood pressure and to serve as an antispasmodic and calmative agent.	• Extracts of the European form have been used as a palliative cancer treatment. There is little evidence supporting effectiveness. • Phase III trials indicated no effect. • Reports of improved quality of life are subjective.	• Berries are poisonous; some evidence suggests the leaves may also be poisonous.	• Not recommended.

(*continued*)

Table 16.5 Herbs and Herbal Products (*continued*)

Herb or Herbal Product	*Claim(s)*	*Efficacy*	*Safety*	*Current Recommendations*
Pau d'arco	• Serves as a powerful tonic and blood builder. • Helps the body fight cancer. • Treats diabetes, rheumatism, and ulcers.	• Has been shown to have anticancer activity in animals but causes severe side effects in humans.	• Toxic; induces nausea, vomiting, anemia, and bleeding. • Potentiates the effects of anticoagulants.	• Not recommended. • Contraindicated with liver disease, hemophilia, thrombocytopenia, and Von Willebrands disease.
Peppermint	• Aids digestion. • Stimulates bile flow. • Decreases tonus of the lower esophageal sphincter.		• Safe for adults. • Not recommended for children because of increased choking reflex with menthol.	• Safe for adults. • Not recommended for children.
Pokeroot	• Induces vomiting. • Alleviates insomnia. • Helps the body fight cancer.	• No efficacy has been demonstrated for any claim except that it is a strong emetic and cathartic.	• Extremely toxic. Causes gastroenteritis, hypotension, decreased respiration. Fatal in children.	• Not recommended.
PC-SPES (a formula consisting of saw palmetto, panax ginseng, chrysanthemum, reishi mushroom, licorice, dyer's wood, rubescens, skull cap)	• Inhibits prostate cancer cell growth and decreases PSA levels.	• PC-SPES may have an active component (baicalein) that suppresses growth of prostate cancer cells.	• Components of warfarin found in some samples, which may increase bleeding time.	• Taken off the market in 2002 because some samples were contaminated with warfarin and DES. • More research is required to determine the bioactive ingredients.
Saw palmetto	• Manages BPH. • Increases sperm production. • Increases breast size. • Decreases spontaneous tumors. • Decreases tumor weight. • Increases estrogenic activity. • Decreases PSA levels. • Decreases pain.	• Improves subjective and objective symptoms of BPH. • More studies needed to delineate role in BPH.	• Use only after diagnosis of BPH. • Obtain baseline PSA before use.	• Safe for adults. No role in prostate cancer.

(*continued*)

Table 16.5 Herbs and Herbal Products (*continued*)

Herb or Herbal Product	*Claim(s)*	*Efficacy*	*Safety*	*Current Recommendations*
Spirulina	• Stimulates the immune system. • Nutrient supplement.	• Contains 47% essential amino acids, iron, vitamins A, E, and B-12. Iron is more absorbable than supplements. • Animal studies have found potential enhanced humoral and cell-mediated immunity.	• No adverse reactions reported.	• Safe for adults.
• St. John's wort	• Treats depression.	• Useful in mild depression.	• Serves as an MAOI. • This herb increases metabolism of many prescription drugs and decreases their effectiveness.	• Safe for use. • Individuals taking antidepressant medication should not take.

Abbreviations: BPH, benign prostatic hyperplasia; GLA, gamma linolenic acid; GRAS, Generally Recognized As Safe; HRT, hormone replacement therapy; MAOI, monamine oxidase inhibitor; PMS, premenstrual syndrome.

*Also found in borage oil.

Source: Data are from references 59–63.

processes are the result of a build-up of toxins and waste products in the body. The assumption follows that when the immune system, respiratory system, liver, and pancreas can no longer rid the body of these toxins, the body's normal metabolic processes are interrupted, and chronic disease may occur (8,10,62). There also can be additional regimen-specific hypotheses for cancer formation (see Table 16.6) (2,14,61–67).

Many metabolic therapies consist of a three-step treatment process of detoxification, fasting, and rejuvenation, which is used in addition to other regimen-specific treatments. For the most part, the diets used in metabolic therapies consist of "natural" and "organic" foods but also include supplements of vitamins, minerals, hormones, enzymes, enemas, laetrile, and various other treatments in their detoxification and rejuvenating process (61). Several metabolic therapies promote the use of large amounts of dietary supplements. For example, the Gonzalez Regimen recommends that individuals diagnosed with cancer consume 130 to 175 supplements a day. Despite attempts to validate the effectiveness of these therapies, none have been documented to show scientific proof of efficacy in the treatment of cancer.

EVALUATING CAM THERAPIES

One evidence-based method for evaluating CAM therapies was proposed by a group of researchers from the Osher Institute of Harvard Medical School (29). They developed four categories to describe the efficacy and safety of the proposed therapy: Recommend, Accept—May Consider Recommending, Accept, and Discourage. Health care practitioners can easily use the guidelines established in this report to evaluate new therapies and to assist in making recommendations to patients. Figure 16.1 (29) describes a process adapted from this report that can guide a practitioner in determining whether a proposed therapy may be recommended, should be recommended with reservations, or

Table 16.6 Metabolic Therapies

Therapy	*Theory*	*Diet Summary*	*Additional Features*
Gerson therapy	• Cancer is caused by an accumulation of toxic waste products in the body.	• Vegetarian meals. Individuals are provided three vegetarian meals made from organically grown fruits, vegetables, and whole grains. A typical meal will consist of salad, cooked vegetables, baked potatoes, vegetable soup, and juice. • Juices prepared and consumed hourly from fresh, organic fruits and vegetables. Individuals are instructed to drink up to 13 glasses of raw carrot/apple and green-leaf juices daily. • Fresh fruit for snacks. Fresh fruit and fresh fruit dessert should be available at all hours for snacking.	• Usually supplemented with potassium compound, Lugol's solution; vitamin B-12; thyroid hormone; injectable crude liver extract; pancreatic enzymes. • Enemas of coffee and/or chamomile are routinely administered.
• Gonzalez regimen	• Pancreatic enzymes, in addition to their digestive function, represent the body's main anticancer defense.	• Diet prescriptions are individualized and range from primarily plant-based diets to diets consisting of red meat 2–3 times/day. • Organic foods are required. • "Synthetic and refined foods," such as white flour and white sugar, must be avoided.	• For cancer patients, the main anticancer supplements are specially manufactured, pig-derived pancreatic enzymes. • Patients can take up to 45 g/day pancreatic enzymes, orally and spread throughout the day. • Additional supplements may include an assortment of vitamins, minerals, trace elements, antioxidants, animal glandular concentrates, and other food concentrates. • Cancer patients will consume 130–175 capsules a day, including nutrients as well as enzymes. • Coffee enemas are recommended to be done twice daily.

(*continued*)

Table 16.6 Metabolic Therapies (*continued*)

Therapy	*Theory*	*Diet Summary*	*Additional Features*
Livingston-Wheeler therapy	• Cancer is caused by bacteria, *P. cryptocides.*	• Predominantly a vegetarian, whole-foods diet.	• In addition to diet therapy, high doses of vitamins and other dietary supplements are recommended with digestive enzymes, vaccines, antibiotics, antiparasite medication, and enemas. • CAM practices integrated in the treatment include psychosocial intervention, group support, and training in relaxation and imagery. • An autogenous (self) vaccine is made from each patient's individual strain of bacteria. The specimen is obtained from the patient's own urine, blood, or tumor tissue and is grown in culture, killed, and processed into a vaccine.

Source: Data are from references 2, 14, and 61–67.

should not be recommended for use. Box 16.2 suggests questions that dietetics professionals can use to assess the efficacy of a CAM therapy in cancer.

WORKING WITH INDIVIDUALS DIAGNOSED WITH CANCER

CAM therapies are becoming common practice for individuals with cancer. Unfortunately, however, patients may be reluctant to discuss the use of these treatments with their physicians or other health care providers (5,57). It is imperative that the health care team routinely attempt to engage individuals in discussions regarding their use of CAM therapies.

Suggestions for working with individuals diagnosed with cancer who are considering or have adopted CAM practices include the following:

- Establish good rapport with your patients. Talk openly and honestly about the therapies they have investigated. Listen to their reasons and understand their need to have an active role in their treatment. Maintain a caring and sensitive attitude. It is important that they know that you are concerned about the impact their nutrition status has on their overall health, not just because of their cancer diagnosis.
- Educate patients about the safety and health concerns related to the treatments they are investigating and how they can evaluate various claims for themselves. If a treatment won't hurt them, even if it has not been proven to be of benefit, it may be worth trying. If there are potential health concerns with a particular product or therapy, you need to let them know those concerns so they will be able to make an educated decision.
- Be knowledgeable about treatments patients are investigating. Make regular visits to health food stores, and ask your patients where they received their information and if you could have a copy of it. Keep a library of books about alter-

Box 16.2

Assessing the Efficacy of Complementary and Alternative Cancer Therapies

- Does an expert body of reputable nutrition experts or scientists support the efficacy of the product or diet? Anecdotal information cannot replace controlled studies. The National Center for Complementary and Alternative Medicine and the National Cancer Institute at the National Institutes of Health can provide current information about products being tested in clinical trials. (Check their Web sites in Appendix B for the most current up-to-date information.)
- Is there documented evidence that this product or diet is safe? The number of subjects who participated in trials and testing is important to note. The word of only a few, or the lack of clinical trial evidence, should be viewed with reservation.
- Does this diet recommend elimination of certain foods or nutrients? If so, what is the rationale? Balance and variety are designed to enhance the synergy of food constituents to promote health. The stress involved in following a restricted diet can be a health risk factor.
- Does the product make singular unfounded claims? A product may act as an antioxidant, yet still produce toxic by-products or imbalances when consumed in large, concentrated quantities.
- Is the cost of the product or diet excessive in comparison to a well-balanced diet?
- Does the product appear to be harmless? If so, even the placebo effect can have positive consequences that cannot be ignored, and the practice should not be necessarily discouraged.

Source: Written by Connie Mobley, PhD, RD.

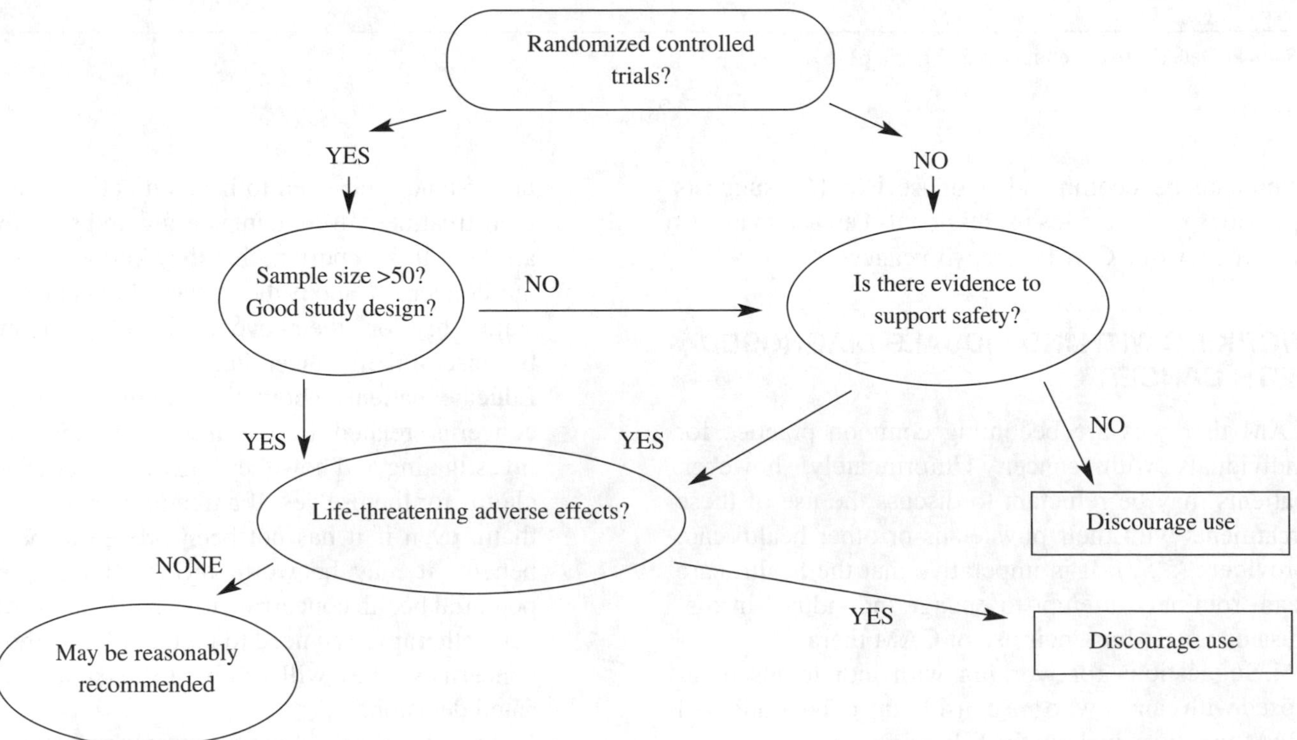

Figure 16.1. Evaluating complementary and alternative medicine therapies. Therapies that have fewer than 3 randomized clinical trials but have evidence to support the safety of the therapy may be recommended with caution or accepted and the patient monitored closely by the health care team for adverse effects or interactions with conventional treatment. Adapted with permission from Weiger WA, Smith M, Boon H, Richardson MA, Kaptchuk TJ, Eisenberg DM. Advising patients who seek complementary and alternative medical therapies for cancer. *Ann Intern Med.* 2002;137:889–903.

native therapies for quick reference. Your patients will respect that you have taken the time to learn about the therapies and know that you are informing them of real concerns.

- Listen to your patient's hopes and desires and understand their need to be an active part of their treatment. Encourage them to read and research treatments and to become knowledgeable about nutrition. Have them bring in articles, books, and newsletters for you to review. Then point out both the potential beneficial aspects of the treatments and any potential harmful effects.

A recent study of health professionals' knowledge about herbal and dietary supplements found that registered dietitians (RDs) had more knowledge about these treatments than other health care providers and communicated more routinely with patients about these treatments (57). This study found, however, that RDs could still improve their knowledge of herbal and dietary supplements, as well as their communication skills with both patients and other health care team members. This study noted that physicians and nurses often defer questions about these treatments to the RD. It is therefore vitally important that dietetics professionals become educated on a variety of CAM modalities and the potential benefits and risks.

REFERENCES

1. Vickers A. Alternative cancer cures: "unproven" or "disproven"? *CA Cancer J Clin.* 2004;54:110–118.
2. Richardson MA, Sanders T, Palmer JL, Greisinger A, Singletary SE. Complementary/alternative medicine use in a comprehensive cancer center and the implications for oncology. *J Clin Oncol.* 2000;18:2505–2514.
3. Richardson MA, Straus SE. Complementary and alternative medicine: opportunities and challenges for cancer management and research. *Semin Oncol.* 2002; 29:531–545.
4. Kaptchuk TJ, Eisenberg DM. The persuasive appeal of alternative medicine. *Ann Intern Med.* 1998;129: 1061–1065.
5. Eisenberg DM, Davis RB, Ettner SL, Appel S, Wilkey S, Van Rompay M, Kessler RC. Trends in alternative medicine use in the United States, 1990–1997: results of a follow-up national survey. *JAMA.* 1998;280: 1569–1575.
6. Kessler RC, Davis RB, Foster DF, Van Rompay MI, Walters EE, Wilkey SA, Kaptchuk TJ, Eisenberg DM. Long-term trends in the use of complementary and alternative medical therapies in the United States. *Ann Intern Med.* 2001;135:262–268.
7. Barnes P, Powell-Griner E, McFann K, Nahin R. CDC Advance Data Report #343. Complementary and alternative medicine use among adults: United States, 2002. May 27, 2004.
8. Yates JS, Mustian KM, Morrow GR, Gillies LJ, Padmanaban D, Atkins JN, Issell B, Kirshner JJ, Colman LK. Prevalence of complementary and alternative medicine use in cancer patients during treatment. *Support Care Cancer.* 2005;13:806–811.
9. Rowan Chlebowski G, Blackburn B, Winters R, Elashoff E, Wynder M, Goodman D, Alberts C, Thompson M, Oken A, Shapiro DN. Long term adherence to dietary fat reduction in the Women's Intervention Nutrition Study (WINS). 2000 American Society of Clinical Oncology Annual Meeting. Abstract 302. Available at: http://www.asco.org/asco/publications/abstract_print_view/1,1148,_12-002643-00_18-002-00_19-00202837,00.html. Accessed September 20, 2005.
10. Ornish D, Weidner G, Fair WR, Marlin R, Pettengill EB, Raisin CJ, Dunn-Emke S, Crutchfield L, Jacobs FN, Barnard RJ, Aronson WJ, McCormac P, McKnight DJ, Fein JD, Dnistrian AM, Weinstein J, Ngo TH, Mendell NR, Carroll PR. Intensive lifestyle changes may affect the progression of prostate cancer. *J Urol.* 2005;174:1065–1069.
11. Byers T, Nestle M, McTiernan A, Doyle C, Currie-Williams A, Gansler T, Thun M; American Cancer Society 2001 Nutrition and Physical Activity Guidelines Advisory Committee. American Cancer Society guidelines on nutrition and physical activity for cancer prevention: reducing the risk of cancer with healthy food choices and physical activity. *CA Cancer J Clin.* 2002;52:92–119.
12. Keeler A. Nutrition quackery and cancer treatment. *On-Line Newsletter of the Oncology Nutrition Dietetic Practice Group.* 1995;3:3–10.
13. Agricultural Marketing Service at USDA. The National Organic Program Web site. Available at: http://www.ams.usda.gov/nop/indexIE.htm. Accessed October 21, 2005.
14. Agricultural Marketing Service at USDA. The Organic Foods Production Act of 1990. Available at: http://www.ams.usda.gov/nop/archive/OFPA.html. Accessed October 21, 2005.

15. Bialy TL, Rothe MJ, Grant-Kels JM. Dietary factors in the prevention and treatment of nonmelanoma skin cancer and melanoma. *Dermatol Surg.* 2002;28: 1143–1152.
16. About.com. The Macrobiotic Diet. Available at: http://altmedicine.about.com/od/popularhealthdiets/a/Macrobiotic.htm. Accessed October 21, 2005.
17. George Ohsawa Macrobiotic Foundation Web site. Available at: http://www.gomf.macrobiotic.net. Accessed September 20, 2005.
18. Kushi Institute Web site. Available at: http://www.kushiinstitute.org. Accessed October 21, 2005.
19. Kushi LH, Cunningham JE, Hebert JR, Lerman RH, Bandera EV, Teas J. The macrobiotic diet in cancer. *J Nutr.* 2001;131(suppl):S3056-S3064.
20. Castle EP, Thrasher JB. The role of soy phytoestrogens in prostate cancer. *Urol Clin N Amer.* 2002;29: 71–81.
21. Seddon JM, Ajani UA, Sperduto RD, Hiller R, Blair N, Burton TC, Farber MD, Gragoudas ES, Haller J, Miller DT, et al. Dietary carotenoids, vitamins A, C, and E, and advanced age-related macular degeneration. Eye Disease Case-Control Study Group. *JAMA.* 1994;272:1413–1420.
22. Cohen JF, Kristal RA, Standford JK. Fruit and vegetable intakes and prostate cancer risk. *J Natl Cancer Inst.* 2003;92:61–68.
23. World Cancer Research Fund Diet and Cancer Project. *Food, Nutrition, and the Prevention of Cancer: A Global Perspective.* Washington, DC: American Institute for Cancer Research; 1997.
24. Thomas CA, Green TL. Cruciferous vegetables and cancer prevention. In: Watson RR, ed. *Functional Foods and Neutraceuticals in Cancer Prevention.* Ames, Iowa: Iowa State Press; 2003:55–86.
25. Mishra SI, Dickerson V, Najm W. Phytoestrogens and breast cancer prevention: what is the evidence? *Am J Obstet Gynecol.* 2003;188:S66-S70.
26. Power KA, Thompson LU. Ligand-induced regulation of ERalpha and ERbeta is indicative of human breast cancer cell proliferation. *Breast Cancer Res Treat.* 2003;81:209–221.
27. Messina MJ, Loprinzi CL. Soy for breast cancer survivors: a critical review of the literature. *J Nutr.* 2001;131(suppl):S3095-S3108.
28. Wagner JD, Anthony MS, Cline JM. Soy phytoestrogens: research on benefits and risks. *Clin Obstet Gynecol.* 2001;44:843–852.
29. Weiger WA, Smith M, Boon H, Richardson MA, Kaptchuk TJ, Eisenberg DM. Advising patients who seek complementary and alternative medical therapies for cancer. *Ann Intern Med.* 2002;137:889–903.
30. United Soybean Board. Soyfoods Guide: Tips and Information for Using Soyfoods. Available at: http://www.soybean.org/sfg.pdf. Accessed September 20, 2005.
31. US Food and Drug Administration. Dietary Supplement Health and Education Act of 1994. Available at: http://www.fda.gov/opacom/laws/dshea.html. Accessed April 28, 2005.
32. Office of Dietary Supplements Web site. Dietary Supplements: Background Information. Available at: http://ods.od.nih.gov/factsheets/dietarysupplements.asp. Accessed February 7, 2006.
33. Committee on the Framework for Evaluating the Safety of the Dietary Supplements, National Research Council. *Dietary Supplements: A Framework for Evaluating Safety.* Washington, DC: National Academies Press; 2005.
34. US Food and Drug Administration. FDA proposes labeling and manufacturing standards for dietary supplements. Available at: http://www.fda.gov/bbs/topics/NEWS/dietarysupp/factsheet.html. Accessed April 28, 2005.
35. About Herbs, Botanicals and other Products. Memorial Sloan Kettering Cancer Center Web site. Available at: http://www.mskcc.org. Accessed September 20, 2005.
36. Institute of Medicine. *Dietary Reference Intakes for Vitamin A, Vitamin K, Arsenic, Boron, Chromium, Copper, Iodine, Iron, Manganese, Molybdenum, Nickel, Silicon, Vanadium, and Zinc.* Washington, DC: National Academies Press; 2001.
37. Drisko JA, Chapman J, Hunter VJ. The use of antioxidants during chemotherapy. *Gynecol Oncol.* 2003;88: 434–439.
38. Institute of Medicine. *Dietary Reference Intakes for Vitamin C, Vitamin E, Selenium, and Carotenoids.* Washington, DC: National Academies Press; 2000.
39. Drisko JA, Chapman J, Hunter VJ. The use of antioxidants with first-line chemotherapy in two cases of ovarian cancer. *J Am Coll Nutr.* 2003;22:118–123.
40. Lesperance ML, Olivotto IA, Forde N, Zhao Y, Speers C, Foster H, Tsao M, MacPherson N, Hoffer A. Megadose vitamins and minerals in the treatment of nonmetastatic breast cancer: an historical cohort study. *Breast Cancer Res Treat.* 2002;76:137–143.
41. Tamayo C, Richardson MA. Vitamin C as a cancer treatment: state of the science and recommendations for research. *Altern Ther Health Med.* 2003;9:94–101.

42. Lee IM, Cook NR, Gaziano JM, Gordon D, Ridker PM, Manson JE, Hennekens CH, Buring JE. Vitamin E in the primary prevention of cardiovascular disease and cancer: the Women's Health Study: a randomized controlled trial. *JAMA*. 2005;294:56–65.
43. Duffield-Lillico AJ, Slate EH, Reid ME, Turnbull BW, Wilkins PA, Combs GF Jr, Park HK, Gross EG, Graham GF, Stratton MS, Marshall JR, Clark LC; Nutritional Prevention of Cancer Study Group. Selenium supplementation and secondary prevention of non-melanoma skin cancer in a randomized trial. *J Natl Cancer Inst*. 2003;95:1477–1481.
44. Anderson PM, Schroeder G, Skubitz KM. Oral glutamine reduces the duration and severity of stomatitis after cytotoxic cancer chemotherapy. *Cancer*. 1998; 83:1433–1439.
45. Bozzetti F, Biganzoli L, Gavazzi C, Cappuzzo F, Carnaghi C, Buzzoni R, Dibartolomeo M, Baietta E. Glutamine supplementation in cancer patients receiving chemotherapy: a double-blind randomized study. *Nutrition*. 1997;12:748–751.
46. Huang EY, Leung SW, Wang CJ, Chen HC, Sun LM, Fang FM, Yeh SA, Hsu HC, Hsiung CY. Oral glutamine to alleviate radiation-induced oral mucositis: a pilot randomized trial. *Int J Radiat Oncol Biol Phys*. 2000;46:535–539.
47. Pytlik R, Benes P, Patorkova M, Chocenska E, Gregora E, Prochazka B, Kozak T. Standardized parenteral alanyl-glutamine dipeptide supplementation is not beneficial in autologous transplant patients: a randomized, double-blind, placebo controlled study. *Bone Marrow Transplant*. 2002;30:953–961.
48. Ziegler TR. Glutamine supplementation in cancer patients receiving bone marrow transplantation and high dose chemotherapy. *J Nutr*. 2001;131:S2578-S2584.
49. van Zaanen HC, van der Lelie H, Timmer JG, Furst P, Sauerwein HP. Parenteral glutamine dipeptide supplementation does not ameliorate chemotherapy-induced toxicity. *Cancer*. 1994;74:2879–2884.
50. Skubitz KM, Anderson PM. Oral glutamine to prevent chemotherapy induced stomatitis: a pilot study. *J Lab Clin Med*. 1996;127:223–228.
51. Kozelsky TF, Meyers GE, Sloan JA, Shanahan TG, Dick SJ, Moore RL, Engeler GP, Frank AR, McKone TK, Urias RE, Pilepich MV, Novotny PJ, Martenson JA; North Central Cancer Treatment Group. Phase III double-blind study of glutamine versus placebo for the prevention of acute diarrhea in patients receiving pelvic radiation therapy. *J Clin Oncol*. 2003;21:1669–1674.
52. Daniele B, Perrone F, Gallo C, Pignata S, De Martino S, De Vivo R, Barletta E, Tambaro R, Abbiati R, D'Agostino L. Oral glutamine in the prevention of fluorouracil induced intestinal toxicity: a double blind, placebo controlled, randomised trial. *Gut*. 2001;48: 28–33.
53. Coghlin Dickson TM, Wong RM, Offrin RS, Shizuru JA, Johnston LJ, Hu WW, Blume KG, Stockerl-Goldstein KE. Effect of oral glutamine supplementation during bone marrow transplantation. *JPEN J Parenter Enteral Nutr*. 2000;24:61–66.
54. Murray SM, Pindoria S. Nutrition support for bone marrow transplant patients *Cochrane Database Syst Rev*. 2002;(2):CD002920.
55. Schloerb PR, Amare M. Total parenteral nutrition with glutamine in bone marrow transplantation and other clinical applications (a randomized, double-blind study). *JPEN J Parenter Enteral Nutr*. 1993;17: 407–413.
56. Piccirillo N, De Matteis S, Laurenti L, Chiusolo P, Sora F, Pittiruti M, Rutella S, Cicconi S, Fiorini A, D'Onofrio G, Leone G, Sica S. Glutamine-enriched parenteral nutrition after autologous peripheral blood stem cell transplantation: effects on immune reconstitution and mucositis. *Haematologica*. 2003;88:192–200.
57. Kemper KJ, Amato-Kynvi A, Dvorkin L, Whelan JJ, Wolff A, Samuels RC, Hibberd P. Herbs and other dietary supplements: healthcare professionals knowledge, attitudes, and practices. *Altern Ther Health Med*. 2003;9:42–49.
58. American Cancer Society. Antioxidants and Cancer: The Jury's Still Out. Available at: http://www.cancer.org/docroot/NWS/content/NWS_2_1x_Antioxidants_and_Cancer_The_Jurys_Still_Out.asp. Accessed April 28, 2005.
59. Foster S, Tyler VE. *The Honest Herbal: A Sensible Guide to the Use of Herbs and Related Remedies*. 4th ed. Binghamton, NY: Haworth Press; 1998.
60. Fetrow CF, Avila JR, eds. *Professional's Handbook of Complementary and Alternative Medicines*. Springhouse, Pa: Springhouse Corporation; 1999.
61. Cassileth BR, Vickers AJ. Complementary and alternative therapies. *Urol Clin North Am*. 2003;30: 369–376.
62. Hamilton K. Complementary and alternative medicine in cancer research. *On-Line Newsletter of the Oncology Nutrition Dietetic Practice Group*. 2001;10:1–9.
63. Plaeger SF. Clinical immunology and traditional herbal medicines. *Clin Diagn Lab Immunol*. 2003;10: 337–338.

64. National Cancer Institute PDQ CAM Summaries. Available at: http://www.cancer.gov/cancertopics/pdq/cam. Accessed September 20, 2005.
65. Gerson Institute Web site. Available at: http://www.gerson.org. Accessed October 21, 2005.
66. Dr. Gonzalez's Nutritional Regimen Web site. Available at: http://www.dr-gonzalez.com. Accessed October 21, 2005.
67. University of California, San Diego, Moores Cancer Center Web site. Available at: http://cancer.ucsd.edu. Accessed October 21, 2005.

Chapter 17

Nutrition in Palliative Care

PAULA DAVIS MCCALLUM, MS, RD, AND ALICE FORNARI, EdD, RD, CDN

NTRODUCTION

For persons with advanced cancer, the maintenance of quality of life is an important goal. Palliative care is the aggressive management of symptoms, with emphasis on quality of life. The objectives of palliative care are to (*a*) relieve physical symptoms; (*b*) alleviate isolation, anxiety, and fear associated with advanced disease; and (*c*) maintain independence as long and as comfortably as possible (1,2). Palliation is usually implemented in cases of advanced cancer; however, it may be extended to a person receiving curative cancer treatment or even to a cancer survivor with long-term side effects or morbidity related to cancer treatment. This chapter distinguishes palliative care from hospice care and identifies the responsibilities of the registered dietitian (RD) in palliative care. This chapter examines the role of oral nutrition as well as artificial nutrition support and hydration for the patient with advanced cancer. Bioethics and decision-making regarding end-of-life feeding are also discussed.

PALLIATIVE CARE VS HOSPICE CARE

The term "palliative care" is often used interchangeably with "hospice care." Hospice care is an organized program encompassing the palliative care philosophies. Hospice care can be provided in the patient's home, a hospital, nursing home, or a free-standing hospice facility (3).

To meet the needs of persons who are not "ready" (medically or emotionally) for hospice, a growing number of organizations provide palliative care services through a variety of mechanisms, often referred to as "bridge services." Services, such as home care, durable medical equipment, and enteral feedings, are provided under the direction of one organization, so that continuity of care is maintained throughout the course of the disease (4).

ROLE OF THE REGISTERED DIETITIAN IN PALLIATIVE CARE

As a member of the multidisciplinary health care team, the RD plays an essential role in providing palliative care. The RD's responsibilities are as follows:

- To understand the symptoms and complications associated with advanced cancer
- To manage symptoms of the disease or treatment side effects
- To implement appropriate medical nutrition therapy (MNT), to prevent further morbidity
- To maintain optimal quality of life and, when possible, provide sufficient dietary intake to maintain energy and strength

SYMPTOMS PREVALENT IN ADVANCED CANCER

Symptom management is the cornerstone of palliative care. Therefore, health care professionals should understand the common symptoms experienced by persons with advanced cancer. Donnelly and associates

Table 17.1 Nutrition-Related Symptoms in Advanced Cancer

		Prevalence, %										
Study (reference)	*No. of Subjects*	*Weight Loss*	*Anorexia*	*Constipa-tion*	*Early Satiety*	*Xero-stomia*	*Nausea*	*Taste Changes*	*Vomiting*	*Dyspepsia*	*Bloating*	*Dysphagia*
Donnelly et al (5)	1000	44	46	31	33	27	16	13	10	N/A	6	5
Komurcu et al (6)	1000	44	46	31	33	27	16	13	10	N/A	6	5
Deeter et al (7)	100	79	67	46	70	41	< 40	40	< 40	< 40	< 40	< 40

Abbreviation: N/A, not available.

(5) published a classic review of the symptoms of 1,000 patients upon their initial referral to a palliative care service. Symptoms experienced by at least 10% of patients surveyed included pain, weakness, anorexia, weight loss, early satiety, constipation, dyspnea, xerostomia, depression, nausea, vomiting, and taste changes. Table 17.1 (5–7) illustrates the prevalence of nutrition-related symptoms in advanced cancer. In general, nutrition-related symptoms worsen with disease progression, as is evidenced by the data. However, many of these symptoms are manageable, further illustrating the need for greater education of health care professionals.

COMORBIDITIES OF ADVANCED CANCER

Advanced cancer often leads to a variety of paraneoplastic syndromes and/or complications, some of which may have nutritional implications (8,9).

Paraneoplastic Syndromes

Paraneoplastic syndromes are caused by substances secreted by the tumor, such as hormones and cytokines (eg, tumor necrosis factor, interleukin-1, gamma interferon), which contribute to metabolic, neurologic, or muscular disorders (9,10). Some of the more common paraneoplastic syndromes with nutritional implications include cachexia, hypercalcemia, hypoglycemia, syndrome of inappropriate secretion of antidiuretic hormone, and Lambert-Eaton syndrome.

Cachexia

The etiology of cachexia is multifactorial (11), and although there is no known treatment to reverse these effects, pharmacological measures and MNT can improve dietary intake and quality of life (12). For information on the pharmacological agents used in cancer treatment, see Chapter 15. For management of cachexia-related symptoms, see Appendix A.

Hypercalcemia

Hypercalcemia of paraneoplastic disease is associated with multiple myeloma, lung cancer, and renal cancer and may be secondary to the release of prostaglandins and osteoclast-activating factor (9,13,14). Hypercalcemia can also occur secondary to bony metastases, although the signs and symptoms are indistinguishable from those of paraneoplastic disease (13,14). Although restriction of dietary calcium is not a treatment for hypercalcemia, it is important to ensure that patients are not taking large amounts of exogenous calcium from supplements or antacids (more than the Dietary Reference Intake [DRI]) (13,14). Hypercalcemia is treated with intravenous (IV) fluids and medication, including bisphosphonates (9,13–16).

Hypoglycemia

Hypoglycemia is most common in patients with insulin-secreting islet-cell tumors, as well as mesenchymal tumors, such as sarcomas, leiomyomas, carcinoids, and mesotheliomas (9,13). Acute episodes of hypoglycemia may be treated with intravenous (IV) dextrose, whereas mild cases of ongoing hypoglycemia may respond to frequent small feedings, emphasizing protein, complex carbohydrates, and fat at each feeding (9,13). Severe cases may benefit from the use of corticosteroids and/or glucagons (9), which can cause vomiting (13).

Syndrome of Inappropriate Secretion of Antidiuretic Hormone

Syndrome of inappropriate secretion of antidiuretic hormone (SIADH) is associated most often with small-cell lung cancer (9,13). Hyponatremia is the most common symptom of SIADH and is treated with diuretics, IV saline with potassium, and/or fluid restriction (usually 500–1,000 mL/day) (9,13,16).

Lambert-Eaton Syndrome

Lambert-Eaton syndrome is a neurologic disorder similar to myasthenia gravis and is associated most often with small-cell lung cancer (9,13,17). Patients can have problems with xerostomia and dysphagia (9), which can be managed with MNT. For tips on managing xerostomia and dysphagia, see Appendix A.

Common Complications of Advanced Cancer

Additional complications commonly seen in advanced cancer include bowel obstruction, steroid-induced hyperglycemia, venous thromboembolic complications, and spinal cord compression.

Bowel Obstruction

Bowel obstruction is associated with pancreatic cancer, gynecological cancers, abdominal carcinomatosis, enlarged retroperitoneal nodes, or pelvic masses (18,19). Prophylaxis may be achieved through MNT (19–21), although further research is necessary to confirm this.

According to gastrointestinal (GI) soft-diet guidelines, foods should be well cooked and well chewed. Additionally, raw fruits and vegetables, nuts, skins or seeds, and whole spices should be avoided. Advanced cancer patients with bowel obstruction may be treated with medications, IV fluids, and gastric decompression (20–23). Parenteral nutrition (PN) is usually inappropriate, although it may be used in certain circumstances. These circumstances may include the patient's desire to live to witness an important life event, such as a birth, a graduation, a wedding, or an anniversary. For PN guidelines, see Chapter 14.

Steroid-Induced Hyperglycemia

Cancer patients frequently are prescribed corticosteroids. One of the common side effects of steroid use is hyperglycemia, which is usually managed successfully with a diet of no added sugar and no concentrated sweets or with medications including oral hypoglycemics. Often patients are eating so poorly that diet is an insignificant contribution to blood sugar levels and, therefore, diet should be liberalized to enhance quality of life.

Venous Thromboembolic Complications

A variety of factors can lead to deep vein thrombosis (DVT) or pulmonary embolism (PE) in patients with cancer. Some patients may be treated with intermittent pneumatic compression, compression stockings, or vena cava filters, although pharmacological management with anticoagulants is common (24). Dosing of anticoagulants is based on the patient's blood clotting time, which reflects his or her average vitamin K intake (24). Therefore, it is usually unnecessary to restrict vitamin K-rich foods from the diet; rather, consistent levels of intake should be maintained.

Spinal Cord Compression

Spinal cord compression is usually, but not exclusively, due to extradural metastasis, in the vertebral column (20,25). Symptoms are determined by the location of the lesion. Treatment of cord compression is vital to prevent complete compression, resulting in paralysis and loss of bowel and bladder function/control. Cord compression is usually treated with spinal field radiation therapy and/or corticosteroids (20,25,26).

Nutrition issues concerning spinal cord compression include constipation secondary to immobility, opiates used for pain management, and dehydration due to poor dietary intake (20). Frequently, patients will self-limit their intake of food and fluids, to avoid embarrassment of urinary or fecal incontinence associated with loss of bladder and bowel control. A multidisciplinary team effort can help alleviate constipation and manage bowel and bladder function, to help preserve the patient's dignity and quality of life. For information on the pharmacological management of constipation, see Chapter 15. Nutrition tips for managing constipation can be found in Appendix A.

ENHANCING ORAL INTAKE TO MAINTAIN STRENGTH

Maintenance of energy and strength is an appropriate goal that directly affects a patient's ability to perform activities of daily living. Oral intake can be enhanced with minor modifications of the patient's usual intake. For guidance, see Appendix A and *Management of Nutrition Impact Symptoms in Cancer and Educational Handouts,* a publication of the American Dietetic Association (27). Additional tips to assist with optimal patient comfort and enjoyment of food include the following (28–31):

- Providing favorite foods
- Providing small, frequent meals, which are often better received
- Using smaller plates and cups to make portions seem less overwhelming
- Making the dining area as appealing as possible (eg, removing bedpans and the like)
- Encouraging the patient to eat at the table when possible
- Encouraging the patient to wash and dress for meals, if possible
- Encouraging eating with others
- Being mindful that preferences and tastes change frequently, and accommodate these changes
- Not forcing food
- Maintaining oral hygiene—rinse patient's mouth with salt and baking soda mouth rinse

(see Appendix A) throughout the day and before meals
- Encouraging activity to stimulate appetite
- Encouraging patient to function independently, to increase feelings of self-worth
- Letting the patient be in control

WHEN DEATH BECOMES IMMINENT

The RD should remain involved in patient care throughout the course of the disease, to serve as a resource to patients, family, and staff for information on nutrition care of the patient with advanced and terminal disease. The RD should assist patients and staff in making informed decisions regarding MNT interventions and in providing ongoing support. It is important to note that, as death approaches, most patients stop taking solid food and may even take very little liquid (20,32). The RD should remain available and supportive to the patient and family members, providing appropriate suggestions to maximize the patient's comfort.

ARTIFICIAL NUTRITION AND HYDRATION

The provision of artificial nutrition and hydration to persons with advanced disease is a difficult and controversial issue (33–35), and such decisions should be made on a case-by-case basis (34–36). It is thought that dehydration at this point in the life cycle is not uncomfortable but rather creates a kind of euphoric state (37). In fact, excess fluids may increase secretions, making breathing more difficult and disturbing to both patient and family members (20).

In some cases, nutrition support does have a place in the treatment of the advanced cancer patient. Enteral nutrition is appropriate for patients with mechanical barriers to achieving oral intake wherein quality of life would suffer and death would be caused by malnutrition rather than the underlying disease (eg, head and neck cancer) (20,38,39). The rationale for implementing PN, however, is less clear. Mercadante (40) and others (39) suggest that PN may be appropriate in cases where oral or enteral nutrition is not possible due to mechanical obstruction or malabsorption. However, Torelli and colleagues (41) found that PN neither influenced the ultimate outcome nor improved the quality of life and, therefore, they conclude that there is little validity to administering PN to terminally ill patients. The authors do admit, however, that there may be subjective rationale to justify the use of PN, such as compassionate, religious, ethical, or emotional reasons. Consideration of the financial cost, the burden on family members, and the potential complications must be weighed against any potential benefit derived from nutrition support, whether it be enteral or parenteral (32,33,42).

Bioethical and Legal Issues

RDs' decisions regarding the provision of artificial nutrition and hydration may be guided by a variety of sources, including advanced directives; case law; and ethical and legal issues in nutrition, hydration, and feeding (43). Consideration should be given to any existing advanced directives that may be in effect. Advance directives in medical care are instructions given by patients to health care providers that define the extent of medical intervention desired in the event of incapacitation or the inability to communicate these desires. Documents under the umbrella of advance directives include the living will, the durable power of attorney (POA) for health care or health care proxy, and the advance medical care directive (44). A living will is a set of instructions documenting a person's wishes about medical care intended to sustain life (45).

A medical power of attorney appoints a person empowered to make health care decisions on behalf of the patient. The advance medical directive is a combination of the living will and the durable health care POA. The advance medical directive is more explicit than the living will and outlines the extent of medical care under specific circumstances and may include the appointment of a health care proxy. Advance directives provide a way for patients to communicate their wishes to family, friends, and health care professionals and to avoid confusion later on, should they become unable to do so (46). Advance directives also allow the health care team, including dietitians, to evaluate the patient's values and goals, a very important first step of providing appropriate care. Each state treats these documents somewhat differently. State-specific documents can be obtained at the Partnership for Sharing Web site (46).

It is the position of the American Dietetic Association (ADA) that "the registered dietitian, as a member of the health care team, has the responsibility to identify the nutritional and hydration needs of each individual patient. Development of ethical guidelines for when feeding may or may not be in the patient's best interest can help the patient and the health care team implement appropriate therapy" (43). The ADA (43) recommends the following considerations be taken with respect to the decisions about artificial feeding:

- The patient's expressed desire for the extent of medical care is a primary guide for determining the level of nutrition intervention.
- The decision to forgo hydration or nutrition should be weighed carefully, because such a decision may be difficult or impossible to reverse within a period of days or weeks.
- The expected benefits, in contrast with the potential burdens, of nonoral feeding must be evaluated by the health care team and discussed with the patient. The focus of care should include the patient's physical and psychological comfort.
- Food and hydration are considered medical interventions.
- Consider whether or not nutrition, either oral or artificial, will improve the patient's quality of life during the final stages of life.
- Consider whether or not nutrition, either oral or artificial, can be expected to provide the patient with emotional comfort, decreased anxiety and cachexia, improved self-esteem with cosmetic benefits, improved interpersonal relationships, or relief from fear of abandonment.
- If death is imminent and feeding will not alter the condition, consider whether or not nutrient support will be burdensome.

REFERENCES

1. Deeter PJ. Palliative care. *Oncol Nutr.* 1993;1:3–10.
2. Komurcu S, Nelson KA, Walsh D, Donnelly SM, Homsi J, Abdullah O. Common symptoms in advanced cancer. *Semin Oncol.* 2000;27:24–33.
3. von Gunten CF, Ferris FD, Portenoy RK, Glajchen M, eds. CAPC manual: how to establish a palliative care program. Available at: http://64.85.16.230/educate/content.html. Accessed May 6, 2005.
4. Walsh D. The Harry R. Horvitz Center for Palliative Medicine (1987–1999): development of a novel comprehensive integrated program. *Am J Hosp Palliat Care.* 2001;18:239–250.
5. Donnelly S, Walsh D, Rybicki L. The symptoms of advanced cancer: identification of clinical and research priorities by assessment of prevalence and severity. *J Palliat Care.* 1995;11:27–32.
6. Komurcu S, Nelson KA, Walsh D. The gastrointestinal symptoms of advanced cancer. *Support Care Cancer.* 2001;9:32–39.
7. Deeter PJ, Goldstein PS, Walsh TD. Nutritional problems in patients with advanced cancer. *Adv Exp Med Biol.* 1994;354:227.
8. Nelson KA, Walsh D, Abdullah O, Mcdonnell F, Homsi J, Komurcu S, Le Grand SB, Zhukovsky DS. Common complications of advanced cancer. *Semin Oncol.* 2000;27:33–44.
9. Alley EW, Schuchter LM. Paraneoplastic syndromes. Available at: http://merck.micromedex.com/index.asp?page=bpm_brief&article_id=CPM03ON015. Accessed May 6, 2005.
10. Lowry SF, Moldawer LL. Tumor necrosis factor and other cytokines in the pathogenesis of cancer cachexia. *Principles Practices Oncol Update.* 1990;4:1–12.
11. Argiles JM, Busquets S, Lopez-Soriano FJ. Cytokines in the pathogenesis of cancer cachexia. *Curr Opin Clin Nutr Metab Care.* 2003;6:401–406.
12. Nelson KA. Modern management of the cancer-anorexia syndrome. *Curr Pain Headache Rep.* 2001;5:250–256.
13. Escalante CP, Manzullo E, Bonin SR. Oncologic emergencies and paraneoplastic syndromes. In: *Cancer Management: A Multidisciplinary Approach.* 8th ed. Available at: http://www.cancernetwork.com. Accessed May 6, 2005.
14. Busick NP, Fretz PC, Galvin JR, Peterson MW. Hypercalcemia. In: *Lung Tumors: A Multidisciplinary Database: Neoplastic and Paraneoplastic Syndromes.* Available at: http://www.vh.org/Providers/Textbooks/LungTumors/ParaneoplasticProcesses/Text/Hypercalcemia.html. Accessed May 6, 2005.
15. Pascual Samaniego M, Torrecilla Garcia-Ripoll JR, Calleja Escudero J, Egea Camacho J, Revera Ferro J, Fernandez del Busto E. Hypercalcemia, leukemoid reaction, and thrombocytosis as paraneoplastic presentation of transitional cell carcinoma of the kidney. *Actas Urol Esp.* 2001;25:400–403.
16. McCloskey EV, Guest JF, Kanis JA. The clinical and cost considerations of biphosphonates in preventing bone complications in patients with metastatic breast cancer or multiple myeloma. *Drugs.* 2001;61:1253–1274.
17. Levin KH. Paraneoplastic neuromuscular syndromes. *Neurol Clin.* 1997;15:597–614.
18. Walsh D. Palliative management of the patient with

advanced pancreatic cancer. *Oncology (Huntingt).* 1996;10(suppl 9):40–44.

19. McCallum P, Nelson KA, Walsh D. Can a soft diet prevent bowel obstruction in advanced pancreatic cancer? *Support Care Cancer.* 2002;10:174–175.
20. Palliative care. In: McCallum PD. *Nutrition in Cancer Treatment* [online course]. Eureka, Calif: Nutrition Dimension; 2003:69–78.
21. Frank C. Medical management of intestinal obstruction in terminal care. *Can Fam Physician.* 1997;43: 259–265.
22. Sason M, Shvartzman P. Management of malignant bowel obstruction in terminal care—is home care possible? *Harefuah.* 1998;134:757–759, 832.
23. Ripamonti C, Twycross R, Baines M, Bozzetti F, Capri S, De Conno F, Gemlo B, Hunt TM, Krebs HB, Mercadante S, Schaerer R, Wilkinson P. Clinical-practice recommendations for the management of bowel obstruction in patients with end-stage cancer. *Support Care Cancer.* 2001;9:223–233.
24. National Heart, Lung, and Blood Institute. Deep Vein Thrombosis. Available at: http://www.nhlbi.nih.gov/health/dci/Diseases/Dvt/DVT_WhatIs.html. Accessed May 6, 2005.
25. Klimo P Jr, Kestle JR, Schmidt MH. Treatment of metastatic spinal epidural disease: a review of the literature. *Neurosurg Focus.* 2003;15:E1.
26. Merimsky O, Kollender Y, Bokstein F, Issakov J, Flusser G, Inbar MJ, Meller I, Bickels J. Radiotherapy for spinal cord compression in patients with soft-tissue sarcoma. *Int J Radiat Oncol Biol Phys.* 2004;58: 1468–1473.
27. Eldridge B, Hamilton K, eds. *Management of Nutrition Impact Symptoms in Cancer and Educational Handouts.* Chicago, Ill: American Dietetic Association; 2004.
28. Gallagher-Allred C, O'Rawe Amenta M, eds. *Nutrition and Hydration in Hospice Care: Needs, Strategies, Ethics.* New York, NY: Haworth Press; 1993.
29. Gallagher-Allred C. *Nutritional Care of the Terminally Ill.* Rockville, Md: Aspen Publishers; 1989.
30. Madioni F, Morales C, Michel JP. Body image and the impact of terminal disease. *Eur J Palliat Care.* 1997; 4:2–5.
31. Stevens EM. Promoting self-worth in the terminally ill. *Eur J Palliat Care.* 1996;3:1–12.
32. Dunlop RJ, Ellershaw JE, Baines MJ, Sykes N, Saunders CM. On withholding nutrition and hydration in the terminally ill: has palliative medicine gone too far? A reply. *J Med Ethics.* 1995;21:141–143.
33. Sharp JW, Roncagli T. Home parenteral nutrition in advanced cancer. *Cancer Pract.* 1993;1:119–124.
34. Sarhill N, Walsh D, Nelson K, Davis M. Evaluation and treatment of cancer-related fluid deficits: volume depletion and dehydration. *Support Care Cancer.* 2001;9:408–419.
35. Torsheim AK, Falkmer U, Kaasa S. Hydration of patients with advanced cancer—is subcutaneous infusion a good solution? *Tidsskr Nor Laegeforen.* 1999; 119:2815–2817.
36. Stagno SJ, Zhukovsky DS, Walsh D. Bioethics: communication and decision-making in advanced disease. *Semin Oncol.* 2000;27:94–100.
37. Bennett JA. Dehydration: hazards and benefits. *Geriatr Nurs.* 2000;21:84–88.
38. Marcy PY, Magne N, Bensadoun RJ, Bentolila F, Bleuse A, Dassonville O, Poissonnet G, Schneider M, Demard F, Bruneton JN. Percutaneous endoscopic gastrostomy: cost/benefit analysis in patients with carcinoma of the upper aero-digestive tract. *Bull Cancer.* 2000;87:329–333.
39. Bachmann P, Marti-Massoud C, Blanc-Vincent MP, Desport JC, Colomb V, Dieu L, Kere D, Melchior JC, Nitenberg G, Raynard B, Roux-Bournay P, Schneider S, Senesse P. Standards, options and recommendations: nutritional support in palliative or terminal care of patients with progressive cancer. *Bull Cancer.* 2001;88:985–1006.
40. Mercadante S. Parenteral nutrition at home in advanced cancer patients. *J Pain Symptom Manage.* 1995;10:475–480.
41. Torelli GF, Campos AC, Meguid MM. Use of TPN in terminally ill cancer patients. *Nutrition.* 1999;15: 665–667.
42. Pironi L, Ruggeri E, Tanneberger S, Giordani S, Pannuti F, Miglioli M. Home artificial nutrition in advanced cancer. *J R Soc Med.* 1997;90:597–603.
43. Position of The American Dietetic Association: ethical and legal issues in nutrition, hydration, and feeding. *J Am Diet Assoc.* 2002;102:837–841.
44. Maxfield CL, Pohl JM, Colling K. Advance directives: a guide for patient discussions. *Nurse Pract.* 2003;28: 38–47.
45. National Cancer Institute. Cancer facts: advance directives. Available at: http://cis.nci.nih.gov/fact/8_12.htm. Accessed May 6, 2005.
46. Partnership for Caring Web site. Available at: http://www.partnershipforcaring.org. Accessed May 6, 2005.

Chapter 18

Nutrition and the Cancer Survivor

SARAH HARDING LAIDLAW, MS, MPA, RD

INTRODUCTION

From 1990 to 2000 the rate of cancer survival increased among most racial/ethnic populations and in most geographic locations in the United States (1). The National Cancer Institute (NCI) estimates that in 2000 there were approximately 9.8 million individuals living with cancer or with no evidence of disease after being diagnosed with cancer and receiving cancer treatment (2). The American Cancer Society defines a cancer survivor as "anyone who has been diagnosed with cancer, from the time of diagnosis through the rest of life" (3). The relative 5-year survival rate for all cancers is estimated at 64%, with rates differing based on the type of cancer and the stage at diagnosis (2). The continuum of cancer survival includes treatment, recovery from treatment, and, for some individuals, living with advanced disease. This chapter explores how nutrition, body weight, and physical activity play roles in reducing the risk of cancer recurrence (secondary prevention), as well as in preventing new primary cancer diagnoses and other chronic diseases (primary prevention) in cancer survivors.

CANCER SURVIVAL AND BODY WEIGHT

It is widely reported that the nutrition needs of persons during cancer treatment and recovery change and differ based on the type of cancer and the stage and treatment of the disease, and that more often than not, persons with cancer often lose weight (4). Although statistics vary regarding weight loss amounts, weight loss has been shown to contribute to poorer response to chemotherapy, as well as decreased quality of life (5,6). Weight loss also results in malnutrition, with approximately 50% of patients with a cancer diagnosis developing malnutrition and 30% of those developing severe wasting and dying as a result (7). Cancers with high risk of nutrition abnormalities, including pancreatic, head and neck, lung, and other digestive tract malignancies, often result in weight loss (8,9).

Other cancers, such as breast and prostate, do not appear to be associated with weight loss but may be associated with weight gain (10,11). Participants in the Nurses' Health Study (12) were evaluated for the effect of weight and weight gain and survival after the diagnosis of breast cancer. Being overweight or obese before diagnosis and gaining weight after diagnosis were positively associated with cancer recurrence and death. Women gaining a median of 6 pounds had a relative risk (RR) of 1.35 (95% confidence interval [CI] = 0.93–1.95), and women gaining a median of 17 pounds had an RR of 1.64 (95% CI = 1.07–2.51) of death due to breast cancer compared with women who maintained their weight. Similar findings were noted for incidence of breast cancer recurrence and all-caused mortality.

Box 18.1

American Cancer Society Guidelines on Nutrition and Physical Activity for Cancer Prevention

Eat a variety of healthful foods, with an emphasis on plant sources.

- Eat five or more servings of a variety of vegetables and fruits each day.
- Choose whole grains in preference to processed (refined) grains and sugars.
- Limit consumption of red meats, especially those high in fat and processed.
- Choose foods that help to maintain a healthful weight.

Adopt a physically active lifestyle.

- Adults: engage in at least moderate activity for 30 minutes or more on 5 or more days of the week; 45 minutes or more of moderate to vigorous activity on 5 or more days per week may further enhance reductions in the risk for breast and colon cancer.
- Children and adolescents: engage in at least 60 minutes per day of moderate to vigorous physical activity at least 5 days per week.

Maintain a healthy weight throughout life.

- Balance caloric intake with physical activity.
- Lose weight if currently overweight or obese.

Limit consumption of alcoholic beverages.

Source: Reprinted with permission from Brown JK, Byers T, Doyle C, Coumeya KS, Demark-Wahnefried W, Kushi LH, McTieman A, Rock CL, Aziz N, Bloch AS, Eldridge B, Hamilton K, Katzin C, Koonce A, Main J, Mobley C, Morra ME, Pierce MS, Sawyer KA; American Cancer Society. Nutrition and physical activity during and after cancer treatment: an American Cancer Society guide for informed choices. *CA Cancer J Clin.* 2003;53:268–291.

Obesity may play a significant role in survival in several types of cancers. A prospective study of patients with colon cancer in Japan suggested that obesity and excessive weight gain are associated with an increased rate of death among Japanese women (13). Women with a normal BMI (≤ 24.9) appeared to have a longer overall survival and disease-free survival than women with a BMI > 25; these effects were the same for pre- and perimenopausal women (14). Additionally, pre- and postmenopausal women with elevated waist to hip ratios (WHR) have been found to be at higher risk of mortality after breast cancer diagnosis, primarily due to hyperinsulinemia and insulin resistance (15). Obesity is known to raise estrogen levels and potentially decrease progesterone levels, both of which increase the risk of estrogen-sensitive cancers (16). In men who have undergone radical prostatectomies for clinically localized prostate cancer, those with severe obesity (BMI ≥ 35) were at a higher risk of PSA failure after the procedure than men of normal weight and even overweight (17). On the basis of these studies and emerging research regarding body weight and cancer, it seems prudent that registered dietitians (RDs) advise cancer survivors to obtain and maintain a healthy body weight, to help reduce their risk for cancer recurrence and other chronic diseases.

NUTRITION AND THE PREVENTION OF CANCER RECURRENCE

Nutrition for cancer survivors should follow the same guidelines as proposed for cancer prevention and risk reduction as for all Americans. Among those recommendations are the American Cancer Society (ACS) Guidelines on Nutrition and Physical Activity for Cancer Prevention (see Box 18.1) (18). These guidelines are similar to those proposed by other health-related organizations for maintaining health and minimizing risk of chronic illness (19).

MACRONUTRIENTS

Cancer survivors may be at risk for other nutrition-related chronic diseases, including heart disease and diabetes (3,20,21), and the type and amount of macronutrients (protein, fat, and carbohydrate) and energy intake can influence long-term health. Therefore, cancer survivors should make sensible food choices with attention to portion sizes and abstain from high-saturated fat, energy-dense foods that offer few protective nutrients. Cancer survivors should select a variety of colorful vegetables and fruits, whole grains, and plant-based foods, and balance energy intake with physical activity (3). Following the ACS prevention guidelines on nutrition and physical activity, which are very similar to those of the American Heart Association (19), can result in a diet that not only promotes sensible weight but may also reduce the risk of comorbidities of obesity, heart disease, diabetes, and other conditions that may present a greater risk of death to patients with cancer than cancer itself (22,23).

Protein

Selection of healthful protein-containing foods, with emphasis on choices that are low in saturated fat (such as lean meats, poultry, and fish; low-fat and nonfat dairy products; and egg whites), and plant-based sources of protein (such as legumes, nuts, and seeds) can help meet the ACS cancer prevention recommendations (3). RDs should note, however, that high-protein, low-carbohydrate diets may not be appropriate for cancer survivors. Such diets may limit important protective nutrients (eg, phytochemicals and naturally occurring vitamins and minerals), and the protein level may increase risk of other complications if not planned carefully to include abundant choices of vegetables and fruits.

Conversely, cancer survivors who choose to follow a vegetarian or vegan lifestyle will need to plan carefully to prevent nutritional deficiencies (24). Regular use of fortified and enriched foods, a multivitamin-mineral supplement containing 100% of the DRIs for vegetarians, and additional vitamin B-12, calcium, iron, and zinc for vegans may be recommended, based on individual assessment (24–26).

Fat

Historically, prospective studies have not supported the association of a high total fat diet contributing to an increased risk of cancer (27,28). However, a recent prospective analysis of dietary fat and breast cancer risk has established a relationship with excessive intake of animal fat, mainly from red meat and high-fat dairy foods in premenopausal women (29). In addition, the recently reported findings of the Women's Interventional Nutrition Study (WINS) researchers concluded that a low-fat diet improved breast cancer survival in postmenopausal women (30). This randomized trial followed 2,347 patients and showed that, after 5 years, women consuming a low-fat diet (daily average fat intake = 33.3 g) had a 24% reduction in cancer recurrence compared with women consuming a typical American diet (average daily fat intake = 51.3 g).

Increased saturated fat intake has been causally related to decreased disease-specific survival in prostate cancer. Men consuming the most saturated fat may have as much as a three times higher risk of death due to prostate cancer (31).

A high intake of *trans* fatty acids has been weakly associated with the development of colon cancer in postmenopausal women who are not taking hormone replacement therapy. Those women who used nonsteroidal anti-inflammatory drugs were at a 50% decreased risk of developing colon cancer when they consumed high levels of *trans* fatty acids. Postmenopausal women not taking hormone replacement therapy and estrogen negative were found to have a twofold increase in risk from high levels of *trans* fatty acids in the diet (29).

For persons who have lost weight and/or are malnourished, careful choices to maximize the number of nutrient-dense calories they consume is important (3,4). These individuals may need to increase the amount of fat they are eating, to maintain current weight or to prevent weight loss (32), with a focus on foods high in n-3 fatty acids (eg, fatty fish, nuts, flaxseed) rather than saturated fatty acids, in order to increase energy density and to improve the ratio between long-chain n-3 to n-6 fatty acid ratio (33) and to potentially decrease the risk of tumor growth, in breast cancer in particular, as has been observed in animal models (34,35). Foods high in n-3 fatty acids have also been associated with a lower risk of cardiovascular disease and diabetes complications (36,37) and seem to be linked with reduced cancer risk and reduced risk of recurrence (28,29).

Carbohydrate

Carbohydrate choices should focus on those foods that provide essential nutrients that are known to help reduce the risk of cancer—whole grains, fruits, vegetables, and legumes (3). These carbohydrates provide fiber, phytochemicals, n-3 fatty acids, and other protective nutrients.

Refined carbohydrates, including white flour and sugar, should be used in moderation. Refined carbohydrates may exacerbate insulin resistance, contributing to obesity, diabetes, and cardiovascular disease, as well as to cancer recurrence (38). This is an area of increasing interest in cancer prevention and survival because mounting evidence points to the relationship between insulin resistance and insulin-like growth factors (IGF) and breast, pancreatic, and other types of cancers (38–42).

Researchers are also paying considerable attention to the glycemic index, the glycemic load of foods, and their relationship to cancer. Glycemic index and glycemic load are measures of the effect of dietary carbohydrate on postprandial blood glucose response and insulin response. With an increase in blood glucose and an elevated insulin response, the risk of endometrial, breast, colorectal, and prostate cancer seems to increase (43–46).

FOOD GROUPS TO ENCOURAGE

Fruits and Vegetables

Vegetables, fruits, botanicals, herbs, and spices have been used for thousands of years for treating and preventing disease (47). Fruits and vegetables contain naturally occurring phytochemicals, many of which have antioxidant and strong anticancer properties (48). Cruciferous vegetables (such as broccoli, cauliflower, and cabbage), members of the Allium family (such as garlic and onion, green tea, citrus fruits, tomatoes, berries, ginger, and ginseng), and some medicinal plants are good sources of phytochemicals (48,49).

Higher consumption of fruits and vegetables may be associated with a reduced risk of cancer, including colorectal, stomach, esophageal, oral, and lung cancers (50). Men younger than 65 years who consumed 28 or more servings of vegetables per week had a 35% decreased risk for prostate cancer than those eating fewer than 14 servings per week (51). Men who consumed three or more servings of cruciferous vegetables per week exhibited a 41% decreased risk of prostate cancer compared with those eating less than one serving per week (52). This relationship was stronger in those men whose intake had spanned at least 10 years, although cruciferous vegetable intake in older men (or elderly men) with advanced cancer appeared to be less relevant (49,51,52).

Consumption of fruits and vegetables appears to be inversely related to risk of colorectal cancer. Populations reportedly consuming higher than average amounts of cereal fibers (13 to 16 g) but low amounts of fruits and vegetables (< 1.5 servings/day) had an RR for developing colorectal cancer of 1.65 (95% CI = 1.23 to 2.2; $P = .001$) compared with those who consumed at least 2.5 or more servings of fruits and vegetables per day (53).

Most studies examining the relationship between nutritional factors, survival, and recurrence after the diagnosis of breast cancer have demonstrated that intakes of nutrients provided by vegetables and fruit were directly related to survival (54–57). Based on what is known about primary prevention and limited knowledge regarding cancer survival, the relationship of fruit and vegetable intake more than likely extends into reducing cancer recurrence, increasing survival, and decreasing risk of secondary tumors.

Fruits and vegetables should be encouraged not only because of their dietary fiber content, but for their phytochemical content (nonnutritive components in plant-based foods), which may play a larger role in cancer risk reduction (3). Brightly colored fruits, especially berries, are rich in polyphenolic compounds, which have been found to have strong anticancer properties and may be combined with other calorie-dense foods, such as dairy products, and are a good choice for those persons who are having difficulty consuming nutrient-dense foods.

Selecting a variety of colorful vegetables and fruits will help ensure that an individual consumes a variety of phytochemicals and micronutrients. One such phytochemical is lycopene, a carotenoid with strong antioxidant properties that gives tomatoes their vibrant red color. Lycopene is not converted to vitamin A. In recent years, the association between the consumption of tomato products and a lower risk of prostate cancer has received considerable attention

(58). Lycopene, consumed primarily from tomato and tomato products, may be the component responsible for lowering the risk of prostate cancer, but it is unknown at this time whether this finding is genuine or causal (59). Thus, many laboratory and clinical studies are now under way with the goal of assessing the ability of pure lycopene to serve as a chemopreventive agent for prostate and other malignancies (58). A study in Italy, where consumption of tomato products is high, consistently showed an inverse relationship between lycopene intake and cancers of the upper digestive tract (60).

An analysis of vegetable, fruit, and legume intake and prostate cancer among white, African-American, and Asian men in the United States showed an inverse relationship between prostate cancer and the intake of all kinds of vegetables, yellow-orange vegetables, cruciferous vegetables, and legumes (including soy products) (61). Neither fruits nor citrus fruits as a subgroup demonstrated any relationship with prostate cancer risk. Given what is known today about the protective benefits of phytochemicals, and lycopene in particular, it is reasonable to recommend eating one serving of tomato products per day or five servings per week, as part of an overall healthy dietary pattern that may reduce the risks of prostate cancer, other malignancies, or other chronic diseases. In addition, this recommendation is consistent with current dietary guidelines to increase vegetable and fruit intake, to lower the risk of heart disease and many types of cancer (62).

Dairy

Evidence is mounting regarding the inverse relationship of calcium intake and a reduced risk of colorectal cancer in men and women, and breast cancer in women. Studies have shown that calcium supplementation of 700 mg/day or more reduces the risk of colorectal cancer (63,64), that dietary calcium has been associated with a reduced risk of colorectal cancer (64,65), and that increased amounts of calcium and vitamin D found in low-fat and nonfat dairy products may reduce the risk of breast cancer in premenopausal women (65). Intake of dairy products and risk reduction was not statistically significant in postmenopausal women, however (65).

The relationship between calcium and cancer may be modified by the amount of vitamin D in the diet or by the amount obtained from sun exposure (66). A study conducted in Norway demonstrated a significant variation in prognosis of breast, colon, and prostate cancer, depending on the season of diagnosis. Fewer cancer deaths were seen in individuals diagnosed in the summer and fall, when the highest amounts of sunlight, and thus vitamin D_3, are available (67).

In addition, mortality from female breast, ovarian, prostate, and colon cancer has been found to be inversely related to exposure to sunlight, both on the job and during leisure (residential) time (68). Exposure to sunlight and dietary vitamin D intake has been associated with reduced risk of breast cancer, with RR ranging from 0.67 to 0.85, and varying by region of residence. The risk reductions were highest for women who lived in United States regions of high solar radiation, with RR ranging from 0.35 to 0.75. Women who lived in regions of low solar radiation, primarily the northeastern region of the country, may experience an increased risk of breast cancer, as well as osteoporosis and fractures, especially during winter months (69,70).

OTHER FOODS AND NUTRIENTS WITH STRONG ANTICANCER PROPERTIES

Soy and Flax

Other plant-based foods, such as soy and flax, contain phytoestrogens (weak estrogens or estrogen-like compounds found in foods) that may reduce the risk of breast, endometrial, and possibly other types of cancers. The phytoestrogens responsible include isoflavones and lignans (71). Although phytoestrogen intake is thought to play a role in breast cancer prevention, recommendations for increasing consumption in breast cancer survivors remains controversial, especially for those with estrogen receptor positive breast cancer (72).

One to two tablespoons of flax, which is also an excellent source of fiber, and some soy foods may be safely consumed. Soy supplements are not recommended, because most research has focused on isoflavones in foods. Evidence for the benefits of isoflavone supplements is not substantiated at this time. Given current knowledge about soy, it is recommended that persons interested in incorporating soy into their diet do so by having up to two servings per day of whole soy foods, tofu, tempeh, soy milk, or soy nuts, which provide an average total of 25 g soy protein (72,73).

Folate

The relationship of dietary folate to the risk of breast, colon, and pancreatic cancer has been receiving considerable attention. Since 1998, folic acid, the more absorbable form of folate, has enriched grain and cereal products in an attempt to reduce the incidence of neural tube defects in infants (74). Since then, researchers have determined greater roles for folic acid in human health.

Higher plasma levels of folate, for example, have been associated with a reduced relative risk of developing breast cancer, when comparing the highest with the lowest quintile (multivariable RR = 0.11; 95% CI = 0.02–0.59). Higher plasma levels of folate may be of particular protective importance in both pre- and postmenopausal women who consume at least 15 g alcohol (approximately one drink) per day (75). Use of multivitamins containing folic acid has an impact on the risk of women with a family history of colon cancer (76). The relative risk of colon cancer in women with a family history of the disease, seems to be reduced (age-adjusted RR = 0.48; 95% CI = 0.28–0.83) by taking daily multivitamins with at least 400 μg folic acid (76).

The association between the intake of folate from food and the incidence of ovarian cancer was studied in the Swedish Mammography Cohort, a population-based prospective cohort of 61,084 Swedish women aged 38 to 76 years. Although the intake of dietary folate was weakly inversely associated with total ovarian cancer risk, there was a strong inverse association between dietary folate intake and ovarian cancer risk in women who consumed two alcoholic drinks per week (77). In a study of 27,000 male smokers between the ages of 50 and 69 years, dietary supplementation with 373 μg or more folic acid per day demonstrated an inverse relationship with pancreatic cancer risk, which was half that of the men with an intake of less than 200 μg/day (78).

n-3 Fatty Acids

n-3 fatty acids from fatty fish, alpha-linolenic acid from plant sources (eg, flaxseed, borage, black currant, and walnuts) have garnered attention recently for their role in reducing the risk of heart disease, inflammation, and chronic disease (79–82). Oils containing n-3 fatty acids are now being considered as therapies for cancer weight loss and cachexia and are being incorporated into specialized high-calorie dietary supplements (83,84).

n-3 fatty acids are also being studied for their role in cancer prevention. Consumption of fatty fish in men with prostate cancer was evaluated; researchers found that eating fish three or more times per week was associated with a reduced risk of prostate cancer, with the strongest association to metastatic cancer (83). The effects of individual fatty acids on breast cancer risk were examined in a prospective study of 35,298 Singapore Chinese women aged 45 to 74 years between 1985 and 1998 (85). Those women who consumed the highest amounts of dietary n-3 fatty acids from fish had a significantly reduced risk of breast cancer compared with women who consumed low levels of fish and higher amounts of n-6 fatty acids. There seemed to be no relationship between the risk of breast cancer and the intake of saturated, polyunsaturated, or monounsaturated fat in this population. The n-6 fatty acids alone did not seem to have an effect on breast cancer risk (84).

Other reviews and studies have offered a less optimistic view about the role of n-3 fatty acids and breast and prostate cancer risk (86,87). Evidence remains unclear. Study of individual fatty acids may provide a clearer and possibly an optimistic picture (88). Despite the inconsistent research, consuming fatty fish is considered a healthful practice for reducing risk of heart disease and possibly cancer and other chronic diseases (85,87,88).

COMPLEMENTARY AND ALTERNATIVE MEDICINE (CAM)

Complementary and alternative medicine (CAM) refers to practices that are used in conjunction with or in place of conventional medicine (see Chapter 16). CAM includes biologically based therapies, of which dietary supplements, antioxidants, herbal medicines, and special diets are examples. Although the availability of research varies widely in the documentation of CAM safety and efficacy, CAM therapies are appealing to cancer patient communities, especially cancer survivors.

Evidence has shown that suboptimal intake or deficiency of vitamins may place a person at risk for chronic disease, including cardiovascular disease, cancer, and osteoporosis. Folate and vitamins D, B-6,

B-12, and C are the vitamins most often associated with suboptimal intake (89).

Cancer survivors, particularly those in the early stages of treatment or remission, may find it difficult to consume a sufficient variety of foods, particularly fruits and vegetables, further increasing their risk of deficiency of these nutrients (12). In addition, those individuals may require supplements, in addition to a good diet, to ensure that nutrition needs are met. A daily multivitamin that provides 100% of the daily value of vitamins B-6, B-12, D, and folate has been recommended for all healthy adults, including cancer survivors (89,90).

DIETARY AND LIFESTYLE MODIFICATIONS

Data regarding cancer survivors who modify their diet and lifestyle are encouraging. Among Finnish and Australian women diagnosed with breast cancer who were surveyed about their experiences and choices after diagnosis, 30% and 39%, respectively, reported changing diet and exercise habits. Both populations identified a high need for diet and lifestyle counseling, and both reported that this need was poorly recognized by physicians (91). In Washington state, 511 adult patients with breast, prostate, and colon cancers were contacted and asked about changes in their diets and physical activity patterns over the past 12 months. Of these, more than 66% made lifestyle changes that included changes in diet, physical activity, and dietary supplement intake (92).

PHYSICAL ACTIVITY

It is well known that moderate physical activity for the cancer survivor, both during and after treatment, can help maintain lean body mass while reducing body fat (3). In addition, increased physical activity may prompt an increase in food consumption by stimulating appetite and decreasing constipation, which contributes to poor appetite (3). Those health care professionals who work with the physical side of treatment, including physical therapists, should reinforce healthy eating, just as nutrition therapists should reinforce physical activity in the patient's care plan.

Patients with cancer can benefit from adopting the ACS guidelines for physical activity (3). These guidelines recommend that adults engage in at least moderate activity for 30 minutes or more, 5 days per week, and that children and adolescents engage in at least 60 minutes per day of moderate to vigorous physical activity at least 5 days per week.

REFERENCES

1. Stewart SL, King JB, Thompson TD, Friedman C, Wingo PA. Cancer Mortality Surveillance—United States, 1990–2000. *MMWR Surveill Summ.* 2004;53: 1–108.
2. American Cancer Society. Cancer Facts and Figures 2005. Available at: http://www.cancer.org/docroot/STT/stt_0.asp. Accessed March 17, 2005.
3. Brown JK, Byers T, Doyle C, Coumeya KS, Demark-Wahnefried W, Kushi LH, McTieman A, Rock CL, Aziz N, Bloch AS, Eldridge B, Hamilton K, Katzin C, Koonce A, Main J, Mobley C, Morra ME, Pierce MS, Sawyer KA; American Cancer Society. Nutrition and physical activity during and after cancer treatment: an American Cancer Society guide for informed choices. *CA Cancer J Clin.* 2003;53:268–291.
4. Shils ME, Olson JA, Ross AC. Prevention and management of cancer. In: *Modern Nutrition in Health and Disease.* 9th ed. Baltimore, Md: Williams & Wilkins; 1999:1235–1325.
5. Wigmore SJ, Plester CE, Richardson RA, Fearon KC. Changes in nutritional status associated with unresectable pancreatic cancer. *Br J Cancer.* 1997;75: 106–109.
6. Fearon KC, von Meyenfeldt MF, Moses AGW, van Geenan R, Roy A, Gouma DJ, Giacosa A, Van Gossum A, Bauer J, Barber MD, Aaronson NK, Voss AC, Tisdale MJ. Effect of a protein and energy dense n-3 fatty acid enriched oral supplement on loss of weight and lean tissue in cancer cachexia: a randomized double blind trial. *Gut.* 2003:52:1479–1486.
7. Palesty JA, Dudrick SJ. What we have learned about cachexia in gastrointestinal cancer. *Dig Dis.* 2003;21: 198–213.
8. Evans WK, Nixon DW, Daly JM, Ellenberg SS, Gardner L, Wolfe E, Shepherd FA, Feld R, Gralla R, Fine S. A randomized study of oral nutritional support versus ad lib nutritional intake during chemotherapy for advanced colorectal and non-small cell lung cancer. *J Clin Oncol.* 1987;5:113–124.
9. Ovesen L, Allingstrup L, Hannibal J, Mortensen EL, Hansen OP. Effect of dietary counseling on food intake, body, response rate, survival, and quality of life in cancer patients undergoing chemotherapy: a prospective, randomized study. *J Clin Oncol.* 1993;11: 2043–2049.

10. Abu-Abid S, Szold A, Klausner J. Obesity and cancer. *J Med.* 2002;33:73–86.
11. Bianchini F, Kaaks R, Vainio H. Overweight, obesity, and cancer risk. *Lancet Oncol.* 2002;3:565–574.
12. Kroenke CH, Chen WY, Rosner B, Holmes MD. Weight, weight gain, and survival after breast cancer diagnosis. *J Clin Oncol.* 2005;23:1370–1378.
13. Tamakoshi K, Wakai K, Kojima M, Watanabe Y, Hayakawa N, Toyoshima H, Yatsuya H, Kondo T, Tokudome S, Hashimoto S, Suzuki K, Ito Y, Tamakoshi A; JACC Study Group. A prospective study of body size and colon cancer mortality in Japan: the JACC study. *Int J Obes Relat Metab Disord.* 2004;28:551–558.
14. Berclaz G, Li S, Price KN, Coates AS, Castiglione-Gertsch M, Rudenstam CM, Holmberg SB, Lindtner J, Erien D, Collins J, Snyder R, Thurlimann B, Fey MF, Mendiola C, Dudley Werner I, Simoncini E, Crivellari D, Gelber RD, Goldhirsch A. Body mass index as a prognostic feature in operable breast cancer: the International Breast Cancer Study Group experience. *Oncology.* 2004;15:875–884.
15. Borugian MJ, Sheps SB, Kim-Sing C, Olivotto IA, Van Patten C, Dunn BP, Coldman AJ, Potter JD, Gallagher RP, Hislop TG. Waist to hip ratio and breast cancer mortality. *Am J Epidemiol.* 2003;15:963–968.
16. Deslypere JP. Obesity and cancer. *Metabolism.* 1995;44:24–27.
17. Freedland SJ, Aronson WJ, Kane CJ, Presti JC, Amling CI, Elashoff D, Terris MK. Impact of obesity on biochemical control after radical prostatectomy for clinically localized prostate cancer: a report shared by the Shared Equal Access Regional Cancer Hospital Database Study Group. *J Clin Oncol.* 2004;22: 446–453.
18. Byers T, Nestle M, McTiernan A, Doyle C, Currie-William A. American Cancer Society guidelines on nutrition and physical activity for cancer prevention: reducing the risk of cancer with healthy food choices and physical activity. *CA Cancer J Clin.* 2002;52; 92–119.
19. Krauss RM, Eckel RH, Howard B, Appel LJ, Daniels SR, Deckelbaum RJ, Erdman JW Jr, Kris-Etherton P, Goldberg IJ, Kotchen TA, Lichtenstein AH, Mitch WE, Mullis R, Robinson K, Wylie-Rosett J, St Jeor S, Suttie J, Tribble DL, Bazzarre TL. AHA Dietary Guidelines: revision 2000: a statement for healthcare professionals from the Nutrition Committee of the American Heart Association. *Circulation.* 2000;102: 2284–2299.
20. Oeffinger KC, Buchanan GR, Eshelman DA, Denke MA, Andrews TC, Germak JA, Tomlinson GE, Snell LE, Foster BM. Cardiovascular risk factors in young adult survivors of childhood acute lymphoblastic leukemia. *J Pediatr Hematol Oncol.* 2001;23:424–430.
21. de Vos FY, Nuver J, Willemse PH, van der Zee AG, Messerschmidt J, Burgerhof JG, de Vries EG, Gietema JA. Long-term survivors of ovarian malignancies after cisplatin-based chemotherapy; cardiovascular risk factors and signs of vascular damage. *Eur J Cancer.* 2004;40:696–700.
22. Khaodhiar L, McCowen KC, Blackburn GL. Obesity and its comorbid conditions. *Clin Cornerstone.* 1999; 2:17–31.
23. Moyad MA. Is obesity a risk factor for prostate cancer, and does it even matter? A hypothesis and different perspective. *Urology.* 2002;59:41–50.
24. American Dietetic Association; Dietitians of Canada. Position of the American Dietetic Association and the Dietitians of Canada: Vegetarian Diets. *J Am Diet Assoc.* 2003;103:748–765.
25. Hunt JR. Bioavailability of iron, zinc, and other trace minerals from vegetarian diets. *Am J Clin Nutr.* 2003; 78:S633-S639.
26. Janelle KC, Barr SI. Nutrient intake and eating behavior scores of vegetarian and nonvegetarian women. *J Am Diet Assoc.* 1995;95:180–186,189.
27. Willet WC, Hunter DJ. Prospective studies of diet and breast cancer. *Cancer.* 1994;74:1085–1089.
28. Silverman DT, Swanson CA, Gridley G, Wocholder S, Greenberg RS, Brown LM, Hayes RB, Swanson GM, Schoenber JB, Pottern LM, Schwartz AG, Fraumeni JF, Hoover RN. Dietary and nutrition factors and pancreatic cancer: a case controlled study based on interviews. *J Natl Cancer Inst.* 1998; 90:1710–1719.
29. Cho E, Spiegelman D, Hunter DJ, Chen WY, Stampfer MJ, Colditz GA, Willett WC. Premenopausal fat intake and risk of breast cancer. *J Natl Cancer Inst.* 2003;95:1079–1085.
30. Chlebowski RT, Blackburn GL, Elashoff RE, Thomson C, Goodman MT, Shapiro A, Giuliano AE, Karanja N, Hoy MK, Nixon DW. The WINS Investigators. Dietary fat reduction in postmenopausal women with primary breast cancer: Phase III Women's Intervention Nutrition Study (WINS). American Society of Clinical Oncology. ASCO 2005 Annual Meeting. (Abstract no.10.) Available at: http://www.asco.org/ac/1,1003,_12–002643–00_18–0034–00_19–0031414,00.asp. Accessed November 27, 2005.
31. Fradet Y, Meyer F, Bairati I, Shadmani R, Moore L.

Dietary fat and prostate cancer progression and survival. *Eur Urol.* 1999;35;388–391.

32. National Cancer Institute. Eating hints for patients: before, during and after treatment. Available at: http://www.nci.nih.gov/cancertopics/eatinghints/page 3. Accessed November 28, 2005.
33. Donaldson MS. Nutrition and cancer: a review of the evidence for an anti-cancer diet. *Nutr J.* 2004;3:19.
34. Rose DP, Connolly JM, Rayburn J, Coleman M. Influence of diets containing eicosapentaenoic or docosahexaenoic acid on growth and metastasis of breast cancer cells in nude mice. *J Natl Cancer Inst.* 1995;87: 587–592.
35. Hardman W. Omega-3 fatty acids to augment cancer therapy. *J Nutr.* 2002;132(suppl):S3508-S3512.
36. Hu FB, Cho E, Rexrode KM, Albert CM, Manson JE. Fish and long-chain omega-3 fatty acid intake and risk of coronary heart disease and total mortality in diabetic women. *Circulation.* 2003;107:1852–1857.
37. Zampelas A, Panagiotakos DB, Pitsavos C, Das UN, Chrysohoou C, Skoumas Y, Stefanadis C. Fish consumption among healthy adults is associated with decreased levels of inflammatory markers related to cardiovascular disease; the ATTICA study. *J Am Coll Cardiol.* 2005;46:120–124.
38. National Heart, Lung, and Blood Institute. *Detection, Evaluation, and Treatment of High Blood Cholesterol in Adults (Adult Treatment Panel III).* Washington, DC: National Institutes of Health; 2002. NIH publication 02–5215.
39. Malin A, Dai Q, Yu H, Shu XO, Jin F, Gao YT, Zheng W. Evaluation of the synergistic effect of insulin and insulin-like growth factors on the risk of breast carcinoma. *Cancer.* 2004;100:694–700.
40. Agurs-Collins T. The role of insulin-like growth factors and breast cancer risk. *On-Line.* 2002;10:1,3–8.
41. Michaud DS, Liu S, Giovannucci E, Willett WC, Colditz GA, Fuchs CS. Dietary sugar, glycemic load, and pancreatic cancer risk in a prospective study. *J Natl Cancer Inst.* 2002;94:1293–1300.
42. Boyd DB. Insulin and cancer. *Integr Cancer Ther.* 2003;2:315–329.
43. LeRoith D, Roberts CT. The insulin-like growth factor system and cancer. *Cancer Lett.* 2003;195:127–137.
44. Augustin LS, Gallus S, Bosetti C, Levi F, Negri E, Franceschi S, Dal Maso L, Jenkins DJ, Kendall CW, LaVecchia C. Glycemic index and glycemic load in endometrial cancer. *Int J Cancer.* 2003;105:404–407.
45. Higginbotham S, Zhang ZF, Lee IM, Cook NR, Giovannucci E, Buring JE, Liu S. Dietary glycemic load and risk of colorectal cancer in the Women's Health Study. *J Natl Cancer Inst.* 2004;96:229–233.
46. Hsing AW, Gao YT, Chua S Jr, Deng J, Stanczyk FZ. Insulin resistance and prostate cancer risk. *J Natl Cancer Inst.* 2003;95:1086–1087.
47. Heber D. *What Color Is Your Diet?* New York, NY: HaperCollins Publishers; 2001.
48. Heber D. Vegetables, fruits and phytoestrogens in the prevention of diseases. *J Postgrad Med.* 2004;50: 145–149.
49. Park EJ, Pezzuto JM. Botanicals in cancer chemoprevention. *Cancer Metastasis Rev.* 2002;21:231–235.
50. World Cancer Research Fund/American Institute for Cancer Research. *Food, Nutrition and the Prevention of Cancer: A Global Perspective.* Washington, DC: American Institute for Cancer Research; 1997.
51. Giovannucci E, Rimm EB, Liu Y, Stampfer MJ, Willett WC. A prospective study of cruciferous vegetables and prostate cancer. *Cancer Epidemiol Biomarkers Prev.* 2003;12:64–67.
52. Cohen JH, Kristal AR, Stanford JL. Fruit and vegetable intake and prostate cancer risk. *J Natl Cancer Inst.* 2003;95:1079–1085.
53. Terry P, Giovannucci E, Michels KB, Bergkvist L, Hansen H, Holmberg L, Wolk A. Fruits, vegetables, dietary fiber intake, and the risk of colorectal cancer. *J Natl Cancer Inst.* 2001;93:525–533.
54. Rock CL, Demark-Wahnefried W. Nutrition and survival after the diagnosis of breast cancer: a review of the evidence. *J Clin Oncol.* 2002;20:3002–3016.
55. Thomson CA, Flatt SW, Rock CL, Ritenbaugh C, Newman V, Pierce JP. Increased fruit, vegetable and fiber intake and lower fat intake reported among women previously treated for invasive breast cancer. *J Am Diet Assoc.* 2002;102:801–808.
56. Rock CL, Demark-Wahnefried W. Can lifestyle modification increase survival in women diagnosed with breast cancer? *J Nutr.* 2002;132(suppl):S3504-S3507.
57. Sieri S, Krogh V, Pala V, Muti P, Micheli A, Evangelista A, Tagliabue G, Berrino F. Dietary patterns and risk of breast cancer in the ORDET cohort. *Cancer Epidemiol Biomarkers Prev.* 2004;13:567–572.
58. Hadley CW, Miller EC, Schwartz SJ, Clinton SK. Tomatoes, lycopene, and prostate cancer: progress and promise. *Exp Biol Med (Maywood).* 2002;227: 869–880.
59. Miller EC, Hadley CW, Schwartz SJ. Lycopene, tomato products, and prostate cancer prevention. Have we established causality? *Pure Applied Chemistry.* 2002;74:1435–1441.

60. LaVecchia C. Tomatoes, lycopene intake, and digestive tract and female hormone-related cancers. *Exp Biol Med.* 2002;227:860–863.
61. Kolonel LN, Hankin JH, Wittemore AS, Wu AH, Gallagher RP, Wilkens LR, John EM, Howe GR, Dreon DM, West DW, Paffenbarger RS. Vegetables, fruits, legumes and prostate cancer: a multiethnic case-control study. *Cancer Epidemiol Biomarkers Prev.* 2000;9:795–804.
62. Miller EC, Giovannucci E, Erdman JW, Bahnson R, Schwartz SJ, Clinton SK. Tomato products, lycopene, and prostate cancer risk. *Urol Clin North Am.* 2002;29:83–93.
63. Wu K, Willett WC, Fuchs CS, Colditz GA, Giovannucci EL. Calcium intake and risk of colon cancer in women and men. *J Natl Cancer Inst.* 2002;94: 437–446.
64. Flood A, Peters U, Chatterjee N, Lacey JV Jr, Schairer C, Schatzkin A. Calcium from diet and supplements is associated with reduced risk of colorectal cancer in a prospective cohort of women. *Cancer Epidemiol Biomarkers Prev.* 2005;14:126–132.
65. Shin MH, Holmes MD, Hankinson SE, Wu K, Colditz GA, Willett WC. Intake of dairy products, calcium, and vitamin D and risk of breast cancer. *J Natl Cancer Inst.* 2002;94:1301–1310.
66. Jacobs ET, Martinez ME, Alberts DS. Research and public health implications of the intricate relationship between calcium and vitamin D in the prevention of colorectal neoplasia. *J Natl Cancer Inst.* 2003;95: 1736–1737.
67. Robsahm TE, Tretli S, Dahlback A, Moen J. Vitamin D_3 from the sunlight may improve the prognosis of breast, colon and prostate cancer (Norway). *Cancer Causes Control.* 2004;15:149–158.
68. Freedman DM, Dosemeci M, McGlynn K. Sunlight and mortality from breast, ovarian, colon, prostate, and non-melanoma skin cancer: a composite death certificate based case-control study. *Occup Environ Med.* 2002;59:257–262.
69. John EM, Schwartz GG, Dreon DM, Koo J. Vitamin D and breast cancer risk: the NHANES I Epidemiologic follow-up study, 1971–1975 to 1992. National Health and Nutrition Examination Survey. *Cancer Epidemiol Biomarkers Prev.* 1999;8:399–406.
70. Holick MF. Vitamin D and bone health. *J Nutr.* 1996;126(suppl):S1159-S1164.
71. Horn-Ross PL, John EM, Canchola AJ, Stewart S, Lee MM. Phytoestrogen intake and endometrial cancer. *J Natl Cancer Inst.* 2003;95:1158–1164.
72. Duffy C, Cyr M. Phytoestrogens: potential benefits and implications for breast cancer survivors. *J Women's Health.* 2003;12:617–631.
73. Messina M, Messina V. Provisional recommended soy protein and isoflavone intake for healthy adults: rationale. *Nutr Today.* 2003;38:100–109.
74. Institute of Medicine. *Dietary Reference Intakes for Thiamin, Riboflavin, Niacin, Vitamin B6, Folate, Vitamin B12, Pantothenic Acid, Biotin, and Choline.* Washington, DC: National Academy Press; 2000.
75. Zhang SM, Willett WC, Selhub J, Hunter DJ, Giovannucci EL, Holmes MD, Colditz GA, Hankinson SE. Plasma folate, vitamin B6, vitamin B12, homocysteine, and risk of breast cancer. *J Natl Cancer Inst.* 2003;95:373–380.
76. Fuchs CS, Willett WC, Colditz GA, Hunter DJ, Stampfer MJ, Speizer FE, Giovannucci EL. The influence of folate and multivitamin use on the familial risk of colon cancer in women. *Cancer Epidemiol Biomarkers Prev.* 2002;11:227–234.
77. Larsson SC, Giovannucci E, Wolk A. Dietary folate intake and incidence of ovarian cancer: the Swedish Mammography Cohort. *J Natl Cancer Inst.* 2004;96: 396–402.
78. Stolzenberg-Solomon RZ, Pietinen P, Barrett MJ, Taylor PR, Virtamo J, Albanes D. Dietary and other methyl-group availability factors and pancreatic cancer risk in a cohort of male smokers. *Am J Epidemiol.* 2001;153:680–687.
79. Simopoulos AP. Essential fatty acids in health and chronic disease. *Am J Clin Nutr.* 1999;70(suppl):S560-S569.
80. Wijendran V, Hayes KC. Dietary n-6 and n-3 fatty acid and cardiovascular health. *Ann Rev Nutr.* 2004;24: 597–615.
81. Harris WS. Fish oil supplementation: evidence for health benefits. *Cleve Clin J Med.* 2004;71: 208–210,212,215–218.
82. Rose DP, Connolly JM. Omega-3 fatty acids as cancer chemoprotective agents. *Pharmacol Ther.* 1999;83: 217–244.
83. Wigmore SJ, Ross JA, Falconer JS, Plester CE, Tisdale MJ, Carter DC, Fearon KC. The effect of polyunsaturated fatty acids on the progress of cachexia in patients with pancreatic cancer. *Nutrition.* 1996;12:S27-S30.
84. Barber MD, Ross JA, Voss AC, Tisdale MJ, Fearon KC. The effect of an oral nutritional supplement enriched with fish oil on weight-loss in patients with cancer cachexia. *Br J Cancer.* 1999;8:80–86.
85. Gago-Dominguez M, Yaun JM, Sun CL, Lee HP, Yu

MC. Opposing effects of dietary n-3 and n-6 fatty acids on mammary carcinogenesis: the Singapore Chinese Health Study. *Br J Cancer.* 2003;89:1686–1692.

86. Willett WC. Specific fatty acids and risks of breast and prostate cancer: dietary intake. *Am J Clin Nutr.* 1997;66(suppl):S1557-S1563.
87. Terry PD, Rohan TE, Wolk A. Intakes of fish and marine fatty acids and the risks of cancer of the breast and prostate and of other hormone-related cancers: a review of the epidemiologic evidence. *Am J Clin Nutr.* 2003;77:532–543.
88. Augustsson K, Michaud DS, Rimm EB, Leitzmann MF, Stampfer MJ, Willett WC, Giovannucci E. A prospective study of intake of fish and marine fatty acids and prostate cancer. *Cancer Epidemiol Biomarkers Prev.* 2003;12:64–67.
89. Fletcher RH, Fairfield KM. Vitamins for chronic disease prevention in adults. *JAMA.* 2002;287: 3127–3129.
90. Willett WC, Stampfer MJ. What vitamins should I be taking, Doctor? *N Engl J Med.* 2001;345: 1819–1824.
91. Salminen E, Bishop M, Poussa T, Drummond R, Salminen S. Dietary attitudes and changes as well as use of supplements and complementary therapies by Australian and Finnish women following the diagnosis of breast cancer. *Eur J Clin Nutr.* 2004;58:137–144.
92. Patterson RE, Neuhouser ML, Hedderson MM, Schwartz SM, Standish LJ, Bowen DJ. Changes in diet, physical activity, and supplement use among adults diagnosed with cancer. *J Am Diet Assoc.* 2003;103:323–328.

Section 3

Clinical Nutrition Management in the Oncology Setting

Chapter 19

Reimbursement for Medical Nutrition Therapy

CAROL FRANKMANN, MS, RD, CNSD

INTRODUCTION

For many years, registered dietitians (RDs) have tried to establish medical nutrition therapy (MNT) as a separate, reimbursable component of health care. This effort was hindered by the lack of billing codes that were specific to the nutrition professional. After a decade of education and lobbying efforts, the American Dietetic Association (ADA), in 2001, established Current Procedure Terminology (CPT) codes for MNT. Although Medicare MNT reimbursement is currently limited to patients with diabetes and chronic renal insufficiency, it is important that dietetics professionals in oncology care understand reimbursement processes. This chapter reviews CPT codes available for MNT, coverage of MNT by Medicare, and Medicare billing and payment procedures. This chapter also examines the Medicare Prescription Drug, Improvement and Modernization Act of 2003.

CODES

CPT-4 is a uniform coding system that is used primarily to identify medical services and procedures provided by physicians and other health care professionals. The CPT-4 codes are updated and published annually by the American Medical Association (AMA). MNT CPT codes, as defined by ADA, AMA, and Centers for Medicare and Medicaid Services (CMS), include the following (1):

- 97802: Medical nutrition therapy; initial assessment and intervention, individual, face-to-face with the patient, each 15 minutes.
- 97803: Reassessment and intervention, individual, face-to-face with the patient, each 15 minutes.
- 97804: Group (two or more individuals), each 30 minutes.

MNT CPT codes best describe nutrition diagnostic, therapy, and counseling services provided by RDs to individuals with chronic diseases or medical conditions. Medicare requires use of the MNT CPT codes, making it inappropriate for health care professionals to bill Medicare beneficiaries for nutrition services with other codes. Use of MNT CPT codes among private insurance plans may vary; many plans now require MNT CPT codes on claims forms.

G codes are temporary Healthcare Common Procedure Coding System (HCPCS) codes that are used to indicate professional health care procedures and services that have not yet been established as permanent CPT codes (2). Effective January 1, 2003, CMS established two new G HCPCS codes for MNT. These new codes should be used when the treating physician determines that there is a change in diagnosis, treatment, or medical condition of the Medicare beneficiary and additional hours of MNT services, beyond the number of hours typically covered by Medicare, are needed in the same calendar year (3,4). An additional physician referral is needed for the extra hours of MNT. The G codes for MNT are as follows (4):

- G0270: Medical Nutrition Therapy; reassessment and subsequent intervention(s) after second referral in same year for change in diagnosis, medical condition, or treatment regimen (including additional hours needed for renal disease), individual, face-to-face with the patient, each 15 minutes.
- G0271: Medical Nutrition Therapy; reassessment and subsequent intervention(s) after second referral in same year for change in diagnosis, medical condition, or treatment regimen (including additional hours needed for renal disease), group (two or more individuals), each 30 minutes.

COVERAGE

The existence of a code does not solely determine whether a specific service is covered. Government, employer, and health-plan coverage for MNT varies nationwide and needs to be determined on a policy-specific basis.

For example, the Tufts Health Plan Web site states that nutrition counseling is reimbursed "based on the member's benefit plan" (5). For services not covered under the members benefit, the member assumes liability and is responsible for paying the provider directly.

Aetna's Clinical Policy Bulletins (6) indicate that nutrition counseling is considered to be "medically necessary for chronic disease states in which dietary adjustment has a therapeutic role, when it is prescribed by a physician and furnished by a provider recognized under the plan." Aetna also states that MNT has been integrated into the treatment guidelines for a number of chronic conditions, including cardiovascular disease, hypertension, eating disorders, gastrointestinal disorders, seizures, and other conditions, based on the efficacy of diet and lifestyle in the treatment of these disease states. Currently, there is no reference to oncology diagnoses within Aetna's nutrition coverage policies.

MEDICARE GUIDELINES

Medicare, the federal insurance program for people 65 years and older and for certain disabled people, consists of two parts: Medicare Part A and Medicare Part B. Medicare Part A pays for inpatient hospital stays, skilled nursing days, hospice care, and some home health care. Medicare Part B is reserved for doctors' services, outpatient hospital care, and other medical services that are not covered by Part A.

Medicare Part B

Medicare Part B guidelines define MNT coverage in terms of treatment setting, diagnosis, and number of visits within a calendar year. Important considerations for Medicare Part B guidelines include the following:

- Medicare Part B provides MNT coverage for outpatient care. MNT is not covered for an inpatient stay in a hospital, skilled nursing care facility, rural health clinic, or federally qualifying health clinic.
- Coverage is restricted to patients with type 1 or type 2 diabetes or gestational diabetes, as well as patients with chronic renal insufficiency, patients with end-stage renal disease when dialysis is not received, and posttransplant care for renal disease for 36 months after discharge from the hospital (7).
- Three hours of MNT may be reimbursed in the initial calendar year and 2 hours in subsequent years. Additional hours are permitted when there is an additional physician referral specifying the need for additional MNT, based on a change in diagnosis, treatment, or medical condition (3).

The following are the general conditions of MNT coverage for Medicare Part B beneficiaries based on CMS regulations and current best practice:

- The treating physician must make a referral and indicate a diagnosis of diabetes or renal disease (7) and include the International Classification of Diseases, 9th Revision, Clinical Modification (ICD-9-CM) code to the highest level of specificity (8).
- A signed copy of the referral is required before providing the service. A physician order is required during each calendar year when nutrition services are needed (3).
- Beneficiaries with diabetes may receive Medicare MNT services and services provided through a Medicare Diabetes Self-Management Training (DSMT) program. Beneficiaries may

Table 19.1 Medical Nutrition Therapy (MNT) Services Provided to Individuals With Cancer

CPT Code	*Example of MNT Provided*
97802	Newly diagnosed esophageal cancer patient referred to RD because of difficulty with swallowing, subsequent decreased oral intake, and 20-pound weight loss. Nutrition assessment performed. Nutrition intervention included recommendation for feeding tube placement. Educated patient on ways to increase energy and protein intake for weight stabilization and ease of swallowing until tube feeding placement.
97803	Esophageal cancer patient seen in follow-up for weight loss after esophagectomy and jejunostomy tube placement. Reassessment and intervention performed. Recommendations made for enteral feeding to provide gradual weight gain of 1 kg/mo.
97804	Breast cancer nutrition education class led by RD: • Small group setting with five patients. • Nutrition intervention included eating strategies for managing treatment-related side effects (eg, fatigue, nausea, and vomiting), recommendations for maintaining and monitoring body weight, education related to nutrition needs during treatment, and suggestions for improving the nutrition quality of daily diet.
G02070	Gastric cancer patient receiving adjuvant chemotherapy referred to RD for dietary intervention for stage 2 hypertension. Patient educated on DASH diet, 2,400-mg sodium intake, and adequate protein/calories for weight maintenance. Patient verbalized ability to make daily food selections consistent with diet plan.
G02071	Weight management class led by RD: • Small group setting with five obese patients who have completed treatment for breast cancer. • Nutrition intervention included assessment of BMI, determination of individual weight, activity, and nutrition goals. Education provided on strategies for changes in diet and physical activity to achieve goals. Goals for next session established.

receive 10 hours of education from Medicare DSMT programs and 3 hours of MNT in the first year. For follow-up DSMT, Medicare allows 2 hours in subsequent years, and for follow-up MNT, Medicare allows 2 hours of MNT in subsequent years, unless the physician indicates additional MNT hours are needed. Comparisons of accredited DSMT programs and of MNT services are available at the ADA Web site (9).

Advanced Beneficiary Notice

RDs who provide MNT to Medicare patients with diabetes and nondialysis kidney disease need to notify patients in advance if they are unsure as to whether the service will be covered (3,10). In these instances, an RD uses an advanced beneficiary notice (ABN) to provide written notice that the patient is responsible for the payment if Medicare denies payment. The ABN must be completed before providing MNT (10). The CMS standardized ABN form (CMS-R-131-G), available online from CMS (11), should be used.

MNT Services Not Covered by Medicare

If MNT is provided to Medicare beneficiaries with any condition other than the renal and diabetes diagnoses described previously, the claim for the nutrition service cannot be billed to Medicare. If no other insurance coverage is available, the patient would pay out-of-pocket for the MNT services provided (12). For examples of MNT services provided to patients with cancer, see Table 19.1.

Documentation

Currently, CMS has not established specific documentation requirements that apply to MNT services

Table 19.2 Documentation Checklist for Medical Nutrition Therapy (MNT)

Documentation Element	*Initial*	*Follow-up*
Receipt of referral	X	X*
Diagnosis	X	
Date of visit and start/stop times	X	X
Demographic data	X	
Clinical and lab data	X	X
Nutrition assessment and history	X	
Learning needs assessment related to MNT	X	
Clinical and behavioral goals—care plan	X	
Interventions—MNT provided	X	
Adherence potential	X	
Scheduling of follow-up appointment	X	X
Progress to goals		X
Adjustments to care plan		X
Interventions—new and reinforcement		X
Barriers and solutions		X
Appointment failures and other ways that the patient is not cooperating with the treatment plan		X
Follow-up plans		X

*A second physician referral is needed for additional MNT provided in the same calendar year, based on a change in diagnosis, medical condition, or treatment regimen.

Source: Adapted with permission from American Dietetic Association. Medical Nutrition Therapy Documentation. Available at: http://www.eatright.org/cps/rde/xchg/SID-5303FFEA-C31F4BB8/ada/hs.xsl/nutrition_mntdoc_ENU_HTML.htm. Accessed November 28, 2005.

provided by RDs. Table 19.2 (13) provides a general guide for documentation of MNT. It is expected that the RD will use nationally established protocols/guides for practice in providing MNT for Medicare beneficiaries (3). In addition, evidence-based practice and the documentation of patient outcomes are essential in demonstrating the benefit of MNT services for all patients.

Becoming a Medicare MNT Provider

RDs or nutrition professionals are eligible to become providers of Medicare MNT. To enroll and receive a Medicare Provider Identification Number (PIN), practitioners may contact their local/state Medicare carrier and receive enrollment forms. Carrier information is available from CMS (14). RDs employed by hospitals or physician clinics must complete a reassignment form along with other enrollment forms. The reassignment form allows the facility to submit claims and collect payment for the MNT services provided by the RD (7). The decision as to whether or not to become a Medicare provider requires careful consideration and should include consultation with others who have compliance, billing, and/or legal expertise.

Opting Out

An RD who chooses not to enroll as a Medicare provider may consider "opting out" of Medicare. "Opting out" of Medicare is a serious decision with substantial administrative responsibilities (10). The practitioner who chooses to "opt out" of Medicare must sign a formal affidavit and mail this detailed statement to the Medicare carrier in the state where the RD's practice is located. The document is effective for 2 years and remains in effect even if the practitioner's place of employment changes (10).

Private practice RDs who are considering opting out of Medicare should consult with a health care lawyer for appropriate counsel and assistance. RDs employed in facilities should consult with the compliance officer and billing experts to assess whether the opt-out provisions may apply at the facility and to review the implications of "opting out" as a Medicare provider. For a discussion of additional considerations, visit the CMS Web site (11).

Billing Medicare

The Medicare Part B MNT benefit is regulated by CMS, and appropriately billing Medicare Part B for service may require learning new claims processing skills. There are several basic principles that should help clarify the Medicare billing requirements:

- Medicare RD providers must either bill Medicare Part B using their own PIN or reassign their Medicare reimbursement to their place of employment who then submits claims to Medicare for MNT services on the RD's behalf.
- Medicare should only be billed for MNT that is provided to qualifying beneficiaries with diabetes or renal disease.
- Medicare cannot be billed for diseases other than the defined diabetes or renal diagnoses.
- For diseases not covered by Medicare, the RD can bill the patient's other insurers, if applicable, but not the Medicare carriers.
- If no other insurance coverage is available, the patient would pay out-of-pocket for MNT services provided.
- MNT should not be billed as an "incident to" physician services (7). MNT codes specifically define professional nutrition services and are to be used for all billing for such services.

The CMS-1500 form (previously called the HCFA-1500 form) is used for billing Medicare for professional services. This claims form is also the accepted billing form with Medicaid and many insurers. This form can be found online at the CMS Web site (11). The Unique Physician Identification Number (UPIN) of the referring physician must be on the claim form submitted by the RD provider (7).

It is important that practitioners establish rates and set-up systems to track billing transactions for the MNT services that they provide. This information and billing process must be established for both private practitioners and RDs working in hospital or physician offices.

Compliance

Most billing companies and health care organizations have compliance officers who are responsible for coordinating activities that safeguard against fraud and abuse, improving the quality of health care, and reducing the costs of care (15). The compliance officer is an important resource for identifying guidelines that affect Medicare MNT and for ensuring that appropriate billing practices are used. The compliance officer, or other designee, may also be involved with the facility or practice's Privacy Rule activities under the Health Insurance Portability and Accountability Act (HIPAA).

To ensure compliance with regulations, audits may be conducted within the organization, as well as by Medicare or other payers. The *ADA Medicare MNT Systems Evaluation* tool, accessible to members through the ADA Web site (9), is helpful for establishing systems that will prepare for Medicare MNT audits. The RD needs to maintain records that show compliance with regulations related to health care benefits for each patient, claims processing, denials and appeals, and HIPAA. Records related to MNT should include complete documentation of physician referral before service, medical record documentation of MNT that is consistent with accepted guides for practice and the components identified in Figure 19.1, and tracking of patient outcomes.

Payment

As a Medicare provider, the RD accepts the payment rate established by Medicare and agrees to collect the co-pay from the Medicare beneficiary (7). Billing additional charges to the patient is illegal.

Medicare payment rates for the MNT-CPT codes are made under the physician fee schedule based on the geographic area where the practitioner provides the service. The physician fee schedule is established annually by CMS and can be accessed from the Medicare carrier's Web page or CMS Web site (11).

Payment rates are a calculation of RVUs (relative value units), a conversion factor, and a geographic location factor. Payment for Medicare MNT is the lesser of the actual charge or 85% of the physician fee schedule amount. Coinsurance is 20% of the lesser of these two amounts (4).

The Medicare beneficiary also is responsible for an annual deductible payment—in 2005, the Medicare Part B deductible was $110. Payment for codes 97802 (initial MNT) and 97803 (follow-up MNT) are the same value; it is assumed that the difference between an initial and a follow-up visit is the time spent performing the service. Group code 97804 is paid at a

Table 19.3 Example of Calculation of Medicare Payment Assignment

*Medicare Payment Assignment**	*Amount†*
Actual bill for MNT	$135
Physician fee schedule amount	$80
MNT approved amount for RDs (85% of assigned physician fee)	$68
Medicare beneficiary payment to RD (20% of approved MNT amount.)	$13.60

*For beneficiary who has met Part B deductible.
†Values are hypothetical.

separate rate and applies to each participant who attends the MNT group session.

Although the RD's usual charge may be a higher amount than the Medicare approved payment rate, Medicare RD providers may collect only the lesser of the Medicare-approved rate or the actual charge for the MNT service provided to qualifying Medicare beneficiaries. Table 19.3 is an example of payment as assigned. RDs who are enrolled as Medicare providers and employed by hospitals or physician clinics must reassign their benefits to their employer in order for the employer to be paid.

MEDICARE PRESCRIPTION DRUG, IMPROVEMENT AND MODERNIZATION ACT OF 2003

Passage of the Medicare Prescription Drug, Improvement and Modernization Act of 2003 (MMA) (16) provided prescription drug benefits to Medicare recipients and altered the Medicare program's structure. Since January 2005, Medicare has covered an initial preventive physical examination to determine physical conditions of new beneficiaries within the first 6 months of becoming eligible for Medicare. The law also provides for screening and other preventive services. Medicare beneficiaries who are diagnosed with diabetes or kidney disease after screening and/or their physical examination and with a physician referral may receive Medicare MNT provided by an RD (17).

The second expansion of MNT is within the establishment of voluntary Chronic Care Improvement (CCI) programs, now called Medicare Health Support programs (18), which began late in 2005 and is to be phased in over 3 to 5 years. Each individual chronic care management plan, as appropriate, will include self-care education through approaches such as disease management or MNT and education for primary caregivers and family members (17).

A CCI organization will provide care management services under contract with Medicare and will receive a fee for each participant per month in the program. Claims for medical services, such as MNT provided to participants, will continue to be covered, administered, and paid under the Medicare fee-for-service program (19). CCI organizations include disease management organizations, health insurers, integrated delivery systems, physician group practices, a consortium of such entities, or any other legal entity that CMS determines appropriate (17). CMS has selected nine programs to offer the pilot Medicare Health Support programs across the country. RDs may be involved in providing MNT services in these designated pilot programs.

Regulations to implement the provisions of the Medicare bill will be written by CMS. As ADA works to contribute to this process, the need to develop and implement new guides for evidence-based practice for diagnosis, such as for chronic obstructive pulmonary disease, will emerge. The MMA offers an opportunity to increase the demand for MNT services (17).

REFERENCES

1. American Medical Association. *CPT 2005 Professional Edition.* Chicago, Ill: AMA Press; 2005.
2. Centers for Medicare and Medicaid Services. Healthcare common procedure coding system (HCPCS) Level II Coding Procedures. Available at: http://www.cms.hhs.gov/medicare/hcpcs/codpayproc.asp. Accessed August 22, 2005.
3. Department of Health and Human Services. *Clarification Regarding Non-physician Practitioners Billing on Behalf of a Diabetes Outpatient Self-Management Training Services (DSMT) Program and the Common Working File Edits for DSMT and Medical Nutrition Therapy (MNT).* Washington, DC: Centers for Medicare and Medicaid Services; October 25, 2002. CMS Pub 60AB, Transmittal AB-02–151, Change Request 2373.
4. Department of Health and Human Services. *Medical Nutrition Therapy (MNT) Services for Beneficiaries with Diabetes or Renal Disease—POLICY CHANGE.*

Washington, DC: Centers for Medicare and Medicaid Services; November 1, 2002. CMS Pub 60A, Transmittal AB-02–115, Change Request 2404.

5. Tufts Health Plan. Nutritional counseling guidelines. Available at: http://www.tufts-healthplan.com/providers/pdf/billing_guidelines/nutr-counseling.pdf. Accessed August 22, 2005.
6. Aetna, Inc. Clinical policy bulletins: nutritional counseling. Available at: http://www.aetna.com/cpb/data/CPBA0049.html. Accessed August 22, 2005.
7. Department of Health and Human Services. *Additional clarification for Medical Nutrition Therapy (MNT) Services.* Washington, DC: Centers for Medicare and Medicaid Services; May 1, 2002. CMS Pub 60AB, Transmittal AB-02–059, Change Request 2142.
8. Practice Management Information Corporation. *International Classification of Diseases, 9th Revision, Clinical Modification.* 6th ed. Los Angeles, Calif: Practice Management Information Corporation; 2003.
9. American Dietetic Association Web site. Available at: http://www.eatright.org. Accessed August 22, 2005.
10. Infante MC, Michael P, Pritchett E. Opting out of Medicare: a serious business decision. *J Am Diet Assoc.* 2002;102:1061–1062.
11. Centers for Medicare & Medicaid Services. CMS Web site. Available at: http://www.cms.hhs.gov. Accessed August 26, 2005.
12. Infante M, Michael P. Medicare Part B coverage and billing for medical nutrition therapy. *J Am Diet Assoc.* 2002;102:32.
13. American Dietetic Association. Medical Nutrition Therapy Documentation. Available at: http://www.eatright.org/cps/rde/xchg/SID-5303FFEA-C31F4BB8/ada/hs.xsl/nutrition_mntdoc_ENU_HTML.htm. Accessed November 28, 2005.
14. Centers for Medicare & Medicaid Services. Medicare fee-for-service provider/supplier enrollment. Available at: http://www.cms.hhs.gov/providers/enrollment/default.asp? Accessed August 22, 2005.
15. American Dietetic Association. Medicare Compliance Program Backgrounder. Available at: http://www.eatright.org/cps/rde/xchg/SID-5303FFEA-C31F4BB8/ada/hs.xsl/nutrition_compbckgrnd_ENU_HTML.htm. Accessed November 28, 2005.
16. Centers for Medicare & Medicaid Services. Medicare Prescription Drug, Improvement and Modernization Act of 2003. Available at: http://www.cms.hhs.gov/medicarereform/MMAactFullText.pdf. Accessed August 22, 2005.
17. Smith R. Medicare reform: what it means to the future of dietetics. *J Am Diet Assoc.* 2004;104:734–735.
18. Centers for Medicare & Medicaid Services. Medicare health support. Available at: http://www.cms.hhs.gov/medicarereform/ccip/overview.asp. Accessed August 22, 2005.
19. Centers for Medicare and Medicaid Services. Medicare program: voluntary chronic care improvement program under traditional fee-for-service Medicare. Available at: http://www.cms.hhs.gov/providerupdate/regs/cms5004n.pdf. Accessed August 26, 2005.

Chapter 20

Incorporating Research Into Oncology Practice

CHRISTINA K. BIESEMEIER, MS, RD, FADA

INTRODUCTION

In Spring 2001, the House of Delegates (HOD) of the American Dietetic Association (ADA) passed a motion recognizing the following research needs for ADA members (1): (*a*) critical evaluation of the research in preparation of evidence-based practice guides, (*b*) integration of research findings into daily practice, and (*c*) participation in research in the practice setting. According to Manore and Myers (1), research is the foundation for evidence-based practice, education of dietetics professionals, and recommendations for public policy related to nutrition, health, and food issues. This chapter describes how dietetics professionals can meet the research needs defined by the HOD, including analyzing evidence, with emphasis given to application in an oncology practice setting.

WHY DIETETICS PROFESSIONALS NEED TO KEEP UP-TO-DATE WITH RESEARCH

Although dietetics professionals may find it difficult to sift through a multitude of articles to determine the merits of applying the recommendations, it is vital, for two reasons, that dietetics professionals in oncology care stay current with research. First, as a result of computer technology, patients seeking answers to their questions have access to the same evidence that is available to their health care providers. Second, patients also access information sources that make unproven but believable claims about treatments and cures. Knowledgeable dietetics professionals can help their patients distinguish evidence-based recommendations from unproven claims (2).

ADA METHOD OF EVIDENCE ANALYSIS

In 2000, the ADA Health Services Research Task Force adopted a method of evidence analysis that is used to develop disease-specific Medical Nutrition Therapy (MNT) Guides for Practice (3). As shown in Figure 20.1 (4,5), the ADA evidence analysis method involves seven steps. Dietetics professionals can use this method to evaluate individual articles they read.

Step 1: Identify a Practice Problem or an Area of Uncertainty in Practice

Questions that oncology dietetics professionals might ask include the following (4,5):

- What is the most effective MNT for patients with cancer who are experiencing side effects from their cancer treatment?
- What is the evidence to support the use of antioxidants before, during, and after chemotherapy and/or radiation therapy?
- What is the evidence to support the use of one type of nutrition intervention rather than an alternate intervention?

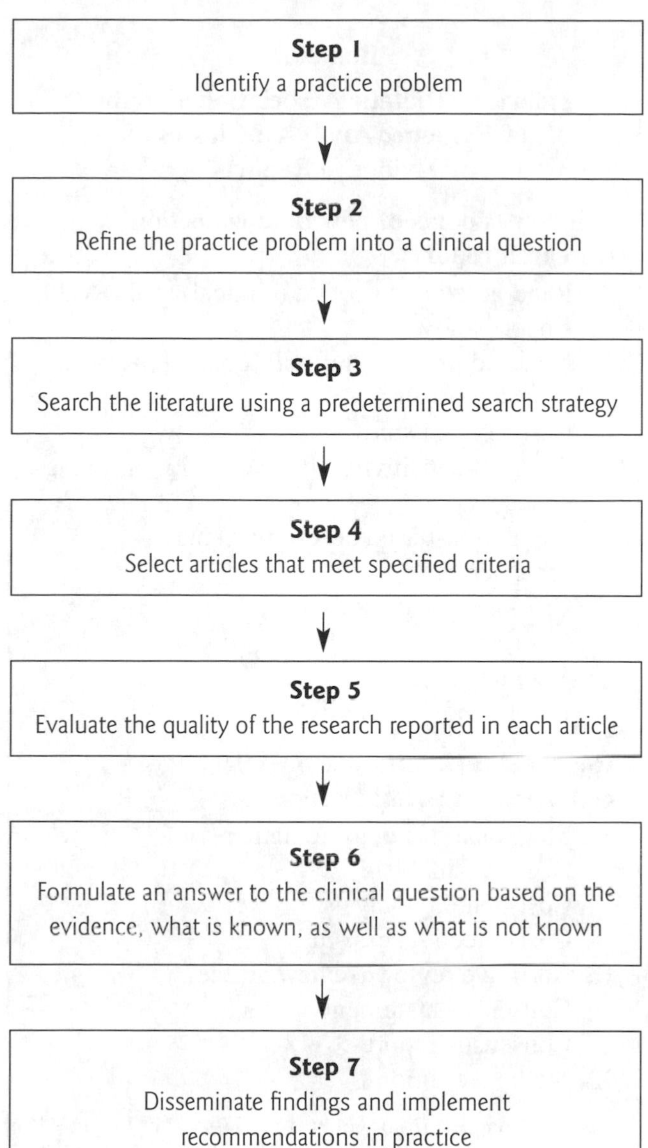

Figure 20.1. American Dietetic Association method of evidence analysis. Data are from references 4 and 5.

- What are the expected nutrition outcomes from MNT in patients with different types of cancer?

At this step, it is appropriate to determine whether other colleagues have had the same practice problem, and if so, whether they have already conducted a systematic review of the literature and published their results. Dietetics professionals should also check the Agency for Healthcare Research and Quality's (AHRQ) National Guideline Clearinghouse Web site (6) and the National Cancer Institute Web site (7), to see whether a systematic review has been completed.

Step 2: Formulate a Clinical Question to Be Answered Based on the Practice Problem or Area of Uncertainty

Clinical questions are refinements of the original practice questions and should include four components (4,5): the patient group, the intervention in question (usually MNT or an MNT recommendation), a comparison intervention, and the outcome. A clinical question related to antioxidant use in patients receiving chemotherapy might be as follows: What is the evidence to support the use of antioxidants during treatment vs not using them, in terms of the impact on the effectiveness of chemotherapy?

Step 3: Search the Professional Literature

To search the literature, dietetics professionals first should define their search strategy (4,5). Defining search strategies requires the following:

- Determining databases to be searched. The National Library of Medicine PubMed Web site (8) is an easily accessed database; however, to avoid narrowing the search focus and missing valuable evidence, dietetics professionals should consider using additional databases.
- Locating other sources of data and evidence. Examples include hand searches of reference lists of articles obtained from database searches, unpublished data from projects conducted at one's own facility, and abstracts presented at national conferences.
- Establishing search terms and keywords.
- Determining whether the terms should be in titles only or if they can be in the abstracts or text of the articles.

The search strategy should also list criteria regarding which types of evidence will be considered in making decisions about practice recommendations. Inclusion criteria define the class or type of research, study population, use of comparison or control groups, sample size of research groups, setting, time frame, and language.

Class or Type of Research

The preferred type of evidence is the randomized controlled trial (RCT) (9). However, if the number of relevant RCTs is limited, the dietetics professional may broaden the criteria to include other types of evidence. Box 20.1 (10) lists the classes or types and strength of evidence used by ADA in systematic reviews of the literature. Dietetics professionals should note that it is important to seek the original evidence or research when possible.

Study Population

Studies should have human participants, not animals, and participants should have a similar condition or disease, disease stage, and age range as the population for which the practice recommendations are intended (4).

Use of Comparison or Control Groups

Use of comparison groups is desirable and a factor in locating research on the evidence hierarchy (4). Random assignment to intervention and comparison groups is preferred.

Sample Size of Research Groups

Each group should contain at least 10 patients (4)—eg, 10 patients in the intervention group and 10 patients in the comparison or control group.

Setting

The setting should be similar to that of the population for which the practice recommendations are intended (4)—eg, inpatient, outpatient, community, or home care.

Time Frame

Research should be recent—ie, conducted within the past 5 years—unless it is considered to be a foundation for the area of practice (4).

Language

To be practical, it is advisable to limit articles to English (4).

Box 20.1

American Dietetic Association's Method of Evidence Analysis: Classes of Evidence Reports

Primary reports of new data collection (research report):

A. Randomized controlled (clinical) trial (RCT)
B. Cohort study
C. Nonrandomized trial with concurrent or historical controls
   Case-control study
   Study of sensitivity and specificity of a diagnostic test
   Population-based descriptive study
   Time series
D. Cross-sectional study
   Case series
   Case report
   Before and after study

Reports that synthesize or reflect on collections of primary reports:

M. Meta-analysis or systematic review
   Decision analysis
   Cost-benefit analysis
   Cost-effectiveness study
R. Narrative review (review article)
   Consensus statement
   Consensus report
X. Medical opinion

Source: Adapted from Greer N, Mosser G, Logan G, Wagstrom Halaas G. A practical approach to evidence grading. *Jt Comm J Qual Improv.* 2000; 26:700–712. Used with permission.

Step 4: Select Articles and Evidence That Meet the Search Criteria

In this step, the dietetics professional uses the search strategy to find articles and determines which ones meet the established search criteria. This is done by (*a*) reviewing a list of titles obtained from the search and omitting any articles that do not appear to meet the criteria, and (*b*) reading the abstracts of the remaining articles and omitting any that do not appear to meet the criteria. Dietetics professionals should keep a list of

Author/Yr	Design Type	Class	Quality (+, –, 0)	Population Studied/ Sample Size	Primary Outcome Measure(s)/Results	Authors' Conclusions/ *Work Group's Comments*

Figure 20.2. Evidence worksheet. Adapted with permission from American Dietetic Association Scientific Affairs and Research. *ADA Evidence Analysis Manual. Edition III*. Chicago, Ill: American Dietetic Association; 2003. Available at: http://www.eatright.org/ada/files/Evidence_Analysis_Manual_ed3a_Jan_26_05.pdf. Accessed November 28, 2005.

the articles that are excluded and the reasons for their exclusion, in case of a question about this later.

Step 5: Evaluate the Quality of the Research in the Articles

In step 5 (which usually takes 1 to 2 hours per article, including reading time), the ADA uses a three-part process to evaluate each article included in a systematic review (4):

1. Abstract or summarize key information from each article. Figure 20.2 (4) is an example that can be used for abstracting information.
2. Determine the class or type of article, and list it on the abstract form. (Refer to Box 20.1 for article classes.)
3. Evaluate the article by answering a set of questions about study validity and relevance to practice. Figures 20.3 and 20.4 are forms used by ADA evidence analysts to score the quality of a study based on an evaluation of the inclusion and exclusion criteria, study results, relevance to practice, and validity of studies (10). Figure 20.3 is used for research articles, and Figure 20.4 is used for summary review articles.

Step 6: Formulate Recommendations for Practice

In this step, the dietetics professional (*a*) creates a table to summarize the evidence from all the articles reviewed, (*b*) develops a conclusion statement that answers the original clinical question, and (*c*) assigns a grade to each conclusion statement, indicating the strength of the recommendation and the supporting evidence. Box 20.2 summarizes the conclusion grades that ADA uses for recommendations in position papers and the MNT Guides for Practice (10).

Step 7: Disseminate Recommendations and Use Them in Practice

In using evidence-based recommendations derived from systematic reviews of the literature, dietetics professionals may consider collecting and summarizing data on the process and the outcomes of MNT for groups of similar patients, eg, patients with the same type of cancer or receiving the same type of treatment (4). By tracking both the process of MNT and the outcomes of the practice recommendations, and by reporting this information in the professional literature, dietetics professionals share valuable evidence.

Plus (+)		Questions—Answer each either yes (Y) or no (N).
Y	N	1. Were the inclusion and exclusion criteria exceptionally well defined?
Y	N	2. Were no serious questions of bias introduced in the study (eg, through the process of subject selection, endpoint selection, observation, or data collection)?
Y	N	3. Does the report show a statistically significant and clinically important treatment effect or, for a negative conclusion, have a high power?
Y	N	4. Are the results widely generalizable to other populations?
Y	N	5. Were other characteristics of a well-designed study clearly addressed in the report (eg, treatment and control groups comparable at baseline, compliance with the intervention, use of intention to treat analysis, all important outcomes measured, and statistics appropriate for study design)?
		If the answer to 2 or more of the above questions is yes, the report may be designated with a plus on the Conclusion Grading Worksheet, depending on the work group's overall evaluation of the report.
Minus (–)		
Y	N	1. Were the inclusion and exclusion criteria unclear, or was there evidence of failure to adhere to defined criteria?
Y	N	2. Were serious questions of bias introduced in the study (eg, through the processes of subject selection, endpoint selection, observation, or data collection)?
Y	N	3. Does the report show a statistically significant but clinically insignificant effect or, for a negative conclusion, lack power and sample size?
Y	N	4. Are the results doubtfully generalizable to other populations?
Y	N	5. Were other characteristics of a poorly designed study clearly evident in the report (eg, treatment and control groups different at baseline, low compliance with intervention, important outcomes not measured, inappropriate statistics for study design)?
		If the answer to 2 or more of the above questions is yes, the report may be designated with a minus symbol on the Conclusion Grading Worksheet, depending on the work group's overall evaluation of the report.
Neutral (Ø)		
		If the answers to the questions pertaining to the PLUS or MINUS criteria do not indicate that the report is exceptionally strong or exceptionally weak, the report should be designated with a neutral symbol on the Conclusion Grading Worksheet

Figure 20.3. Research report quality scoring form. Reprinted from Greer N, Mosser G, Logan G, Wagstrom Halaas G. A practical approach to evidence grading. *Jt Comm J Qual Improv.* 2000;26:700–712. Used with permission.

Determine Relevance—Based on the conclusion of the article:		
Y	N	1. Is the article proposing to answer a specific clinical question?
Y	N	2. Will the answer, if true, have a direct bearing on the health of your patients, and is it something that they will care about?
Y	N	3. Is the problem addressed in the review one that is common to your practice, and is the intervention feasible?
Y	N	4. Will the information, if true, require you to change your practice?
		If the answer to all of the above questions is yes, the report may be designated with a **plus** on the Conclusion Grading Worksheet, depending on the work group's overall evaluation of the report.
Determine Validity:		
Y	N	1. Were methods used to locate relevant studies comprehensive and clearly stated?
Y	N	2. Were explicit methods used to select studies to include in the overview?
Y	N	3. Was the validity of the original studies included in the overview appropriately assessed?
Y	N	4. Was the assessment of the relevance and validity of the original studies reproducible and free from bias?
Y	N	5. Was variation between the results of the relevant studies analyzed (test of homogeneity)?
Y	N	6. Is there adequate documentation? Are references current? Do they refer to primary research studies rather than other review articles? Are supporting references provided?
Y	N	7. Is quantitative information presented in an appropriate way? Can you judge not only the statistical significance but also the clinical significance?
Y	N	8. If specific interventions are described, is the target population defined? Is the outcome clearly indicated?
Y	N	9. Were the results combined appropriately (apples to apples)?
		If the answer to any of the first three validity questions is no, the report may be designated with a **minus** symbol on the Conclusion Grading Worksheet, depending on the work group's overall evaluation of the report.
NEUTRAL (Ø)		
If the answers to the validity questions 4–9 do not indicate that the report is exceptionally strong, the report should be designated with a **neutral** symbol on the Conclusion Grading Worksheet.		

Figure 20.4. Review article quality scoring form. Adapted from Greer N, Mosser G, Logan G, Wagstrom Halaas G. A practical approach to evidence grading. *Jt Comm J Qual Improv.* 2000;26:700–712. Used with permission.

Box 20.2

Methods of Evidence Analysis: Conclusion Statement Grades

Grade I: Good

The evidence consists of results from studies of strong design for answering the question addressed. The results are both clinically important and consistent, with minor exceptions at most. The results are free of serious doubts about generalizability, bias, and flaws in research design. Studies with negative results have sufficiently large samples to have adequate statistical power.

Grade II: Fair

The evidence consists of results from studies of strong design answering the question addressed, but there is uncertainty attached to the conclusion, because of inconsistencies among the results from different studies or because of doubts about generalizability, bias, research design flaws, or adequacy of sample size. Alternatively, the evidence consists solely of results from weaker designs for the questions addressed, but the results have been confirmed in separate studies and are consistent, with minor exceptions at most.

Grade III: Limited

The evidence consists of results from a limited number of studies of weak design for answering the questions addressed. Evidence from studies of strong design is unavailable, either because no studies of strong design have been done or because studies that have been done are inconclusive due to lack of generalizability, bias, design flaws, or inadequate sample sizes.

Grade IV: Expert Opinion Only

The support of the conclusion consists solely of the statement of informed medical commentators based on their clinical experience, unsubstantiated by the results of any research studies.

Grade V: Not Assignable

There is no evidence available that directly supports or refutes the conclusion.

Source: Greer N, Mosser G, Logan G, Wagstrom Halaas G. A practical approach to evidence grading. *Jt Comm J Qual Improv.* 2000;26:700–712. Used with permission.

EVIDENCE ANALYSIS IN PRACTICE

Here is a practical application of the evidence analysis process in an oncology setting.

Step 1: Identify a Practice Problem

An RD receives a nutrition consult requesting recommendations for parenteral nutrition support for a 71-year-old man diagnosed with primary colon cancer, with metastasis to the liver. In addition to right upper quadrant pain, he has experienced anorexia and a 15-pound weight loss. Palliative chemotherapy is planned. The RD is concerned that parenteral nutrition may not achieve desired clinical outcomes and may in fact produce undesired side effects and complications. Similar consults have been received in the past. The RD identifies the following practice problem: Is parenteral nutrition support appropriate under these circumstances?

Step 2: Refine the Practice Problem Into a Clinical Question

Posing the practice problem as a clinical question, the RD asks: In patients with colon cancer undergoing chemotherapy, is initiation of parenteral nutrition support more effective in terms of maintaining or improving nutritional status (prevention of weight loss, preservation of muscle mass, and immunocompetence) than not initiating parenteral nutrition support?

Step 3: Search the Literature Using a Predetermined Search Strategy

The RD's first step was to look for existing practice guidelines, protocols, and structured abstracts, by searching the National Guideline Clearinghouse Web site, MNT Guides for Practice and Protocols, and publications of the American Society for Parenteral and Enteral Nutrition.

After doing this, the RD defined a strategy for searching the professional literature that included conducting a search of the Medline database for articles reporting the results of RCTs studying the use of parenteral nutrition support in human adult patients with cancer, preferably colon cancer (search terms: parenteral nutrition, chemotherapy, and nutritional status; subset—cancer), and a hand search of the reference lists of articles obtained through the Medline search. Studies selected were required to have a research design with control or comparison groups and a minimum of 10 patients randomly assigned to the intervention and comparison groups.

Step 4: Select Articles That Meet Specified Criteria

Numerous randomized trials have been conducted to evaluate the impact of parenteral nutrition support on patients with cancer; however, many of the articles were published before 1990. One clinical trial was specific to patients with colon cancer. Other references were identified: American College of Physicians (ACP) position statement and a systematic review conducted jointly by the National Institutes of Health (NIH), the American Society for Parenteral and Enteral Nutrition, and the American Society for Clinical Nutrition.

Step 5: Evaluate the Quality of the Research Reported in Each Article

Overall, the quality of the clinical trials was limited. In low-quality studies, the benefits of treatment tend to be overstated, and lack of effect or negative effects may be understated. Only one clinical trial was conducted in patients with colon cancer.

The ACP Position Statement and the NIH systematic review reported no benefit from the use of parenteral nutrition support. In addition, they reported an increased rate of infection. Clinical trial data did not support benefit from the use of parenteral nutrition support in terms of prognosis. In addition, the possibility of increased tumor growth as a result of parenteral nutrition support was identified.

Step 6: Formulate an Answer to the Clinical Question Based on the Evidence (What Is Known as Well as What Is Not Known)

The conclusion reached, based on limited evidence, is that parenteral nutrition support is generally not recommended for patients with end-stage cancer, because of the lack of data to support benefit, the possibility of increased infections resulting from this therapy, and the lack of favorable impact on prognosis.

Step 7: Disseminate Findings and Implement Recommendations in Practice

The RD presented the results of the systematic review at Oncology Grand Rounds. The data collected from this review were used to develop an institutional practice guideline for the appropriate use of parenteral nutrition support in patients with end-stage cancer.

INTEGRATING RESEARCH FINDINGS INTO DAILY PRACTICE

If the HOD's second research need is going to be achieved, dietetics professionals need to know how to incorporate research and the recommendations generated from systematic reviews of the literature into their care of patients. Dietetics professionals can incorporate evidence-based recommendations into all four steps of the Nutrition Care Process (NCP), as described in Chapter 5, by following these guidelines (11):

1. Assessment: Collect pertinent information, using valid and reliable methods for data collection; compare gathered data to evidence-based standards, norms, and ideals.
2. Nutrition diagnosis: Identify nutrition problems accurately and consistently, focusing on the primary problems associated with diseases and conditions.
3. Nutrition intervention: Select evidenced-based interventions that target actual or potential causes of the identified nutrition problems.

4. Monitoring and evaluation: Collect and review serial data, to evaluate how chosen interventions have altered the signs and symptoms associated with nutrition problems.

EVIDENCE-BASED TOOLS

Dietetics professionals can use evidence-based tools that were developed using the systematic review process, to incorporate research findings into their daily practice. Evidence-based tools include interdisciplinary guidelines, which can be accessed via the AHRQ National Guideline Clearinghouse (6) and the National Cancer Institute Web site (7). Dietetics professionals should read guidelines from these sites carefully, first to understand the process used in their development, and second to determine for whom their use is intended. For example, guidelines for one type of cancer do not necessarily apply to another type of cancer. Nor do guidelines for adults with cancer automatically apply to children with cancer. In addition, interdisciplinary guidelines may be limited in their nutrition recommendations. For these reasons, MNT Protocols, including the MNT protocols for cancer (12) and Guides for Practice (13,14), may be more useful when making decisions about MNT interventions. A revision of the MNT protocols for cancer patients is under development, using the more stringent systematic review process that ADA has since implemented, to ensure that the recommendations included are evidence based.

For many dietetics professionals, the challenge is implementing the protocols and guidelines in day-to-day practice. Issues that affect implementation include:

- Identifying patients at nutritional risk and patients with nutrition problems early in their course of treatment, rather than after substantial nutritional deficits have occurred.
- Developing referral mechanisms once risk has been identified.
- Defining the components of the nutrition assessment, to ensure that all relevant nutrition problems are identified and addressed.
- Finding data needed for nutrition assessment and reassessment (eg, laboratory data) and limited ability to order needed tests when not already available.
- Establishing systems for ongoing monitoring and evaluation of patients with nutrition problems.
- Implementing data collection processes for the outcomes, in order to evaluate the effectiveness of interventions in patients with the same diagnosis or nutrition problems.
- Providing care across the continuum and ensuring continuity in care, as patients move back and forth between inpatient and outpatient settings.
- Finding dietetics professionals to provide needed MNT intervention, and, in the outpatient setting, obtaining reimbursement for their services.

The issues hindering implementation of the oncology MNT protocol and other practice guidelines vary from one practice setting or clinic to another. Inclusion of managers and other health care team members in problem analysis and procedure development promotes acceptance of any procedures established and increases the likelihood that they will be followed.

PARTICIPATION IN RESEARCH IN THE PRACTICE SETTING

Collecting outcomes data for individual patients and summarizing the data for groups of similar patients help prepare dietetics professionals to conduct practice-based research. Developing and implementing systems for routine data collection allows some of the barriers to conducting research to be addressed.

For dietetics professionals who have not conducted research before, it may be helpful to begin by participating in a research project led by an experienced investigator or joining a cooperative research group. Participating in projects led by others allows opportunities for learning research methods in small segments.

Participating on a project also allows dietetics professionals to become accustomed to the time requirements for research and the commitment that is involved. This is important because for many, if not most, dietetics professionals in clinical practice settings, research activities must be completed in addition to their regular job duties, often on their own time.

Ideally, dietetics professionals will be able to participate in the planning of the projects led by others, in order to ensure collection and analysis of data related to MNT interventions in the research proposal. Principal investigators may be very interested in the effect of nutrition on the outcomes they are studying and may want to include a dietetics professional on their research team, but may not consider tracking the amount, type, and duration of MNT, which is the effect of having a dietetics professional who provides MNT on the outcomes of interest.

The steps in conducting a research project include the following:

1. Define the research question—ie, the question the research is intended to answer.
2. Review the literature relevant to the research question, to provide background for the project and help in defining the types of outcomes to collect and the data collection methods.
3. Specify the study design—the characteristics of the population to be studied, the sample size and sampling method, and use of a control or comparison group.
4. Select data and define data collection methods. Determine which data will be collected, how data will be collected and by whom, and how data will be analyzed; make plans to check for missing data during the project.
5. Develop a project timeline and plan for dissemination of results.
6. Write the research proposal and obtain approval from the Institutional Review Board (IRB).
7. Conduct a pilot study. Revisions may be needed based on the results of the pilot. If significant revisions are made, the proposal will need to be resubmitted to the IRB.
8. Implement the research project. Collect and analyze data; disseminate results; and identify opportunities for further research.

DIETETICS PRACTICE-BASED RESEARCH NETWORK

Understanding that limitations exist while seeking to promote practice-based research, ADA created a Dietetics Practice-Based Research Network (DPRN) (15), to assist dietetics professionals in clinical practice with conducting well-designed research projects. The DPRN is intended to bring practicing dietetics professionals together with experienced researchers in initiatives that identify needed research, based on common questions that arise in practice settings; design top-class research to answer these questions; and obtain funding to support the research. The experienced researchers will provide the technical support for dietetics professionals who conduct the much-needed multisite research to investigate nutrition issues within specific patient populations and in designated practice settings around the country (16). Dietetics professionals can obtain more information about the DPRN on the Research page of the ADA Web site (15). They can become DPRN members by completing the survey on this Web site.

REFERENCES

1. Manore MM, Myers EM. Research and the dietetics profession: making a bigger impact. *J Am Diet Assoc.* 2003;103:108–112.
2. Ayoob KT, Duyff RL, Quagliani D; American Dietetic Association. Position of the American Dietetic Association: food and nutrition misinformation. *J Am Diet Assoc.* 2002;102:260–266.
3. Myers EF, Pritchett E, Johnson EQ. Evidence-based practice guides vs. protocols: what's the difference? *J Am Diet Assoc.* 2001;101:1085–1090.
4. American Dietetic Association Scientific Affairs and Research. *ADA Evidence Analysis Manual.* 3rd ed. Chicago, Ill: American Dietetic Association; 2003. Available at: http://www.eatright.org/ada/files/Evidence_Analysis_Manual_ed3a_Jan_26_05.pdf. Accessed November 28, 2005.
5. Myers EF, Splett PL. Research in evidence-based practice. In: Monsen ER, ed. *Research: Successful Approaches.* 2nd ed. Chicago, Ill: American Dietetic Association; 2003:164–184.
6. Agency for Healthcare Quality and Research. National Guideline Clearinghouse. Available at: http://www.guideline.gov. Accessed May 16, 2005.
7. National Cancer Institute. Cancer information. Available at: http://www.nci.nih.gov/cancerinfo. Accessed May 16, 2005.
8. National Library of Medicine. PubMed Search Service. Available at: www.ncbi.nlm.nih.gov/entrez/query.fcgi. Accessed May 11, 2005.
9. Gray GE, Gray LK. Evidence-based medicine: applications in dietetic practice. *J Am Diet Assoc.* 2002; 102:1263–1271.

10. Greer N, Mosser G, Logan G, Wagstrom Halaas G. A practical approach to evidence grading. *Jt Comm J Qual Improv.* 2000;26:700–712.
11. Lacey K, Pritchett E. Nutrition Care Process and Model: ADA adopts road map to quality care and outcomes management. *J Am Diet Assoc*. 2003;103: 1061–1072.
12. American Dietetic Association. *Medical Nutrition Therapy Across the Continuum of Care.* 2nd ed. Chicago, Ill: American Dietetic Association; 1998.
13. American Dietetic Association. *American Dietetic Association Medical Nutrition Therapy Evidence Based Guides for Practice: Hyperlipidemia Medical Nutrition Therapy Protocol* [CD-ROM]. Chicago, Ill: American Dietetic Association; 2001.
14. American Dietetic Association. *American Dietetic Association Medical Nutrition Therapy Evidence Based Guides for Practice: Chronic Kidney Disease (Non-dialysis) Medical Nutrition Therapy Protocol* [CD-ROM]. Chicago, Ill: American Dietetic Association; 2002.
15. American Dietetic Association. Research activity: Dietetics Practice Based Research Network. Available at: http://www.eatright.org/cps/rde/xchg/SID-5303FFEA-5175E2A8/ada/hs.xsl/career_1698_ENU_HTML.htm. Accessed November 28, 2005.
16. Trostler N, Meyers EM. Blending practice and research: practice-based research networks an opportunity for dietetics professionals. *J Am Diet Assoc.* 2003;103:626–632.

Appendixes

Appendix A

Tips for Managing Nutrition Impact Symptoms

Symptom	*Potential Secondary Problems*	*Tips for Symptom Management*
Nausea	Vomiting, anorexia, weight loss, dehydration, electrolyte imbalances	• Try small, frequent feedings • Take liquids between meals/sips throughout the day/ice chips • Try room temperature or cold foods • Try dry, starchy, and/or salty foods (pretzels, saltines, potatoes, noodles, cooked cereals) • Try sips of ginger ale or candied dried ginger • Try peppermint candies • Try light exercise and cleansing breaths of fresh air • Avoid sweet, rich, greasy, and/or spicy foods • Avoid strong odors • Avoid favorite foods when nauseated to decrease potential aversions • Avoid liquids on an empty stomach • Avoid lying down for about an hour after eating

Vomiting	Anorexia, weight loss, dehydration, electrolyte imbalances	• If nausea precedes vomiting, try nausea management tips
		• If gagging on secretions is triggering vomiting, consider the following:
		  • Increase fluid intake to thin secretions (oral, pharyngeal, and respiratory)
		  • Rinse and gargle frequently with baking soda solution (1 Tbsp baking soda/1 quart water) to clean oropharynx and temporarily remove thick, ropey secretions
		  • Eat fresh pineapple, which might help thin oral and pharyngeal secretions
		  • Limit caffeine, as it is dehydrating
		  • Use a cool mist humidifier
		  • Avoid mouthwashes that contain alcohol, which can dry the mouth

Symptom	*Potential Secondary Problems*	*Tips for Symptom Management*
Anorexia	Weight loss, cachexia, dehydration, electrolyte imbalances	• Eat nutrient-dense meals and snacks frequently • Add protein and calories to favorite foods • Eat meals and snacks in pleasant atmosphere • Drink nutrient-dense beverages between meals to avoid feeling too full with meals • Try a small amount of wine, beer or aperitif to stimulate the appetite, if approved by the physician • Try light exercise to stimulate appetite • Capitalize on the times when feeling best (breakfast is often the best meal of the day)

Weight loss/cachexia	Electrolyte imbalances, impaired organ function, immunosuppression	• If cause of weight loss can be determined, treat appropriately
		• If cause cannot be determined, the patient may consider the following:
		  • Eat small, frequent, nutrient-dense meals and snacks
		  • Add protein and calories to favorite foods
		  • Take meals in snacks in pleasant atmosphere
		  • Keep nutrient-dense snacks close at hand and snack frequently
		  • Try a small amount of wine, beer, or aperitif to stimulate the appetite, if approved by the physician
		  • Capitalize on the times when feeling best (breakfast is often the best meal of the day)

Early satiety	Anorexia, weight loss, cachexia, electrolyte imbalances, bloating, nausea	• Eat small, frequent, nutrient-dense meals and snacks • Add protein and calories to favorite foods • Drink a nutrient-dense liquid diet, which may be more quickly digested and absorbed than solid food • Drink nutrient-dense liquids between meals to avoid feeling too full with meals • Avoid fried, greasy, or rich foods, which take longer to digest • Avoid gaseous foods, which can cause bloating • Capitalize on the times when feeling best (breakfast is often the best meal of the day) • Try light exercise to stimulate digestion
Constipation	Nausea, bloating, anorexia, weight loss	• Eat at regular intervals throughout the day • Increase fluid intake to 8–10 cup/day • Avoid caffeine • Increase dietary fiber, if able to take adequate fluids • Try hot beverages as a bowel stimulant • Try prune juice, preferably hot, as a bowel stimulant • Try to increase physical activity, as able • Try to establish a schedule for having bowel movements

Symptom	*Potential Secondary Problems*	*Tips for Symptom Management*
Diarrhea	Dehydration, electrolyte imbalances, malabsorption, anorexia, weight loss	• Add soluble fiber to diet at regular intervals throughout the day • Limit/avoid insoluble fiber • Eat small, frequent meals and snacks throughout the day • Avoid greasy, fried, spicy, or very rich foods • Avoid alcohol and caffeine • Avoid dairy products, or use lactase enzyme, if lactose intolerant • Avoid excessive amounts of sweetened beverages (fruit juice cocktails, fruit drinks, sodas, teas) and juices that might contribute to osmotic diarrhea • Avoid sugar-free gum and candy made with sorbitol • Increase fluid intake (1 cup water for each diarrheal stool) • Increase consumption of high-potassium foods if diarrhea is severe (potatoes and bananas are especially good, since they are also sources of soluble fiber) • Increase consumption of high-sodium foods if diarrhea is severe (commercially prepared broths and soups are good sources of fluid and sodium)
Malabsorption	Nutrient deficiencies	• Eat several small, frequent meals throughout the day • Avoid fluids and foods that promote diarrhea (intake and output should be monitored, along with the number, color, and consistency of stools to determine foods that are problematic) • Increase fluid intake (1 cup water/diarrheal or steatorrheal stool)
Lactose intolerance	Avoidance of dairy products without diet instruction or supplementation could lead to calcium and vitamin D deficiencies	• Try lactase enzyme supplement to help digest dairy products; dosage should be titrated to alleviate symptoms • Try dairy products treated with lactase enzyme • Limit/avoid dairy products; substitute milk with soy or rice milk or Vita Mite nondairy beverage; increase consumption of nondairy high-calcium foods
Xerostomia	Difficulty chewing and swallowing, decreased intake of food	• Try tart foods to stimulate saliva • Sip on liquids or suck on ice chips throughout the day (aim for 8–10 cups of fluid per day) • Try sipping fruit nectars throughout the day • Try drinking through a straw • Rinse the mouth frequently with baking soda solution (1 Tbsp baking soda/1 quart water) • Try sucking on lemon drops, eating frozen grapes, popsicles or chewing sugar-free gum • Avoid caffeine • Avoid alcohol and tobacco • Avoid alcohol-containing mouthwashes • Try soft and/or moist foods with extra sauce, dressings, or gravies • Try using a cool mist humidifier

Symptom	*Potential Secondary Problems*	*Tips for Symptom Management*
Taste changes	Anorexia, decreased intake of food, weight loss	• Try different protein source—like poultry, fish, eggs, dairy products, beans, and soy products—if red meat is unappealing • Try marinades and spices to mask strange tastes • Use plastic utensils rather than stainless steel to help alleviate metal taste • Try to eat foods at room temperature or chilled • Add lemon, lime, vinegar, or salt to foods that seem too sweet • Try adding lemon, lime, instant decaffeinated coffee powder, or mint to milkshakes or commercially prepared supplements that taste too sweet • Rinse the mouth frequently with baking soda solution (1 Tbsp baking soda/1 Quart water) • Try sipping pleasant-tasting beverages, sucking popsicles or hard candy, or eating sherbet or sorbet to mask bad taste between meals • Try fresh or frozen foods rather than canned
Dysphagia	Decreased intake, weight loss	• Follow instructions regarding diet consistency and swallowing techniques provided by the speech pathologist • Try soft, moist, or pureed foods—uniform consistency is best, as opposed to chunky soups and stews • Eat smaller, more frequent meals and snacks • Use commercially prepared food thickeners, tapioca, flour, instant mashed potatoes, infant rice cereal, and/or cornstarch to thicken liquids, as advised by the speech pathologist • Avoid breads, cakes, cookies, and crackers, or soak in milk, juice, gravy, or sauce before eating • Try ice, sherbet/sorbet, or popsicles before a meal to stimulate the swallowing reflex, as advised by the speech pathologist
Mucositis	Decreased intake, weight loss	• Try soft, moist foods with extra sauce, dressings, and gravies (watch for acidic ingredients like tomatoes, citrus, or vinegar, however) • Use a straw to direct fluid away from the painful parts of the mouth • Avoid alcohol, citrus, caffeine, tomatoes, vinegar, and hot peppers • Avoid dry, coarse, or rough foods • Avoid spicy foods • Try foods at room temperature or chilled • Try sucking popsicles or ice chips to numb the mouth • Rinse the mouth frequently with baking soda solution (1 Tbsp baking soda/1 quart water) • Avoid alcohol-containing mouthwashes

Symptom	*Potential Secondary Problems*	*Tips for Symptom Management*
Esophagitis	Decreased intake, weight loss	• Try soft, moist foods with extra sauce, dressings, and gravies (watch for acidic ingredients like tomatoes, citrus, or vinegar, however) • Use a straw to direct fluid away from the painful parts of the mouth • Avoid alcohol, citrus, caffeine, tomatoes, vinegar, and hot peppers • Avoid dry, coarse, or rough foods • Avoid spicy foods • Try foods at room temperature or chilled • Try sucking popsicles or ice chips to numb the mouth • Rinse the mouth and gargle frequently with baking soda solution (1 Tbsp baking soda/1 quart water) • Avoid alcohol-containing mouthwashes
Oral candidiasis	Taste changes, sore mouth, decreased intake, weight loss; can spread to the pharynx and esophagus, causing and sore throat and dysphagia	• Try soft, moist foods with extra sauce, dressings, and gravies (watch for acidic ingredients like tomatoes, citrus, or vinegar, however) • Use a straw to direct fluid away from the painful parts of the mouth • Avoid alcohol, citrus, caffeine, tomatoes, vinegar, and hot peppers • Avoid dry, coarse, or rough foods • Avoid spicy foods • Try foods at room temperature or chilled • Try sucking popsicles or ice chips to numb the mouth • Rinse the mouth and gargle frequently with baking soda solution (1 Tbsp baking soda/1 quart water) • Avoid alcohol-containing mouthwashes
Pain (not specific to the alimentary tract)	Anorexia, nausea and vomiting, weight loss	• Try small frequent feedings • Try soft foods at room temperature or chilled • Try deep cleansing breaths of fresh air • Try to eat dry, starchy, and/or salty foods frequently throughout the day to manage nausea • Take sips of cool, soothing beverages between meals • Try peppermint candy or gum to relieve nausea • Try candied dried ginger to relieve nausea • Take pain medications as ordered (usually around the clock, rather than PRN), to avoid "catching up with the pain"

References

1. American Cancer Society. *Nutrition for the Person with Cancer*. Atlanta, Ga: American Cancer Society; 2002.
2. American Institute for Cancer Research. *Nutrition of the Cancer Patient*. Washington, DC: American Institute for Cancer Research; 2000.
3. Dobbin M, Hartmuller VW. Suggested management of nutrition-related symptoms. In: McCallum PD, Polisena CG, eds. *The Clinical Guide to Oncology Nutrition.* Chicago, Ill: American Dietetic Association; 2000:164–167.
4. National Cancer Institute. Physician Data Query, Supportive Care. Available at: http://www.cancer.gov/cancerinfo/pdq/supportivecare. Accessed May 17, 2005.
5. Walker MS, Masino K. *Oncology Nutrition Patient Education Materials*. Chicago, Ill: American Dietetic Association; 1998.
6. McCallum PD. Management of nutrition impact symptoms. In: *Nutrition in Cancer Treatment.* Eureka, Calif: Nutrition Dimension, Inc; 2003.

Appendix B

Resources

DEE GABBARD, RD

INTRODUCTION

Compiling a list of resources for both public and professional use is a monumental task. This list is not guaranteed to be comprehensive, but it is thorough. The following criteria were used to select the resources:

- Authored by a medical professional
- Endorsed by a nationally recognized professional organization
- Based on research or science
- Available or accessible at the time of publication

The resources are categorized by the type of media, including books, journals, brochures/audiovisual/other, and agencies/Web sites. These categories are arranged by the subspecialties encountered in the spectrum of oncology practice ranging from prevention to palliative care.

AGENCIES/WEB SITES

General Oncology

AMERICAN CANCER SOCIETY (ACS)

http://wwww.cancer.org

Provides information on all aspects of cancer and cancer support.

AMERICAN INSTITUTE FOR CANCER RESEARCH (AICR)

http://www.aicr.org

Offers a variety of services, from a nutrition hotline to healthful living tips.

THE ASSOCIATION OF CANCER ONLINE RESOURCES (ACOR)

http://www.acor.org

Offers access to mailing lists that provide support, information, and community to everyone affected by cancer and related disorders.

CANCER NEWS ON THE NET

http://www.cancernews.com

Brings patients and their families the latest news and information on cancer diagnosis, treatment, and prevention.

CANCER SOURCE

http://cancersource.com

Offers current cancer information and resources for professionals and consumers, including interactive tools and programming.

CURE Magazine

http://curetoday.com

Offers cancer information for patients and their loved ones. *CURE* stands for Cancer Updates, Research, and Education. This is a good educational magazine. Readers can get back issues online.

Food and Drug Administration

http://www.fda.gov

Provides food and drug safety information and recalls.

Guide to Internet Resources for Cancer

http://www.cancerindex.org

Provides more than 100 pages and more than 4,000 links to cancer-related information.

MEDLINEplus

http://www.nlm.nih.gov/medlineplus

Provides links to current, trustworthy health care information. Links are compiled by the National Library of Medicine at the National Institutes of Health (NIH). Topics include health and nutrition, drug information, and directories of doctors and hospitals.

National Cancer Institute (NCI)

http://www.cancer.gov

Provides information on cancer diagnosis, treatment, and supportive care, including nutrition information and PDQ summaries.

National Cancer Institute Cancer Information Service/PDQ

http://cancernet.nci.nih.gov

Provides current, comprehensive information on all major types of cancer, treatments, and clinical trials, plus referrals to treatment facilities and doctors, via telephone, fax, online, and print.

Oncolink

http://cancer.med.upenn.edu

Provides information on different types of cancer, treatment options, clinical trials, and resources, and a library. Oncolink is sponsored by the Abramson Cancer Center of the University of Pennsylvania.

Oncology Nursing Society

http://ons.org

Provides information for health care providers, people with cancer, and their caregivers.

The University of Texas MD Anderson Cancer Center

http://www.mdanderson.org

Examines the latest cancer news and information.

Oncology Nutrition

Cancer Nutrition Info

http://www.cancernutritioninfo.com

Provides information on cancer prevention and symptom management. Research summaries and educational materials available through subscription. Written by Suzanne Dixon, MPH, MS, RD.

Diana Dyer's Web Site

http://cancerRD.com

Provides information and inspiration for cancer survivors regarding nutrition and lifestyle choices from a three-time cancer survivor.

Oncology Nutrition Dietetic Practice Group Web Site

http://oncologynutrition.org

Includes valuable resources for patients, dietitians, and other health care professionals.

Caregivers

National Family Caregivers' Association

http://www.nfcacares.org

Provides counseling support, toll-free line, education, respite care, and advocacy for caregivers.

Today's Caregiver Magazine

http://www.caregiver.com

Bimonthly, national magazine for family and professional caregivers.

Well Spouse Foundation

http://www.wellspouse.org

Provides support groups, newsletters, conferences, and bereavement counseling for partners of the chronically ill or disabled.

Complementary and Alternative Medicine

About Herbs from Memorial Sloan Kettering Cancer Center

http://www.mskcc.org/mskcc/html/11570.cfm

The consumer version is available to help the general public sift through the confusing claims made for over-the-counter products and programs.

American Botanical Council

http://www.herbalgram.org

Nonprofit organization devoted to promoting responsible use of herbal medicine.

American Cancer Society, Dietary Supplements

http://www.cancer.org/docroot/MBC/MBC_6_1_DietarySupplements.asp

Offers information on dietary supplements, vitamins, minerals, and herbal products.

American Dietetic Association Complementary Care Practice Group

http://www.complementarynutrition.org

Web site of the Complementary Care Dietetic Practice Group, which promotes the integration of conventional nutrition practices with evidence-based alternatives through education, research, and practice. Links to Web sites, books, and resources.

American Herbal Products Association

http://ahpa.org

Certifies companies with good manufacturing processes.

Columbia University Rosenthal Center, Carol Ann Schwartz Cancer Initiative

http://www.rosenthal.hs.columbia.edu

Provides information about current complementary research studies and findings.

Consumer Lab

http://www.consumerlabs.com

Offers independent reviews of dietary supplements.

FDA Center for Food Safety and Applied Nutrition: Dietary Supplements—Tips for the Savvy Supplement User

http://www.cfsan.fda.gov/~dms/ds-savvy.html

Gives tips for making informed decisions and evaluating information about dietary supplements.

FDA Center for Food Safety and Applied Nutrition: Dietary Supplements—Warnings and Safety Information

http://www.cfsan.fda.gov/~dms/ds-warn.html

Provides warnings and safety information about dietary supplements (vitamins, minerals, herbs, botanicals, and enzymes).

FDA MedWatch

http://www.fda.gov/medwatch/index.html

Program for FDA safety information and for reporting adverse effects.

Herb Research Foundation

http://www.herbs.org

A source of accurate and science-based information on health benefits and safety of herbs; available through subscription.

Integrative Therapies Program for Children with Cancer

http://carolann.hs.columbia.edu

Provides information on pediatric cancer and alternative medicine.

International Bibliographic Information on Dietary Supplements (IBIDS)

http://ods.od.nih.gov/Health_Information/IBIDS.aspx

Access to bibliographic citations and abstracts.

Longwood Herbal Task Force

http://www.longwoodherbal.org

Gives information about herbal supplements, monographs, toxicity information, fact sheets, and clinical information summaries.

Memorial Sloan Kettering Cancer Center Integrative Medicine Service

http://www.mskcc.org/mskcc/html/11917.cfm

Provides answers to frequently asked questions regarding herbs, botanicals, and other products.

National Cancer Institute: Summary of Complementary Therapies

http://www.cancer.gov/cancerinfo/pdq/cam

Offers summaries of substances promoted to cancer patients.

National Center for Complementary and Alternative Medicine

http://altmed.od.nih.gov

Provides health information, alerts, advisories, and research information on complementary therapies.

National Council Against Health Fraud

http://www.ncahf.org

Provides science-based opinions of health information and quackery.

Natural Medicines Comprehensive Database

http://www.naturaldatabase.com

A database available by subscription, which includes the safety and efficacy of herbal supplements.

Office of Dietary Supplements

http://dietary-supplements.info.nih.gov

NIH site about dietary supplements.

Quackwatch

http://www.quackwatch.org

Quackwatch, Inc, a member of Consumer Federation of America, is a nonprofit corporation whose purpose is to combat health-related frauds, myths, fads, and fallacies. Hundreds of articles, reviews, and opinions.

Steve Dunn's Cancer Guide

http://cancerguide.org/index.html

Helps find the answers to questions about cancer, and helps find the questions patients need to ask. Includes good information on alternative therapies.

Hospice

California State Hospice and Palliative Care Association

http://www.calhospice.org

Provides technical resources to its membership, monitors state legislative and regulatory activities, and works closely with other organizations that have an interest in end-of-life care. It partners with the California Hospice Foundation to offer public and professional educational programs and materials to enhance understanding and availability of hospice and palliative care.

Growth House

http://www.growthhouse.org

Provides resources for life-threatening illness and end-of-life care. Provides information on palliative care and grief.

Hospice Association of America

http://www.hospice-america.org

Offers general information about hospice, including consumer guides, fact sheets, historical perspectives, and other background information.

Hospice Education Institute

http://www.hospiceworld.org

An independent, not-for-profit organization serving members of the public and health care professionals with information and education about the many facets of caring for the dying and the bereaved.

Hospice Foundation of America

http://www.hospicefoundation.org

A nonprofit organization that promotes hospice care and works to educate professionals and the families they serve in issues relating to care giving, terminal illness, loss, and bereavement.

Hospice Net

http://www.hospicenet.org

Provides support for patients with life-threatening illness and their children, family members, and caregivers.

National Cancer Institute, Advanced Directives

http://www.cancer.gov/cancertopics/factsheet/support/advance-directives

This fact sheet provides patients with an outline for thinking about end-of-life issues and some guidelines for discussion with their doctors, families, and loved ones.

National Hospice and Palliative Care Organization

http://www.nhpco.org

A nonprofit organization representing hospice and palliative care programs and professionals in the United States.

Pediatrics

Bandaides and Blackboards

http://www.lehman.cuny.edu/faculty/jfleitas/bandaides

A site about growing up with medical problems. Its goal is to help people understand what it is like, from the perspective of the children and teens who are doing just that.

Childhood Cancer Foundation

http://www.candlelighters.ca

A national volunteer charitable organization dedicated to improving the quality of life for families experiencing the effects of childhood cancer through the provision of resources, parent support, and the promotion of research. This organization has put a large resource catalog online at their Web site, including categories for "When a Parent Dies," "When a Parent Has Cancer," "Coping with Childhood Cancer," "Siblings," "Bereavement," and "Adolescents."

Children's Oncology Group

http://www.childrensoncologygroup.org

Provides information about clinical trials for pediatric cancers.

National Children's Cancer Society

http://www.children-cancer.com

Helps children with cancer through nationwide programs and services.

Pediatric Oncology Resource Center

http://www.acor.org/diseases/ped-onc

Provides information on childhood cancers, treatment, family issues, and activism.

Special Love

http://www.speciallove.org

Provides camps, day trips, and fun programs for kids with cancer.

Prevention

American Institute for Cancer Research

http://www.aicr.org

This site provides the latest research-based advice regarding nutrition practices to reduce the risk for cancer.

Cancer Research Foundation of America

http://www.preventcancer.org

Provides information on cancer that may be prevented by lifestyle, screening, and early treatment. Includes breast, colon, prostate, lung, cervical, and testicular cancers.

National Cancer Institute, Division of Cancer Prevention

http://www3.cancer.gov/prevention/lifestyle.html

This site addresses lifestyle factors, including good nutrition, to help reduce the risk of cancer. It also offers sound information regarding artificial sweeteners and food additives.

Research

Cancer Nutrition Info

http://www.cancernutritioninfo.com

Cancer Nutrition Info provides up-to-date and comprehensive information on the connection between nutrition and cancer. This site is useful both for individuals living with cancer and their friends, family, and health care providers. Nutrition information is provided both for treatment and prevention of cancer.

CRISP (Computer Retrieval of Information on Scientific Projects)—National Institutes of Health

http://crisp.cit.nih.gov

A searchable database of federally funded biomedical research projects conducted at universities, hospitals, and other research institutions.

TheDataWeb

http://thedataweb.org

An online network of data libraries created by the US Census Bureau and the Centers for Disease Control and Prevention.

Finding Clinical Trials (National Cancer Institute)

http://cancer.gov/clinicaltrials/finding

This Web site provides comprehensive information for the lay reader about participating in clinical research trials. From the National Cancer Institute.

Institute of Medicine: Dietary Reference Intakes Tables and Food and Nutrition Board

http://www.iom.edu/board.asp?id=3788

This site offers links to Food and Nutrition Board and Institute of Medicine reports, including the Dietary Reference Intakes series.

NATIONAL HEALTH AND NUTRITION EXAMINATION SURVEY, NATIONAL CENTER FOR HEALTH STATISTICS

http://www.cdc.gov/nchs/nhanes.htm

This site provides information about the health and diet of people in the United States, with data from home interviews and health tests that are done in a mobile examination center. The current NHANES is the eighth in a series of national examination studies conducted in the United States since 1960.

ONCOLINK

http://www.oncolink.com

The University of Pennsylvania's resource center on clinical trials, cancer treatments, and cancer research.

ONCOLINK LIBRARY

http://cancer.med.upenn.edu/library/index.cfm

This Web site is a collection of book, music, and video reviews related to cancer. It also provides links to medical journals and medical literature databases.

PUBMED (MEDLINE)/NATIONAL LIBRARY OF MEDICINE

http://www.ncbi.nlm.nih.gov/entrez/query.fcgi

Free online access to MedLine. Includes links to online journals when available.

USDA NUTRIENT DATA LABORATORY

http://www.nal.usda.gov/fnic/foodcomp

This Web site offers one-stop shopping for the USDA's nutrient data. The USDA National Nutrient Database can be downloaded from this site, as well as the Nutritive Value of Foods (Home and Garden Bulletin no. 72), and many other single-nutrient food composition tables.

Specific Cancers

Lung Cancer

ALLIANCE FOR LUNG CANCER ADVOCACY, SUPPORT AND EDUCATION (ALCASE)

http://www.alcase.org

ALCASE is a national not-for-profit organization dedicated solely to helping people with lung cancer, and those who are at risk for the disease, improve the quality of their lives through advocacy, support, and education.

LUNG CANCER ONLINE

http://wwwlungcanceronline.org

A gateway to lung cancer resources for the benefit of people with lung cancer and their families. Site is intended to facilitate the time-consuming and often frustrating process of learning about lung cancer, treatment options, and support services.

Colorectal Cancer

COLON CANCER ALLIANCE

http://www.ccalliance.org

The Colon Cancer Alliance is an organization of colon and rectal cancer survivors, caregivers, people with a genetic predisposition to the disease, and other individuals touched by colorectal cancer. Colorectal cancer is the second leading cancer killer in the United States. The Colon Cancer Alliance is committed to ending the suffering caused by cancers of the colon, rectum, appendix, and anus.

OSTOMY ASSOCIATION OF SOUTHWESTERN INDIANA

http://www.ostomy.evansville.net

Provides support and education for individuals with ostomies.

Breast Cancer

CANCER INDEX, BREAST CANCER RESOURCES DIRECTORY

http://www.cancerindex.org/clinks3.htm

Includes breast cancer resources such as Breast Cancer Organizations, Information for Patients and the Public, Information for Health Professionals, Personal Experiences, Paget's Disease of the Breast, Breast Cancer Screening and Self Examination, Hereditary Breast Cancer, Molecular Biology of Breast Cancer, Multimedia Breast Cancer Resources, Male Breast Cancer, Lymphedema.

Y-ME-NATIONAL BREAST CANCER ORGANIZATION

http://www.y-me.org

Provides hotline counseling, educational programs, and support and self-help meetings for breast cancer survivors and families.

Blood-Related Cancers/Disorders

BLOOD AND MARROW TRANSPLANT INFORMATION NETWORK

http://www.bmtinfonet.org

A not-for-profit organization dedicated exclusively to serving the needs of persons facing a bone marrow, blood stem cell, or umbilical cord blood transplant.

LEUKEMIA AND LYMPHOMA SOCIETY

http://www.leukemia.org

The world's largest voluntary health organization dedicated to funding blood cancer research, education, and patient services. The society's mission is to cure leukemia, lymphoma, Hodgkin's disease, and myeloma, and to improve the quality of life of patients and their families.

Head and Neck Cancers

GUIDE TO INTERNET RESOURCES FOR HEAD AND NECK CANCER

http://www.cancerindex.org/clinks2h.htm

Resources on head and neck cancer, molecular biology of head and neck cancers, oral cancer, laryngeal cancer, and nasopharyngeal cancer.

LET'S FACE IT

http://www.faceit.org

A nonprofit network that links people with facial disfigurement to resources that can enrich their lives.

SUPPORTING PEOPLE WITH ORAL AND HEAD AND NECK CANCER

http://www.spohnc.org

A patient-directed, self-help organization dedicated to meeting the needs of oral and head and neck cancer patients. SPOHNC addresses the broad emotional, physical, and humanistic needs of this population.

Pancreatic Cancer

THE PANCREATIC CANCER ACTION NETWORK (PANCAN)

http://www.pancan.org

Works to focus national attention on the need to find the cure for pancreatic cancer. Provides public and professional education that embraces the urgent need for more research, effective treatments, prevention programs, and early detection methods.

Brain Tumors

BRAIN TUMOR SOCIETY

http://www.braintumorsociety.org

A resource for patients with a new diagnosis, survivors, and health care professionals.

National Brain Tumor Foundation

http://www.braintumor.org
Provides support, referrals, treatment information, and a newsletter; raises funds for brain tumor research.

Lymphoma

Lymphoma Research Foundation of America

http://www.lymphoma.org
Provides educational materials, support groups and help-line, a national "buddy" system, and a quarterly newsletter.

Gynecological Cancer

Gynecologic Cancer Foundation/Women's Cancer Network

http://www.wcn.org
Offers support programs to benefit women who have or are at risk for developing a gynecological cancer. The Women's Cancer Network is an interactive Web site providing information about the disease, treatment options, and new therapies.

Prostate Cancer

Prostate Cancer Foundation

http://www.prostatecancerfoundation.org
Has information on nutrition and lifestyle recommendations.

US-TOO

http://www.ustoo.com
Provides support groups and a newsletter for prostate cancer survivors.

Thyroid Cancer

American Thyroid Association

http://www.thyroid.org
Provides patient education material, support, a newsletter, and research for people with thyroid cancer and other diseases of the thyroid.

Support Groups and Survivors

American Cancer Society, The Cancer Survivors Network

http://www.acscsn.org
A forum for people whose lives have been touched by cancer. Includes personal stories, discussions, and expressions of caring.

American Institute for Cancer Research: Survivor Area

http://www.aicr.org/survivor
Section of the American Institute for Cancer Research Web site for individuals who are cancer survivors.

Cancer Care

http://www.cancercare.org
A nonprofit social service agency that helps survivors and families cope with the emotional, psychological, and financial consequences of cancer. Individual, family, or group counseling is available in Connecticut, New York, and New Jersey, and referrals are provided in other states. Callers to the toll-free counseling hotline speak with a social worker.

Cancer Supportive Care

http://www.cancersupportivecare.com
Coping tips and support for the survivor undergoing therapy.

Diana Dyer, A Dietitian's Cancer Story

http://www.cancerrd.com
Diana Dyer is a three-time cancer survivor and registered dietitian. Her Web site provides nutrition and general information to cancer survivors. There is a useful list of links to other Web sites.

Lance Armstrong Foundation

http://www.laf.org
Aims to enhance the quality of life for those living with, through, and beyond cancer. The Web site contains a useful list of resources.

National Coalition for Cancer Survivorship

http://www.canceradvocacy.org

A network of organizations and individuals concerned with the support of cancer survivors and their families. It serves as a clearinghouse for information on services and materials for survivors, advocates the rights and interests of survivors, encourages the study of survivorship, and promotes the development of support activities.

People Living With Cancer

http://www.plwc.org

Current cancer news with live chats on timely topics.

The Wellness Community

http://www.thewellnesscommunity.org

A national support program devoted solely to providing free psychological and emotional support to cancer survivors at all stages and their families. There are more than 20 facilities in the United States.

Symptom Management

General Suggestions

American Cancer Society: When Treatment Causes Eating Problems

http://www.cancer.org/docroot/MBC/MBC_6_1_when_treatment_causes_eating_problems.asp

Suggestions for dealing with the problems that can occur due to treatment.

Cancer Nutrition Info

http://www.cancernutritioninfo.com

Medical nutrition therapy and recipes to prevent and relieve side effects of cancer and cancer treatments.

National Cancer Institute: Coping With Side Effects

http://www.cancer.gov/cancer_information/coping

Information and strategies to help deal with the side effects of cancer treatment.

National Cancer Institute: Patient Information on Nutrition During Cancer Treatment

http://cancer.gov/cancerinfo/pdq/supportivecare/nutrition/patient

Resource on cancer treatments and effects on nutrition status as well as nutrition assessment and treatment guidelines.

Swallowing Problems

Dysphagia Online

http://www.dysphagiaonline.com

Provides information on dysphagia, treatment options, and eating tips.

Dysphagia Resource Center

http://www.dysphagia.com

Contains a vendor list that is helpful for purchasing thickeners and devices to make swallowing easier.

Diarrhea

National Cancer Institute: Gastrointestinal Complications PDQ®—Patient Version

http://www.cancer.gov/cancertopics/pdq/supportivecare/gastrointestinalcomplications/Patient

Suggestions on dealing with both acute and chronic diarrhea due to radiation therapy.

Food Safety

American Cancer Society: Food Handling Tips

http://www.cancer.org/docroot/MBC/content/MBC_6_2X_Food_Handling_Tips.asp?sitearea=MBC

Safe food handling tips to help prevent food-borne illness.

Treatment Modalities

Surgery

American Cancer Society: When You Have Cancer Surgery

http://www.cancer.org/docroot/MBC/content/MBC_6_2X_When_You_Have_Cancer_Surgery.asp?sitearea=MBC

Information on general side effects of surgery and effects on nutrition.

Radiation Therapy

American Cancer Society: When You Have Radiation Therapy

http://www.cancer.org/docroot/MBC/content/MBC_6_2X_When_You_Have_Radiation_Therapy.asp?sitearea=MBC

Information about radiation therapy and the side effects associated with this type of treatment.

Radiology

RadiologyInfo

http://www.radiologyinfo.org

Answers questions related to the many radiologic procedures and therapies, including how various x-ray, CT, MRI, ultrasound, radiation therapy, and other procedures are performed, what the patient may experience, and how to prepare for examinations. The Web site does not cover all radiologic procedures and therapies, but it is frequently updated. All material on the Web site is reviewed and approved by experts in the field of radiology.

Chemotherapy

American Cancer Society: When You Have Chemotherapy

http://www.cancer.org/docroot/MBC/content/MBC_6_2X_When_You_Have_Chemotherapy.asp?sitearea=MBC

Information on chemotherapy and the side effects that affect nutrition.

Tirgan Oncology Associates: List of Chemotherapy Drugs and Side Effects

http://www.tirgan.com/chemolst.htm

This Web site is under the supervision of Dr. Tirgan, a practicing hematologist-oncologist affiliated with St. Luke's-Roosevelt Hospital Center in New York. The list of chemotherapy drugs is written in layperson's language and includes side effects.

Tube Feedings

Cincinnati Children's Hospital Medical Center: Home Care

http://www.cincinnatichildrens.org/health/info/abdomen/home

This Web page gives an overview of pediatric gastrostomy-jejunostomy tube care. It contains a handy list of supplies needed to maintain the care of the feeding tube, procedure for cleaning and dressing the wound, flushing the g-tube, giving medications or feedings, giving medicines, protecting the tube, and problem-solving.

Horizon Health Care Home Services: Educational Resources

http://www.horizonhealthcareservices.com/resources/enteral_therapy_tube.htm

Step-by-step instructions for care of the feeding tube, care of the tube site, mouth care, proper positioning, and when to notify your home health nurse of problems.

Oley Foundation

http://oley.org

A nonprofit organization that provides information and support for home tube feeding and parenteral nutrition patients, caregivers, and professionals.

Oral Cancer Foundation: Feeding Tubes

http://www.oralcancerfoundation.org/dental/tube_feeding.htm

Brief overview about feeding tubes.

UNIVERSITY OF NEW YORK—SUNY UPSTATE MEDICAL UNIVERSITY HOSPITAL: PATIENT EDUCATION ON GASTROSTOMY FEEDINGS

http://www.upstate.edu/uhpated/pdf/peds/gastrogravitysyringe.pdf

Three pages of instructions for the care and use of the gastrostomy feedings—gravity drip or syringe method of feeding a child—in a downloadable PDF format.

BOOKS AND OTHER PUBLICATIONS

Prevention

American Institute for Cancer Research. *Food, Nutrition, and the Prevention of Cancer: A Global Perspective*. Washington, DC: American Institute for Cancer Research; 1997.

Heber D, Bowerman S. *What Color Is Your Diet? The 7 Colors of Health*. New York, NY: Regan Books; 2001.

Joseph J, Nadeau D, Underwood A. *The Color Code. A Revolutionary Eating Plan for Optimum Health.* New York, NY: Hyperion Books; 2003.

National Cancer Institute. 5-a-day program. Available at: http://www.5aday.gov. Accessed November 7, 2005.

Complementary and Alternative Medicine

American Cancer Society. *American Cancer Society's Guide to Complementary and Alternative Cancer Methods*. Atlanta, Ga: American Cancer Society; 2000.

Blumenthal M, ed. *Herbal Medicine: Expanded Commission E Monographs*. Philadelphia, Pa: Lippincott Williams and Wilkins; 2000.

Fetrow CF, Avila JR, eds. *Professionals Handbook of Complementary and Alternative Medicines.* 2nd ed. Springhouse Corporation; 2001.

Fragakis AS. *The Health Professional's Guide to Popular Dietary Supplements.* 3rd ed. Chicago, Ill; American Dietetic Association; 2006.

Herr SM, Ernst E, Young VS. *Herb-Drug Interaction Handbook.* 2nd ed. Nassau, NY: Church Street Books; 2002.

PDR for Herbal Medicines by Medical Economics. 3rd ed. Montvale, NJ: Thompson Healthcare; 2004.

Rakel D, ed. *Integrative Medicine*. Philadelphia, Pa: WB Saunders; 2002.

United States Pharmacopoeia. USP-24/NF-19. Rockville, Md: Stationery Office Books; 1999.

Medical Nutrition Therapy

ASPEN. *Oncology Diet and Nutrition Patient and Education Resource Manual.* Gaithersburg, Md: Aspen Publishers; 2001.

Byers T, Nestle M, McTiernan A, Doyle C, Currie-Williams A, Gansler T, Thun M; American Cancer Society 2001 Nutrition and Physical Activity Guidelines Advisory Committee. American Cancer Society guidelines on nutrition and physical activity for cancer prevention: reducing the risk of cancer with healthy food choices and physical activity. *CA Cancer J Clin.* 2002;52: 92–119.

Eldridge B. Medical nutrition therapy and neoplastic disease. In: Mahan LK, ed. *Krause's Food, Nutrition, and Diet Therapy*. 11th ed. Philadelphia, Pa: WB Saunders; 2003.

Eldridge B, Hamilton K. *Management of Nutrition Impact Symptoms in Cancer and Educational Handouts.* Chicago, Ill: American Dietetic Association; 2004.

Heber D, Blackburn GL, Go VL, Holland JF. *Nutritional Oncology.* San Diego, Calif: Academic Press; 1999.

McCallum P, Polisena C. *Patient Generated Subjective Global Assessment Video.* Chicago, Ill: American Dietetic Association; 2001.

Nevino-Folino N, ed. *Pediatric Manual of Clinical Dietetics.* 2nd ed. Chicago, Ill: American Dietetic Association; 2003.

Wilkes GM. *Cancer and HIV Clinical Nutrition Pocket Guide.* 2nd ed. Sudbury, Mass: Jones and Bartlett Publishers; 1999.

Client Education

ASPEN. *Dietitian's Patient Education Resource Manual.* 2nd ed. Gaithersburg, Md: Aspen Publishers; 2001.

Eldridge B, Hamilton K. *Management of Nutrition Impact Symptoms in Cancer and Educational Handouts.* Chicago, Ill: American Dietetic Association; 2004.

Eating Well During Cancer Treatment

Aker SN, Lenssen P, eds. *A Guide to Good Nutrition During Cancer Treatment.* 4th ed. Seattle, Wash: Seattle Cancer Care Alliance; 2000.

American Cancer Society. *American Cancer Society's Healthy Eating Cookbook: A Celebration of Food, Friends, and Healthy Living.* 2nd ed. Atlanta, Ga: American Cancer Society; 2001.

Clegg H, Miletello G. *Eating Well Through Cancer.* Memphis, Tenn: Wimmer Cookbooks; 2001.

Dalzell K. *Challenge Cancer and Win! Step-by-Step Nutrition Action Plans for Your Specific Cancer.* Round Lake, Ill: Nutriquest; 2002.

Dyer D. *A Dietitian's Cancer Story: Information and Inspiration From a Three-Time Cancer Survivor.* Ann Arbor Mich: Swan Press; 2000. Also available in Spanish.

Ghosh K, Carson L, Cohen E. *Betty Crocker's Living with Cancer Cookbook.* New York, NY: John Wiley and Sons; 2001.

Keim R, Smith G. *What to Eat Now: The Cancer Lifeline Cookbook. An Easy to Use Nutrition Guide to Delicious and Healthy Eating for Cancer Patients, Survivors and Caregivers.* Seattle, Wash: Sasquatch Books; 1996.

Thigpen PR. *Dinner Through a Straw.* Murfeesboro, Tenn: Dinner Through a Straw; 2002.

Weihofen DL, Marino C. *The Cancer Survival Cookbook: 200 Quick and Easy Recipes With Helpful Eating Hints.* New York, NY: John Wiley and Sons; 2002.

Weihofen DL, Robbins J, Sullivan P. *Easy-to-Swallow, Easy-to-Chew Cookbook: Over 150 Tasty and Nutritious recipes for People Who Have Difficulty Swallowing.* New York, NY: John Wiley and Sons; 2002.

Weldon G. *Dietary Options for Cancer Survivors: A Guide to Research on Food, Food Substances, Herbals, and Dietary Regimens That May Affect Cancer.* Washington, DC: American Institute for Cancer Research; 2002.

Palliative Care

ASPEN Reference Group, Eutsey D, DiLima S. *Palliative Care Patient and Family Counseling Manual.* 2nd ed. Gaithersburg, Md: Aspen; 2002.

Gallagher-Allred C, Amenta M. *Nutrition and Hydration in Hospice Care: Needs, Strategies, Ethics.* Binghamton, NY: Haworth Press; 1997.

JOURNALS FOR HEALTH CARE PROFESSIONALS

CA: A Cancer Journal for Clinicians

Peer-reviewed journal published by American Cancer Society with current information on all aspects of cancer. Available at: caonline.amcancersoc.org.

Nutrition Connection

Published by the Oncology Nutrition Dietetic Practice Group (ON DPG), this quarterly newsletter highlights timely oncology topics and their application to the dietetics professional. For ordering information, contact the American Dietetic Association at 800/877-1600, ext. 5000, or visit the ON DPG Web site at http://www.oncologynutrition.org.

Nutrition in Clinical Practice
Journal of Parenteral and Enteral Nutrition

Peer-reviewed journals published by the American Society for Parenteral and Enteral Nutrition (ASPEN). Available at: http://www.nutritioncare.org.

Index

Page numbers with *f* indicate figures; page numbers with *t* indicate tables.